# Lecture Notes in Artificial Intelligence 9441

Subseries of Lecture Notes in Computer Science

## LNAI Series Editors

Randy Goebel
*University of Alberta, Edmonton, Canada*
Yuzuru Tanaka
*Hokkaido University, Sapporo, Japan*
Wolfgang Wahlster
*DFKI and Saarland University, Saarbrücken, Germany*

## LNAI Founding Series Editor

Joerg Siekmann
*DFKI and Saarland University, Saarbrücken, Germany*

More information about this series at http://www.springer.com/series/1244

Xiao-Li Li · Tru Cao
Ee-Peng Lim · Zhi-Hua Zhou
Tu-Bao Ho · David Cheung
Hiroshi Motoda (Eds.)

# Trends and Applications in Knowledge Discovery and Data Mining

PAKDD 2015 Workshops: BigPMA, VLSP, QIMIE, DAEBH
Ho Chi Minh City, Vietnam, May 19–21, 2015
Revised Selected Papers

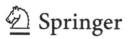 Springer

*Editors*
Xiao-Li Li
Institute for Infocomm Research
Singapore
Singapore

Tru Cao
Ho Chi Minh City University of Technology
Ho Chi Minh City
Vietnam

Ee-Peng Lim
School of Information Systems
Singapore Management University
Singapore
Singapore

Zhi-Hua Zhou
Nanjing University
Nanjing
China

Tu-Bao Ho
Japan Advanced Institute of Science and
    Technology
Nomi-shi, Ishikawa
Japan

David Cheung
The University of Hong Kong
Hong Kong
China

Hiroshi Motoda
AOARD
Tokyo
Japan

ISSN 0302-9743          ISSN 1611-3349  (electronic)
Lecture Notes in Artificial Intelligence
ISBN 978-3-319-25659-7          ISBN 978-3-319-25660-3  (eBook)
DOI 10.1007/978-3-319-25660-3

Library of Congress Control Number: 2015952758

LNCS Sublibrary: SL7 – Artificial Intelligence

Springer Cham Heidelberg New York Dordrecht London

Printed on acid-free paper

Springer International Publishing AG Switzerland is part of Springer Science+Business Media
(www.springer.com)

# Preface

This volume contains papers presented at PAKDD Workshops 2015 in conjunction with the 19th Pacific-Asia Conference on Knowledge Discovery and Data Mining, which was held on May 19, 2015, in Ho Chi Minh City, Vietnam. PAKDD has established itself as the premier event for data mining researchers in the Pacific-Asia region. This year, PAKDD 2015 had five workshops, including Pattern Mining and Application of Big Data (BigPMA), Quality Issues, Measures of Interestingness and Evaluation of Data Mining Models (QIMIE), Data Analytics for Evidence-Based Healthcare (DAEBH), Vietnamese Language and Speech Processing (VLSP), and Intelligence and Security Informatics (PAISI). This volume includes the revised workshop papers from the first four workshops, while the papers from PAISI are included in a separate proceedings volume.

The PAKDD 2015 workshops received 57 submissions. All the papers were reviewed by at least three reviewers, and only 23 papers were accepted for publication in this volume. The acceptance rate was approximately 40.35 %. The general quality of submissions was high and the competition was tough. We would like to thank all the authors who submitted their papers on many exciting and important research topics to the PAKDD workshops. We also thank all the workshop participants and presenters for attending these workshops. It is our hope that the workshops will provide a lasting platform for disseminating the latest research results and practice of data-mining approaches and applications. Our heartfelt thanks go to the Program Committee members and external reviewers for their timely reviews working to a tight schedule. Last but not least, we thank the members of the Organizing Committees for managing the paper submission, review, discussion, feedback, and final submission phases. We appreciate the professional service provided by Springer's LNCS editorial and publishing teams, and in particular Anna Kramer's assistance.

August 2015

Xiao-Li Li
Tru Cao
Ee-Peng Lim
Zhi-Hua Zhou
Tu-Bao Ho
David Cheung
Hiroshi Motoda

# Organization

## Organizing Committee and Program Committee

### Workshop Chair

Xiao-Li Li        Institute for Infocomm Research, A*Star, Singapore

## BigPMA Workshop (The Second Workshop on Pattern Mining and Application of Big Data)

### Workshop Organizers:

| | |
|---|---|
| Keith C.C. Chan | Hong Kong Polytechnic University, Hong Kong, SAR China |
| Hui-Huang Hsu | Tamkang University, Taiwan |
| Jiun-Long Huang | National Chiao Tung University, Taiwan |
| Yi-Cheng Chen | Tamkang University, Taiwan |

### Program Committee Members

| | |
|---|---|
| Philip S. Yu | University of Illinois at Chicago, USA |
| Vincent S. Tseng | National Chiao Tung University, Taiwan |
| Joshua Zhexue Huang | Shenzhen University, China |
| Jiannong Cao | Hong Kong Polytechnic University, Hong Kong, SAR China |
| Yan Huang | University of North Texas, USA |
| Wang-Chien Lee | The Pennsylvania State University, USA |
| Xing Xie | Microsoft Research Asia |
| Suh-Yin Lee | National Chiao Tung University, Taiwan |
| Xiaohua Tony Hu | Drexel University, USA |
| Jun Ma | Shandong University, China |
| Wei-Shinn Ku | Auburn University, USA |
| Guanling Lee | National Dong Hwa University, Taiwan |
| Xiang Zhang | Case Western Reserve University, USA |
| Kun-Ta Chuang | National Cheng Kung University, Taiwan |
| Dai Bing Tian | Singapore Management University, Singapore |
| Lin Hui | Tamkang University, Taiwan |
| Julia T.Y. Weng | Yuan Ze University, Taiwan |
| Meng-Fen Chiang | Singapore Management University, Singapore |
| Wei-Guang Teng | National Cheng Kung University, Taiwan |
| Kuo-Wei (David) Hsu | National Chengchi University, Taiwan |

Hsiao-Ping Tsai          National Chung Hsing University, Taiwan
Shan-Hung Wu             National Tsing Hua University, Taiwan
Chih-Hua Tai             National Taipei University, Taiwan
Chen-Yi Lin              National Taichung University of Science and
                         Technology, Taiwan

## QIMIE Workshop (Quality Issues, Measures of Interestingness and Evaluation of Data Mining Models)

**Workshop Organizers:**

| | |
|---|---|
| Stéphane Lallich | ERIC, Université Lyon, France |
| Philippe Lenca | Lab-STICC, Telecom Bretagne, France |
| Thanh-Nghi Do | College of Information Technology, Can Tho University, Vietnam |

**Program Committee Members**

| | |
|---|---|
| Hidenao Abe | Bunkyo University, Japan |
| Komate Amphawan | Faculty of Informatics, Burapha University, Thailand |
| Jérôme Azé | Université de Montpellier, LIRMM, France |
| Jose Balcazar | Universitat Politècnica de Catalunya, Spain |
| Cecile Bothorel | Telecom Bretagne, France |
| Paulo Cortez | University of Minho, Portugal |
| Jean Diatta | Université de la Réunion, France, New Caledonia |
| Thanh-Nghi Do | College of Information Technology, Can Tho University, Vietnam |
| Dominique Gay | Orange Labs, France |
| Fabrice Guillet | LINA - CNRS UMR 6241 - Polytech'Nantes, France |
| Fedja Hadzic | Digital Ecosystems and Business Intelligence Institute, DEBII, Curtin Univeristy of Technology, Australia |
| Michael Hahsler | Southern Methodist University, USA |
| Martin Holena | Institute of Computer Science, Czech Republic |
| Stéphane Lallich | University of Lyon 2, France |
| Jean-Charles Lamirel | LORIA Nancy, France |
| Ludovic Lebart | TeLecom-ParisTech, France |
| Philippe Lenca | Telecom Bretagne, France |
| Sorin Moga | Telecom Bretagne, France |
| Amedeo Napoli | LORIA Nancy, France |
| David Olson | University of Nebraska-Lincoln Lincoln, USA |
| Krishna Reddy Polepalli | IIIT-H, India |
| Zbigniew Ras | University of North Carolina, USA |
| Julie Soulas | Telecom Bretagne, France |
| Jerzy Stefanowski | Poznan Univeristy of Technology, Poland |
| Izabela Szczech | Poznan University of Technology, Poland |
| Bay Vo | Ton Duc Thang University, Vietnam |
| Kitsana Waiyamai | Kasetsart University, Thailand |
| Dianhui Wang | La Trobe University, Australia |
| Gary Weiss | Fordham University, USA |
| Albrecht Zimmermann | INSA Lyon, France |
| Guangfei Yang | Dalian University of Technology, China |

# DAEBH Workshop (Data Analytics for Evidence-Based Healthcare)

## Workshop Organizers:

| | |
|---|---|
| Xujuan Zhou | Australian Institute of Health Innovation (AIHI), Macquarie University, Australia |
| Diego Mollá Aliod | Macquarie University, Australia |
| Oscar Perez Concha | Australian Institute of Health Innovation (AIHI), Macquarie University, Australia |

## Program Committee Members

| | |
|---|---|
| Miew Keen Choong | AIHI Macquarie University, Australia |
| Adam Dunn | AIHI Macquarie University, Australia |
| Peter Dolog | Aalborg University, Denmark |
| Tudor Groza | Garvan Institute, Australia |
| Antonio Jimeno-Yepes | IBM Research Australia, Australia |
| Ritu Khare | The Children's Hospital of Philadelphia, USA |
| Simon Kocbek | RMIT University, Australia |
| Blanca Gallego Luxan | AIHI Macquarie University, Australia |
| David Martinez | MedWhat.com, Australia |
| Abdul Mateen | Federal Urdu University of Arts, Science and Technology, Pakistan |
| Mohd Saberi Mohamad | Universiti Teknologi Malaysia, Malaysia |
| Anthony Nguyen | CSIRO, Australia |
| Abeed Sarker | Arizona State University, USA |
| Weifeng Su | United International College, Hong Kong, SAR China |
| Laurianne Sitbon | Queensland University of Technology, Australia |
| Shusaku Tsumoto | Shimane University, Japan |
| Karin Verspoor | The University of Melbourne, Australia |
| Xin Wang | University of Calgary, Canada |
| Zhiang Wu | Nanjing University of Finance and Economics, China |
| Neil Yen | The University of Aizu, Japan |
| Ji Zhang | University of Southern Queensland, Australia |
| Yanchang Zhao | RDataMining.com, Australia |

# VLSP Workshop (The Third International Workshop on Vietnamese Language and Speech Processing)

**Workshop Organizers:**

| | |
|---|---|
| Nguyen Thi Minh Huyen | VNU University of Science, Hanoi, Vietnam |
| Luong Chi Mai | Institute of Information Technology, Vietnam Academy of Science and Technology |
| Le Hai Son | Institute of Information Technology, Vietnam Academy of Science and Technology |

**Program Committee Members**

| | |
|---|---|
| Cao Hoang Tru | University of Technology, VNU-HCM, Vietnam |
| Dinh Dien | University of Science, VNU-HCM, Vietnam |
| Ho Bao Quoc | University of Science, VNU-HCM, Vietnam |
| Ho Tu Bao | JAIST, Japan |
| Le Anh Cuong | University of Engineering and Technology, VNU, Hanoi, Vietnam |
| Le Hai Son | Institute of Information Technology, VAST, Vietnam |
| Le Hong Phuong | University of Science, VNU, Hanoi, Vietnam |
| Le Thanh Huong | Hanoi University of Science and Technology, Vietnam |
| Luong Chi Mai | Institute of Information Technology, VAST, Vietnam |
| Nguyen Le Minh | JAIST, Japan |
| Nguyen Phuong Thai | University of Engineering and Technology, VNU, Hanoi, Vietnam |
| Nguyen Thi Minh Huyen | University of Science, VNU, Hanoi, Vietnam |
| Pham Bao Son | University of Engineering and Technology, VNU, Hanoi, Vietnam |
| Phan Thi Tuoi | University of Technology, VNU-HCM, Vietnam |
| Phan Xuan Hieu | University of Engineering and Technology, VNU, Hanoi, Vietnam |
| Tran Do Dat | Hanoi University of Science and Technology, Vietnam |
| Vu Hai Quan | University of Science, VNU-HCM, Vietnam |
| Vu Tat Thang | Institute of Information Technology, VAST, Vietnam |
| Phung Trung Nghia | Thai Nguyen University of Information and Communication Technology, Vietnam |
| Nguyen Quoc Cuong | Hanoi University of Science and Technology, Vietnam |
| Dang Ngoc Duc | Acaltel Vietnam, Vietnam |

# Contents

## Quality Issues, Measures of Interestingness and Evaluation of Data Mining Models

## Data Analytics for Evidence-Based Healthcare

# Vietnamese Language and Speech Processing

# Pattern Mining and Application
# of Big Data

# ProbitUCB: A Novel Method
# for Review Ranking

Wanying Ding[1]([⊠]), Yue Shang[1], Dae Hoon Park[2], Lifan Guo[3],
and Xiaohua Hu[1]

[1] College and Computing and Informatics,
Drexel University, Philadelphia, PA, USA
{wd78,ys439,xh29}@drexel.edu
[2] Department of Computer Science,
University of Illinois at Urbana-Champaign,
Champaign, IL, USA
dpark34@illinois.edu
[3] TCL Research America, San Jose, CA, USA
GuoLifan@tcl.com

**Abstract.** Online reviews play an important role in facilitating customers in making online purchase decisions. But with the dramatic increase in volume, it will cost customers hours going through all the reviews. This paper proposes a review ranking algorithm to present the most helpful reviews ahead, saving consumers' plenty of time in review hunting. Our ProbitUCB model implements a probabilistic kernel embedded UCB (Upper Confident Bound) ranking framework, and adopts a self-learning mechanism to distinguish out helpful reviews. Comparing to the current models, ProbitUCB's advantage is listing as follows: (1) it ranks under the exploit and explore mechanism, reducing the error brought from probability estimation inaccuracy; (2) it is training dataset free, saving users enormous amount of time in labeling data, which is required for most supervised methods; (3) it considers various potential features to rank, remedying the defect of only using word information in most unsupervised methods; (4) it adjusts the values of hyper parameters automatically, solving the intuitively value setting problem in many related work. Finally, we experiment our model on 6 datasets, and compare its performance with 10 other classical learn to rank algorithms, and the results show that our algorithm outperform all of them.

**Keywords:** Review ranking · Multi-armed bandit · Restricted Boltzmann machine · Probabilistic kernel

## 1 Introduction and Related Work

In order to attract potential consumers, good e-commerce websites provide users with not only reliable product descriptions, but also informative user-generated reviews. Online reviews are becoming more and more imperative in facilitating consumers to make their purchase decisions. However, with the dramatically proliferating in the

© Springer International Publishing Switzerland 2015
X.-L. Li et al. (Eds.): PAKDD 2015, LNCS 9441, pp. 3–15, 2015.
DOI: 10.1007/978-3-319-25660-3_1

amount of online reviews, one consumer might need to spend tens of hours going through the reviews in order to get a whole picture about the target product. In addition, among the reviews, there are a considerable number of spams, which might confuse or even mislead consumers. Thus, how to provide online consumers with trustful and informative reviews has caught a lot of attentions.

Some e-commerce websites, like Amazon and Yelp, provide *vote* mechanism to present customers with most helpful-voted reviews ahead. This method has alleviated the problem, but it has evoked some new challenges, such as cold start problem, imbalance vote bias, winner circle bias, and early bird bias [1]. Thus, researchers in academia also get involved to help detect the helpful reviews.

Generally speaking, there are mainly three genres in academia to detect helpful reviews, namely, Explorative Methods, Supervised Methods and Unsupervised Methods. *Exploratory Method* tends to use survey and correlation tests to explore features that contribute one review's helpfulness [2–5]. However, exploratory study is time consuming and hard to re-conduct, so it is inadequate in social media environment. *Supervised Method* is the mainstream to solve review ranking problems, and has achieved considerable success. Regression models are widely used to detect features which contribute one review's helpfulness, like timeliness, writing style, and so on [5–9]. SVM based models [1, 10–12] are also deeply studied to classify reviews into helpful and unhelpful, and recommend the helpful ones to consumers. Besides, models based on Radial Basis Functions (RBF) kernels [13–16] or Entropy Theory [17, 18] are also introduced to detect helpful reviews. The limitation of supervised methods is that they heavily rely on the training dataset. However, with online information exploration, it turns out to be harder and harder to obtain a good enough training dataset which conveys all possibilities in the real world. *Unsupervised Method* aims to free researchers from training dataset construction. Most existing unsupervised methods utilize the relationship between words to differentiate reviews [19–21], but ignores the information like syntax and sentiment, which are also essential for helpfulness detection. Besides, unsupervised methods are totally uncontrollable, but in some situations, we indeed want to exert controls to get a better result.

Considering all the problems mentioned above, this paper has proposed a novel review ranking model—ProbitUCB. ProbitUCB implements a probabilistic kernel embedded UCB ranking framework, and adopts a self-learning mechanism to distinguish out helpful reviews. Figure 1 represents a brief overview about ProbitUCB.

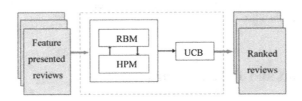

**Fig. 1.** Overview of ProbitUCB

Comparing to previous works, ProbitUCB has the following advantages:

(1) It adopts Upper Confidence Bound (UCB) [9, 22] framework to rank. UCB takes both of the expectation and derivation into consideration, reducing the errors brought from probability estimation.
(2) It implements a Helpfulness Probabilistic Model (HPM) to infer each review's probability to be helpful. HPM can help to estimate one review's helpfulness directly from the dataset itself, and does not depend on training dataset. Thus it frees users from training dataset construction.
(3) It uses the Restricted Boltzmann Machine (RBM) [23] to adjust the hyper-parameters for HPM, alleviating the inaccuracies associated with hyper-parameters which are always set manually and intuitively.
(4) It allows users to take various features into consideration, not just words, making this model able and flexible to incorporate as much useful information as possible.

## 2   Model Description

ProbitUCB implements an Upper Confidence Bound (UCB) framework for rank. UCB framework is a realization of Multi-Armed Bandit, which deals with gambling problem and aims to provide gamblers with a sequence to play the gambling machines in order to maximize their final rewards. Thus, UCB is natural for a ranking problem. Comparing to rank natively according to helpfulness probability, which might lead to poor results because of the ineluctable inaccuracies in probability estimation, UCB not only exploits the entities with high estimated expectations, but also explores the ones with low estimated expectation but high uncertainty, since their true expectation might be higher, and thus provides a more reliable ranking result.

In UCB framework, reviews are deemed as a series of gambling machines to play, and our goal is to generate an order with which the customers can get the maximum reward. In our case, we treat the helpfulness of each review as its reward. We use a Beta distribution to describe each review's reward distribution, since each review only distributes on two parameters: helpfulness and unhelpfulness. For review $r$, its real reward is $\mu_r$, and estimated reward is $\widehat{\mu}_r$. The standard deviation of this Beta distribution is denoted as $\widehat{\sigma}_r$. According to Chebyshev's inequality, with a proper $\lambda$

$$\mu_r \leq \widehat{\mu}_r + \lambda \widehat{\sigma}_r \tag{1}$$

So, the upper confidence bound for review $r$'s reward is $\widehat{\mu}_r + \lambda \widehat{\sigma}_r$. Because each review is represented by a Beta distribution $Beta(\pi_r)$ with parameter vector $\pi_r(\pi_{r,\alpha}, \pi_{r,\beta})$, in which $\pi_{r,\alpha}$ indicates the probability to be helpful, and $\pi_{r,\beta}$ indicates the probability to be unhelpful. The corresponding estimated expectation and standard deviation are easy to calculate as formula 2 and formula 3.

$$\widehat{u}_r = \frac{\pi_{r,\alpha}}{\pi_{r,\alpha} + \pi_{r,\beta}} \tag{2}$$

$$\widehat{\sigma_r} = \sqrt{\frac{\pi_{r,\alpha} * \pi_{r,\beta}}{\left(\pi_{r,\alpha} + \pi_{r,\beta}\right)^2 * \left(\pi_{r,\alpha} + \pi_{r,\beta} + 1\right)}} \tag{3}$$

How to estimate a review's parameter vector $\boldsymbol{\pi_r}\left(\pi_{r,\alpha}, \pi_{r,\beta}\right)$ becomes the core issue we need to consider about. Most current related methods tend to choose supervised methods, like linear or logic regression, to make such estimations [9, 24]. Just as we mentioned above, the supervised methods heavily rely on the training dataset, but in many cases, a well labeled dataset is not available. Thus, we create a probabilistic model—Helpfulness Prediction Model (HPM), which can help to make estimations without the support from training dataset.

In order to find each review's distribution on helpfulness/unhelpfulness, a latent variable $l \in \{\alpha, \beta\}$ is introduced. Assume we have $R$ reviews, and have $F$ features in total, and each review has a Beta distribution $\pi$ on the latent variables, namely help-fulness ($l_\alpha$) and unhelpfulness ($l_\beta$). For each label, it has a distribution over all the features. Because there might be multiple features, we assume each latent variable has a Multinomial distribution on the features. The model can be shown in Fig. 1.

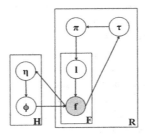

**Fig. 2.** Graphical model of HPM

The generate process of this model can be described as follows:

**Step 1:** For each latent label $l$, generate a distribution $\phi_l \sim Dirichlet(\boldsymbol{\eta})$ according to hyper-parameter $\boldsymbol{\eta}$.
**Step 2:** For each review $r$, generate a helpful distribution $\pi_r \sim Beta(\boldsymbol{\tau})$ according to hyper-parameter $\boldsymbol{\tau}$.

(2.1) For each feature position $f$ in the review, generate a helpfulness label $l_{r,f} \sim Bernoulli(\pi_r)$
(2.2) For each feature position, generate a feature according to $l_{r,f}$ and $\phi_l$, $f \sim Multinomial\left(\phi_l, l_{r,f}\right)$

We use the Gibbs Sampling to conduct inference. Following the model described above, the full joint distribution for the model can be represented as formula (4).

$$p(f, l, \pi, \phi | \tau, \eta) = Beta(\pi|\tau) * Dir(\phi|\eta) * Bern(l|\pi) * Mult(f|l, \phi)$$

$$= \frac{\Gamma(\tau_\alpha, \tau_\beta)}{\Gamma(\tau_1) * \Gamma(\tau_2)} * \pi^{\tau_\alpha - 1} * (1 - \pi)^{\tau_\beta - 1} * \prod_{i=1}^{F} \prod_{l=1}^{H} \phi_{i,l}^{\eta_{i,l} - 1} * \frac{\Gamma(\sum_{i=1}^{F} \eta_i)}{\prod_{i=1}^{F} \Gamma(\eta_i)} * \pi^{N_{r,l\alpha}} *$$

$$(1 - \pi)^{N_{r,l\beta}} * \prod_{i=1}^{F} \prod_{l=1}^{H} \phi_{f_i}^{N_l}$$

$$(4)$$

After Bayesian Transformation, we get formula (5) to infer the label assignment.

$$p(f_i = l | f_{-i}, l, \pi, \phi, \tau, \eta) \propto \frac{N_{r,l} + \tau_{r,l}}{\sum_{l=1}^{H} (N_{r,l} + \tau_{r,l})} * \frac{N_{l,f_i} + \eta_{l,i}}{\sum_{i=1}^{F} (N_{l,f_i} + \eta_{l,i})} \qquad (5)$$

Where $N_{r,l}$ is the number of features in review $r$ those have been assigned to $l$, $\tau_{r,l}$ is the hyper parameter for $r^{th}$ review on $l$, $N_{l,f_i}$ is the number of feature $i$ that has been assigned to $l$, and $\eta_{l,i}$ is the hyper parameter of the $i^{th}$ feature of label $l$.

HPM has two hyper parameters, $\tau$ and $\eta$. Most probabilistic models just ask users to manually set the values of hyper parameters, and most researchers just give the values intuitively, reducing the reliability of the models. We implement Restricted Boltzmann Machine (RBM) to help adjust the values of the hyper parameters. The reason we choose RBM is that, first it is a binary model, and suitable to solve our binary distribution problem, and second, it can fit any discrete distribution, and thus easy to combine with our probabilistic model (Fig. 2).

We set $v_1$ as the observed features of each review, $v_2$ as the estimated feature distribution generated from RBM. We use $w_{i,j}$ to represent the weight between visible feature $v_i$ and hidden variable $h_j$, and initiate it according to a normal distribution $N$ $(0,0.01)$. Along with the default setting rules, we initiate hidden bias $a_i$ as $1.0/F$, where $F$ is the number of visible features, and visible bias $b_j$ is set to 0. We set the number of hidden variables as 2 to represent helpfulness and unhelpfulness respectively. For each iteration, it calculates the parameters as follows, where $\sigma(*)$ represents the sigmoid function.

**Step 1:** for each hidden unit j: $P(h_{1,j} = 1 | v_1) = \sigma(a_i + \sum_i v_{1,i} * w_{i,j})$

**Step 2:** for each visible unit i: $P(v_{2,i} = 1 | h_1) = \sigma(b_j + \sum_j h_{1,j} * w_{i,j})$

**Step 3:** for each hidden unit j: $P(h_{2,j} = 1 | v_2) = \sigma(a_i + \sum_i v_{2,i} * w_{i,j})$

So, the updated latent variables can be represented as formula (6)

$$W = W + lr * (P(h_1 = 1 | v_1)v_1^T - P(h_2 = 1 | v_2)v_2^T)$$

$$a = a + lr * (v_1 - v_2) \qquad (6)$$

$$b = b + lr * (P(h_1 = 1 | v_1) - P(h_2 = 1 | v_2))$$

We use $W$ to infer the hyper parameter $\eta$ for feature-helpfulness distribution. For a feature $f_i$, its prior distribution on a helpful label $l_j$ is calculated as:

$$\eta_{i,j} = e^{w_{i,j}*\kappa} \tag{7}$$

where $\kappa$ is the magnification coefficient to range $\eta_{i,j}$ to a suitable magnitude.

We use the value of $(P(h_1 = 1|v_1)$ and $P(h_2 = 1|v_2))$ to infer the hyper parameter $\tau$. For a review $r$, its prior distribution on a helpful label $l_j$ can be calculated as:

$$\tau_{r,j} = \frac{P(h_{rj,1} = 1|v_{r,1}) + P(h_{rj,2} = 1|v_{r,2})}{2} \tag{8}$$

## 3  Feature Definition

ProbitUCB is a feature driven model, which, on one hand, can provide users with maximum freedom to define features that they believe will denote to a review's helpfulness, and on the other hand, can incorporate as much meaningful information as possible to guide a better helpfulness ranking. Although some previous work [8, 10, 13, 16, 25–28] has provided many kinds of features, most of them just make analysis from a single perspective, like content or author only. In order to incorporate as much information as possible, this paper has defines 3 kinds of features: *Author Features*, *Descriptive Features* and *Semantic Features*, aiming to make a comprehensive explore to see which features will affect a review's helpfulness, and how they affect.

### 3.1  Author Feature

Author Features include *Author Rating Deviation* (ARD), *Author Review Entropy* (ARE) and *Repeatedly Review Times* (RRT).

ARD is used to measure whether one author's voting score dramatically differ from other users. A greater deviation might indicate that this author might be a spammer. We calculate ARD as formula (9):

$$ARD(a) = \frac{\sqrt{\sum_p (R_p - \bar{R})^2}}{n} \tag{9}$$

Where $a$ represents an author, $R_p$ indicates the rating value given by a certain author to the $p$th product, $\bar{R}$ is the average rating of the product, and $n$ is the number of ratings given by the author.

ARE is used to measure the similarities among reviews written by one author. A spammer tends to write high similar reviews. ARE is calculated as in formula (10), where $a$ indicates an author, $i$ denotes the $i^{th}$ word $w_i$ in this author's lexicon, $C_i$ is the count of $w_i$, and $N$ is total count of all the words in this author's lexicon.

$$ARE(a) = -\sum_i \frac{C_i}{N} log \frac{C_i}{N} \tag{10}$$

RRT is used to measure one author's review publication frequency. A normal author will have a comparatively lower frequency than the spammers. We use the maximum number of repeated reviews that one author publishes at one time as the feature.

## 3.2   Descriptive Features

Descriptive Features consist of *Review Length* (RL), *Review Readability* (RED), *Conjunction Count* (CC), and *Product Rating Bias* (PRB).

RL is the length of one review. Generally speaking, long reviews will contain more information, and should be more helpful.

RED is used to measure that whether a review is easy to be understood. In formula (11), #char is the number of characters, #word denotes the number of words, #sentence indicates the number of sentences, and #para the number of paragraphs.

$$RED(r) = \frac{\#char}{\#word} + \frac{\#word}{\#sentence} + \frac{\#sentence}{\#para} \tag{11}$$

CC is used to count the number of conjunction words in one review. Conjunction words often connect two levels of semantics, like "The color of this shirt is cool, but the design is terrible", so if a review contains a reasonable number of conjunctions, it might be informative.

PRB is used to measure the difference between a review's rating and the average rating the certain product gets. A large PRB might indicate this review is a spam. We use formula (12) to calculate this feature:

$$PRB(r) = |R_r - \bar{R}| \tag{12}$$

Where $R_r$ is the rating given by a review of one product, $\bar{R}$ denotes the average rating this product gets.

## 3.3   Semantic Feature

Semantic Features include *KL-Divergence of Reviews* (RKL), *Sentiment in Title* (SIT) and *Reviews* (SIR), *Name Entity* (NE) and *Relation* (NER), and *Information Gain* (IG).

RKL is used to measure the semantic distance between a review $r$ and all the other reviews of a certain product. A very deviated review might be a spam. KL-divergence is used to measure this difference.

$$RKL(r) = D_{KL}(\vec{r}|\vec{R}) = \sum_{i=1}^{m} p_{i,r} * \log\left(\frac{p_{i,r}}{p_{i,\bar{R}}}\right) \tag{13}$$

Where $r$ indicates a review, $\vec{r}$ is this review's distribution on words, $\bar{R}$ is the all the reviews' average distribution on words. $p_{i,r}$ is the probability of the $i^{th}$ word in review r. and $p_{i,\bar{R}}$ is the $i^{th}$ word's average probability in all the reviews.

SIT is used to measure the sentiment words in the title, and SIR measures the sentiment words in the review body. A good review should contain a considerable number of sentiment words.

$$SIR(r) = \frac{\#sentiment_{words}\,in\ review}{review\ length} \qquad (14)$$

$$SIT(r) = \frac{\#sentiment_{words}\,in\ title}{title\ length} \qquad (15)$$

NE is used to count the number of entities mentioned in the review, and NER is used to count the number of entity relationships among one review. A comprehensive review may describe more than one aspect about a product.

IG is used to measure how much new information one can get from a review after one has read all the other reviews about a product. We assume that, the more new information one can get from one review, the more likely this review is helpful. Information Gain could be calculated as in formula (16)

$$IG(r) = -\sum_i p_i^{(R+r)} log p_i^{(R+r)} + \sum_i p_i^R log p_i^R \qquad (16)$$

$r$ is used to indicate a review, R is all the other reviews except r. $p_i^{(R+r)}$ is the probability of the $i^{th}$ word in the collection of all reviews, and $p_i^R$ is the probability of the $i^{th}$ in all the reviews except review $r$.

As shown above, all the feature values are continuous, but the input of HPM should be concrete. Thus, we map the feature values to [1, 10]. Taking RL (Review Length) as an example, we use a normal distribution to simulate all the reviews' length distribution, and then we get the corresponding cumulative distribution function(CDF). With the CDF, given a review length, we can get the corresponding probability $p$, and then we round up $(10*p)$ as the input of this feature value.

## 4    Experiments and Evaluation

### 4.1    Dataset and Parameter Settings

The dataset we use is provided by [29]. We randomly choose six products containing in this dataset to conduct our experiment. The six products are (1) Air Conditioner (AirCon), (2) MP3 Player (Mp3Ply), (3) Space Heater (SpaHea), (4) Vaccum Cleaner (CanVac), (5) Coffee Machine (CofMak), and (6) Lap Top (Lap Top).

There are three parameters need to be set in the model: the learning rate $lr$, lambda $\lambda$, and the magnification coefficients $\kappa$. We employ the standard and out of box settings without any tuning to our data, and set learning rate $lr$ as 1E-3, $\lambda$ as 1 to balance the estimated expectation and derivation, and $\kappa$ as 10.

The reviews with less than 5 votes are removed from the dataset. Then, we define the users' helpful vote ratio (formula (17)) as the ground truth for ranking evaluation.

$$\text{vote ratio} = \frac{\textit{number of helpful votes}}{\textit{number of votes}} \tag{17}$$

## 4.2 Experimental Settings

We employ ten popular learn to rank algorithms as our benchmarks: Linear Regression (LR), Multiple Additive Regression Tree(MT), RankNet(RN), RankBoost(RB), AdaRank(AR), LAMBDARANK(LRK), LAMBDAMART(LAR), LiseNet(LN), Coordination Ascent(CA), and Random Forest(RF). In order to keep consistent with our models, the features used by these ten models are the same as the ones we use for our models. Besides, we want to test whether RBM has improved the performance, so we compare the model with RBM (P(R)) learned hyper parameters, to the model without RBM(P (S). For P(S), we set its hyper parameters manually and uniformly as $\tau = 0.2$ and $\eta = 0.1$.

We use 10-fold cross validation methods to evaluate the performance of each method. The evaluation indexes are Mean Average Precision (MAP), F-Measure, P@5, P@10. Different from the traditional F-Measure, which takes use of precision and recall, instead, we use sensitivity and specificity, because our task is ranking but not retrieving. We take the top 10 records as relative ones, and bottom 10 as unrelated ones provided by this ranking system.

Tables 1, 2, 3 and 4 show our results. P(R) outperforms all other models in most cases, and performs just a slightly worse in very limited cases. Comparing P(R) and P (S), P(R) outperforms P(S) in most situations, indicating hyper parameter self-learning is helpful to improve the performance of probabilistic model.

**Table 1.** Comparison result based on MAP

|        | P (R) | P (S) | LR    | MT    | RN    | RB    | RA    | CA    | LRK   | LAR   | LN    | RF    |
|--------|-------|-------|-------|-------|-------|-------|-------|-------|-------|-------|-------|-------|
| AirCon | 0.886 | 0.858 | 0.798 | 0.796 | 0.800 | 0.803 | 0.803 | 0.816 | 0.813 | 0.820 | 0.798 | 0.787 |
| Mp3Ply | 0.741 | 0.697 | 0.704 | 0.730 | 0.734 | 0.727 | 0.390 | 0.676 | 0.451 | 0.467 | 0.477 | 0.730 |
| SpaHea | 0.839 | 0.812 | 0.771 | 0.774 | 0.821 | 0.806 | 0.608 | 0.766 | 0.667 | 0.653 | 0.691 | 0.809 |
| CanVac | 0.849 | 0.754 | 0.805 | 0.800 | 0.773 | 0.858 | 0.594 | 0.848 | 0.575 | 0.606 | 0.658 | 0.842 |
| CofMak | 0.839 | 0.771 | 0.758 | 0.785 | 0.790 | 0.813 | 0.541 | 0.766 | 0.600 | 0.641 | 0.608 | 0.837 |
| LapTop | 0.805 | 0.783 | 0.845 | 0.861 | 0.806 | 0.833 | 0.482 | 0.813 | 0.570 | 0.613 | 0.520 | 0.894 |

**Table 2.** Comparison result based on F-measure

|        | P (R) | P (S) | LR    | MT    | RN    | RB    | RA    | CA    | LRK   | LAR   | LN    | RF    |
|--------|-------|-------|-------|-------|-------|-------|-------|-------|-------|-------|-------|-------|
| AirCon | 0.715 | 0.643 | 0.504 | 0.508 | 0.534 | 0.507 | 0.562 | 0.586 | 0.422 | 0.461 | 0.550 | 0.553 |
| Mp3Ply | 0.852 | 0.706 | 0.807 | 0.804 | 0.842 | 0.910 | 0.445 | 0.821 | 0.588 | 0.629 | 0.607 | 0.792 |
| SpaHea | 0.852 | 0.651 | 0.646 | 0.735 | 0.693 | 0.677 | 0.650 | 0.685 | 0.612 | 0.629 | 0.430 | 0.681 |
| CanVac | 0.930 | 0.852 | 0.675 | 0.746 | 0.742 | 0.780 | 0.559 | 0.778 | 0.522 | 0.745 | 0.619 | 0.744 |
| CofMak | 0.814 | 0.683 | 0.684 | 0.792 | 0.537 | 0.641 | 0.467 | 0.694 | 0.670 | 0.536 | 0.603 | 0.715 |
| LapTop | 0.875 | 0.718 | 0.934 | **0.940** | 0.611 | 0.468 | 0.370 | 0.898 | 0.371 | 0.610 | 0.835 | 0.900 |

**Table 3.** Comparison result based on P@5

|        | P (R) | P (S) | LR   | MT   | RN   | RB   | RA   | CA   | LRK  | LAR  | LN   | RF   |
|--------|-------|-------|------|------|------|------|------|------|------|------|------|------|
| AirCon | 1.0   | 1     | 0.8  | 0.78 | 0.74 | 0.76 | 0.86 | 0.8  | 0.84 | 0.9  | 0.72 | 0.82 |
| Mp3Ply | 1.0   | 0.8   | 0.78 | 0.78 | 0.82 | 0.78 | 0.42 | 0.72 | 0.48 | 0.66 | 0.46 | 0.8  |
| SpaHea | 0.8   | 0.6   | 0.82 | 0.8  | 0.86 | 0.88 | 0.62 | 0.68 | 0.68 | 0.66 | 0.52 | 0.88 |
| CanVac | 0.8   | 0.8   | 0.84 | 0.8  | 0.74 | 0.86 | 0.5  | 0.56 | 0.52 | 0.66 | 0.46 | 0.84 |
| CofMak | 1.0   | 0.8   | 0.8  | 0.82 | 0.78 | 0.8  | 0.56 | 0.6  | 0.58 | 0.64 | 0.6  | 0.92 |
| LapTop | 1.0   | 0.6   | 0.88 | 0.92 | 0.88 | 0.84 | 0.5  | 0.72 | 0.6  | 0.68 | 0.44 | 1.0  |

**Table 4.** Comparison result based on P@10

|        | P (R) | P (S) | LR   | MT   | RN   | RB   | RA   | CA   | LRK  | LAR  | LN   | RF   |
|--------|-------|-------|------|------|------|------|------|------|------|------|------|------|
| AirCon | 0.9   | 0.8   | 0.74 | 0.78 | 0.81 | 0.84 | 0.82 | 0.75 | 0.73 | 0.75 | 0.8  | 0.82 |
| Mp3Ply | 0.9   | 0.8   | 0.73 | 0.76 | 0.78 | 0.77 | 0.46 | 0.64 | 0.47 | 0.65 | 0.53 | 0.79 |
| SpaHea | 0.9   | 0.6   | 0.77 | 0.8  | 0.81 | 0.77 | 0.68 | 0.67 | 0.67 | 0.68 | 0.61 | 0.84 |
| CanVac | 0.9   | 0.9   | 0.73 | 0.71 | 0.67 | 0.76 | 0.51 | 0.58 | 0.57 | 0.68 | 0.54 | 0.75 |
| CofMak | 0.9   | 0.8   | 0.75 | 0.78 | 0.76 | 0.79 | 0.51 | 0.67 | 0.52 | 0.71 | 0.5  | 0.84 |
| LapTop | 1.0   | 0.7   | 0.91 | 0.93 | 0.84 | 0.89 | 0.52 | 0.75 | 0.49 | 0.74 | 0.47 | 0.97 |

The possible reason that our models can outperform other models is that we learn the parameters directly from the dataset itself, not from training dataset or manually set. So the parameters can fit the data well, and generate a better ranking result.

## 5   Result Analysis

ProbitUCB generates a feature-helpfulness distribution, and from this distribution, we can infer each feature's contribution to helpfulness. The result is shown in Fig. 3. In Fig. 3, the horizontal axis represents the feature value, from 1 to 10, and vertical axis represents the feature's contribution to helpfulness. If the value is greater than 0, it means this feature contribute positively, otherwise negatively (Fig. 3).

**Descriptive Features:** Figure 3(a) tells us the most helpful reviews have a medium length, not too long or too short. Short reviews often cannot attract other users, while longs ones consume too much time to read. Figure 3(h) shows the result of coordinating conjunction count. A reasonable number of coordinating conjunction can contribute to a helpful review. Figure 3(g) shows the result of readability. The larger the value is, the harder this review to be understood. We find that a high score in readability doesn't mean a low helpfulness, but low score in often contribute to high helpfulness. Figure 3(j) shows the positive correlation between product rating biases with the review quality.

**Semantics Features:** Figure 3(e) shows the result of name entity feature and Fig. 3(f) shows the result of relation count. The vibrate line in Fig. 3(e) indicates a considerable number of name entities and relations appear in the review will improve the helpfulness

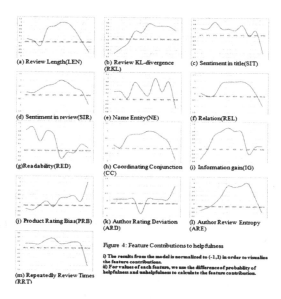

(a) Review Length(LEN)

(b) Review KL-divergence (RKL)

(c) Sentiment in title(SIT)

(d) Sentiment in review(SIR)

(e) Name Entity(NE)

(f) Relation(REL)

(g)Readability(RED)

(h) Coordinating Conjunction (CC)

(i) Information gain(IG)

(j) Product Rating Bias(PRB)

(k) Author Rating Deviation (ARD)

(l) Author Review Entropy (ARE)

(m) Repeatedly Review Times (RRT)

Figure 4: Feature Contributions to helpfulness

i) The results from the model is normalized to (-1,1) in order to visualize the feature contributions.
ii) For values of each feature, we use the difference of probability of helpfulness and unhelpfulness to calculate the feature contribution.

**Fig. 3.** Effects of features to helpfulness

of the reviews, but too much semantic information may make the idea of review unclear and distract users' attentions. Figure 3(i) indicates that if a review states the ideas that have been expressed by previous reviewers, it would not be helpful, but if a review contains too much different information, it would not be useful as well because it be a spam. From the results in Fig. 3(c) and (d), the trends of the line goes down as the feature values become larger. This means readers may be sick of reviews with high sentiment polarity or too many sentiment words. Figure 3(b) shows that reviews with novel, distinctive ideas are more likely to be voted as helpful by other users.

**Author Features:** If an author does not have spam behavior, such as publishing many similar reviews or always rating differently, this reviewer is more trustful. The reviews written by him/her will be more helpful according to the results shown in Fig. 3(k), (l) and (m).

## 6    Conclusion

This paper proposes a novel model – ProbitUCB for review ranking. ProbitUCB implements a UCB ranking framework, considering both the exploit and explore characteristics of a review. In addition, ProbitUCB applies a probabilistic kernel HPM to estimate each review's distribution on helpfulness and unhelpfulness. HPM learns the parameters directly from the dataset, and thus frees from training dataset construction. Moreover, ProbitUCB combines a self-learning mechanism to adjust the value of hyper parameters automatically, and experiments shows such self-learning mechanism indeed help to improve the performance. To construct the experiment, this paper extracts 13 features to describe a review's potential helpfulness, including 3 author features, 4 descriptive features, and 6 semantic features, and experiment to 10 classical ranking algorithms on 6 datasets. The result indicates that ProbitUCB is a promising model for review ranking and review recommendation.

# References

1. Liu, J., et al.: Low-quality product review detection in opinion summarization. In: Proceedings of the Joint Conference on Empirical Methods in Natural Language Processing and Computational Natural Language Learning EMNLP-CoNLL2007, pp. 334–342
2. Dubey, W.H.: The Principles of Readability. Impact Information, Costa Mesa (2004)
3. Tintarev, N., Masthoff, J.: A survey of explanations in recommender systems. In: 2007 IEEE 23rd International Conference on Data Engineering Workshop. IEEE (2007)
4. Tintarev, N., Masthoff, J.: The effectiveness of personalized movie explanations: an experiment using commercial meta-data. In: Nejdl, W., Kay, J., Pu, P., Herder, E. (eds.) AH 2008. LNCS, vol. 5149, pp. 204–213. Springer, Heidelberg (2008)
5. Mudambi, S.M., Schuff, D.: What makes a helpful online review? A study of customer reviews on amazon.com. MIS Q. **34**(1), 185–200 (2010)
6. Ghose, A., Ipeirotis, P.G.: Designing novel review ranking systems: predicting the usefulness and impact of reviews. In: Proceedings of the Ninth International Conference on Electronic Commerce, pp. 303–310 . ACM, Minneapolis, MN, USA (2007)
7. Lu, Y., et al.: Exploiting social context for review quality prediction. In: Proceedings of the 19th International Conference on World Wide Web. ACM (2010)
8. Cao, Q., Duan, W., Gan, Q.: Exploring determinants of voting for the "helpfulness" of online user reviews: a text mining approach. Decis. Support Syst. **50**, 511–521 (2011)
9. Mahajan, D.K., et al.: LogUCB: an explore-exploit algorithm for comments recommendation. In: Proceedings of the 21st ACM International Conference on Information and Knowledge Management. ACM (2012)
10. Kim, S.-M., et al.: Automatically assessing review helpfulness. In: Proceedings of the 2006 Conference on Empirical Methods in Natural Language Processing, pp. 423–430. Association for Computational Linguistics, Sydney, Australia (2006)
11. Chen, C.C., Tseng, Y.-D.: Quality evaluation of product reviews using an information quality framework. Decis. Support Syst. **50**(4), 755–768 (2011)
12. Yu, X., et al.: Mining online reviews for predicting sales performance: a case study in the movie domain. IEEE Trans. Knowl. Data Eng. **24**(4), 720–734 (2012)
13. Liu, Y., et al.: Modeling and predicting the helpfulness of online review. In: 2008 Eighth IEEE International Conference on Data Mining (2008)
14. Zhang, Z.: Weighing stars: aggregating online product reviews for intelligent e-commerce applications. IEEE Intell. Syst. **23**(5), 42–49 (2008)
15. Zhang, Z., Varadarajan, B.: Utility scoring of product reviews. In: Proceedings of the 15th ACM International Conference on Information and Knowledge Management. ACM (2006)
16. Liu, Y., et al.: HelpMeter: a nonlinear model for predicting the helpfulness of online reviews. In: IEEE/WIC/ACM International Conference on Web Intelligence and Intelligent Agent Technology, 2008. WI-IAT 2008. IEEE (2008)
17. Zhang, R., Tran, T.: An entropy-based model for discovering the usefulness of online product reviews. In: IEEE/WIC/ACM International Conference on Web Intelligence and Intelligent Agent Technology, 2008. WI-IAT 2008. IEEE (2008)

18. Hoang, L., Lee, J.-T., Song, Y.-I., Rim, H.-C.: A model for evaluating the quality of user-created documents. In: Li, H., Liu, T., Ma, W.-Y., Sakai, T., Wong, K.-F., Zhou, G. (eds.) AIRS 2008. LNCS, vol. 4993, pp. 496–501. Springer, Heidelberg (2008)

19. Wu, J., Xu, B., Li, S.: An unsupervised approach to rank product reviews. In: 2011 Eighth International Conference on Fuzzy Systems and Knowledge Discovery (FSKD). IEEE (2011)

20. Tsur, O., Rappoport, A.: RevRank: a fully unsupervised algorithm for selecting the most helpful book reviews. In: Adar, E., et al. (eds.) ICWSM. The AAAI Press, Menlo Park (2009)

21. Moghaddam, S., Ester, M.: Opinion digger: an unsupervised opinion miner from unstructured product reviews. In: Proceedings of the 19th ACM International Conference on Information and Knowledge Management. ACM (2010)

22. Agrawal, R.: Sample mean based index policies with O (log n) regret for the multi-armed bandit problem. Adv. Appl. Probab. 1054–1078 (1995)

23. Hinton, G.E., Sejnowski, T.J.: Learning and Relearning in Boltzmann Machines, vol. 1, pp. 282–317. MIT Press, Cambridge (1986)

24. Li, L., et al.: A contextual-bandit approach to personalized news article recommendation. In: Proceedings of the 19th International Conference on World Wide Web. ACM (2010)

25. Conners, L., Mudambi, S.M., Schuff, D.: Is it the review or the reviewer? A multi-method approach to determine the antecedents of online review helpfulness. In: Proceedings of the 44th Hawaii International Conference on System Sciences (2011)

26. Ghose, A., Ipeirotis, P.G.: Estimating the helpfulness and economic impact of product reviews: mining text and reviewer characteristics. IEEE Trans. Knowl. Data Eng. 23(10), 1498–1512 (2011)

27. Wu, P.F., van derHeijden, H., Korfiatis, N.T.: The influences of negativity and review quality on the helpfulness of online reviews. In: The Second International Conference on Information System, Shanghai, China (2011)

28. Korfiatis, N., Bariocanal, E.G., Alonso, S.S.: Evaluating content quality and helpfulness of online product reviews: the interplay of review helpfulness vs. review content. Electron. Commer. Res. Appl. 11, 205–217 (2012)

29. Jo, Y., Oh A.H.: Aspect and sentiment unification model for online review analysis. In: Proceedings of the Fourth ACM International Conference on Web Search and Data Mining. ACM (2011)

# From Cluster-Based Outlier Detection to Time Series Discord Discovery

Nguyen Huy Kha and Duong Tuan Anh[(✉)]

Faculty of Computer Science and Engineering,
Ho Chi Minh City University of Technology,
Ho Chi Minh City, Vietnam
dtanh@cse.hcmut.edu.vn

**Abstract.** Anomalous patterns or discords are just the kind of outliers in time series. In this paper, we present a new approach for time series discord discovery which is based on cluster-based outlier detection. In this approach, first, subsequence candidates are extracted from the time series using a segmentation method, then these candidates are transformed into the same length and are input for an appropriate clustering algorithm, and finally, we identify discords by using a measure suggested in the cluster-based outlier detection method given by He et al. 2003. The experimental results show that our approach is much more efficient than the HOTSAX algorithm in detecting time series discords while the anomalous patterns discovered by the two methods perfectly match with each other.

**Keywords:** Time series discord · Discord discovery · Segmentation · Important extreme points · Outlier detection · Cluster-based outlier detection

## 1 Introduction

Time series data are ubiquitous, touching almost every aspect of human life, in domains such as business, finance, industry, medicine, science or government. The problem of detecting unusual (abnormal, novel, deviant, anomalous, *discord*) time series has recently attracted much attention. Time series discord discovery brings out the "most unusual subsequence" in a time series. Areas that explore such time series discords are, for example, fault diagnostics, intrusion detection and data cleansing.

Some popular algorithms for discord discovery include window-based methods such as HOT SAX by Keogh et al. [14] and WAT by Bu et al. [1]; hidden Markov model-based such as TARZAN by Keogh et al. [13]; a method based on neural-network by Oliveira et al. [18] and a method based on one-class support vector machine by Ma et al. [17]. However, these methods still have two major limitations. First, they require the user to supply the length of the discord subsequence which is always unknown. Second, these algorithms involve high computational cost in the case of working with very large time series datasets.

Outlier detection is the process of detecting the data objects which are grossly different from or inconsistent with the remaining set of data. Searching for outliers is an important area of research in the world of data mining with numerous applications.

© Springer International Publishing Switzerland 2015
X.-L. Li et al. (Eds.): PAKDD 2015, LNCS 9441, pp. 16–28, 2015.
DOI: 10.1007/978-3-319-25660-3_2

Approaches for outlier detection can be classified into five major classes: distribution-based, distance-based, depth-based, density-based and cluster-based. Among all these classes of outlier detection, cluster-based is the latest and the most promising approach. The cluster-based approach considers outlier detection as by-product of clustering algorithm. This approach regards small clusters resulting from clustering as outliers and defines a measure for identifying the degree of each object being an outlier.

In this work, we address the second limitation of previous time series discord discovery algorithms by introducing a novel algorithm inspired by recent advances in the problem of outlier detection in the field of data mining. Anomalous patterns or discords are just the kind of outliers in time series. This work is the first of our attempt to apply outlier detection techniques in discord discovery for time series data. The main idea of our proposed method is to combine segmentation and cluster-based outlier detection. In this approach, first, pattern candidates are extracted from the time series using a segmentation method which is based on important extreme points, then these candidates are transformed into the same length and are input for an appropriate clustering algorithm, and finally, we identify discords by using a measure suggested in the cluster-based outlier detection method given by He et al. [9]. We experimented our proposed method for time series discord discovery on several real world datasets. The experimental results show that our approach is much more efficient than the HOTSAX algorithm in detecting time series discords while the anomalous patterns discovered by the two methods perfectly match with each other.

The rest of the paper is organized as follows. In Sect. 2 we give some essential definitions and explain briefly some basic ideas of cluster-based outlier detection algorithm. Section 3 introduces our proposed method for time series discord discovery. Section 4 reports the experiments on the proposed algorithm in comparison to HOT-SAX. Section 5 gives some conclusions and remarks for future work.

## 2  Background

### 2.1  Time Series Discord

Intuitively a time series discord is a subsequence that is very different from its closest matching subsequence. However, in general, the best matches of a given subsequence (apart from itself) tend to be very close to the subsequence under consideration. For example, given a certain subsequence at position $p$, its closest match will be the subsequence at the position $q$ where $q$ is far from $p$ just a few points. Such matches are called *trivial matches* and are not interesting [14].

**Definition 1:** (*Non-self Match*) Given a time series $T$ containing a subsequence $C$ of length $n$ beginning at position $p$ and a matching subsequence $M$ beginning at the position $q$, we say that $M$ is a non-self match to $C$ if $|p - q| \geq n$.

**Definition 2:** (*Time Series Discord*) Given a time series $T$, the subsequence $C$ of length $n$ beginning at position $p$ is said to be a discord of $T$ if $C$ has the largest distance to its nearest non-self match.

We may be interested in examining the top $K$ discords, which is defined as:

**Definition 3: ($K$-th Time Series Discord)** Given a time series $T$, the subsequence $D$ of length $n$ beginning at position $p$ is the $K$-th discord of $T$ if $D$ has the $K$-th largest distance to its nearest non-self match, with no overlapping region to the $i$-th discord beginning at position $p_i$, for all $1 \leq i \leq K$.

## 2.2    Related Works on Outlier Detection

Intuitively, outlier can be defined as given by Hawkins [10]:

*"An outlier in a dataset is an observation that deviates so much from other observations as to arouse suspicion that it is generated from a different mechanism".*

Many data mining algorithms in literature find outliers as side-product of clustering algorithm, such as DBSCAN by Ester et al. [5], BIRCH by Zhang et al. [21], CURE by Guha et al. [6]. But these techniques define outliers as points which do not lie in clusters. Thus these techniques implicitly define outliers as the background noise in which the clusters are embedded.

Jiang et al. [11] regard *small* clusters as outliers, but a measure for identifying the degree of each object being outlier and how to distinguish small clusters from the rest are not presented in their work. He et al. [9], for the first time, not only regard small clusters as outliers but also define a measure for identifying the degree of each object being an outlier which is called CBLOF (Cluster-based local outlier factor) and present an efficient algorithm for mining outliers. Duan et al. [4] proposed another cluster-based outlier detection method which applies a new defined cluster-based outlier factor and use LDBSCAN algorithm (Duan et al. [3]) for clustering. One improvement in the method of Duan et al. 2009 is that it can evaluate the outlier factor for each cluster as a whole.

## 2.3    Cluster-Based Outlier Detection

The main ideas in the cluster-based outlier detection method proposed by He et al. [9] can be reviewed as follows.

It is reasonable to define the outliers from the point of view of clusters and identify those objects that do not lie in any large clusters as outliers. The algorithm for detecting outliers has two main parts: (1) clustering the dataset and (2) computing the value of *cluster-based local outlier factor* (CBLOF) for each object.

The clustering algorithm used is the Squeezer algorithm (He et al. [8]), which can produce good clustering results and at the same time preserves good scalability. The process of mining outliers is tightly coupled with the clustering algorithm.

The outlier factor CBLOF of each object which identifies the physical significance of an outlier is measured by both the size of the cluster the object belongs to and the distance between the object and its closest cluster (if the object lies in a small cluster) or the distance between the object and the cluster it belongs to (if the object lies in a large cluster).

# 3   From Cluster-Based Outlier Detection to Time Series Discord Discovery

This work is the first of our attempt to employ cluster-based outlier detection approach in time series discord discovery. The main idea of our proposed method is to combine segmentation and cluster-based outlier detection in the problem of time series discord discovery. Our proposed method for discovering discord is called FindCBD (Finding Cluster-based Discord). The FindCBD algorithm consists of the following steps:

Step 1.   Divide the time series into segments (pattern candidates) using important extreme points method.

Step 2.   Transform the pattern candidates to the same length by using homothetic transformation and discretize them using Symbolic Aggregate Approximation (SAX) discretization.

Step 3:   Cluster the discretized pattern candidates using the Squeezer algorithm and calculate the anomaly scores of all the candidates using CBLOF factors.

Step 4:   Identify the pattern candidate with the largest CBLOF score as the top discord of the time series. And the pattern with the $K$-th largest CBLOF score will be the $K$-th discord of the time series.

The details of all four steps are explained in the following subsections.

## 3.1   Time Series Segmentation Using Significant Extreme Points

In this work, we assume that the anomaly within a time series begins and ends at characteristic points such as maxima or minima. In Step 1, to extract a temporally ordered sequence of pattern candidates, significant extreme points of a time series have to be found. The definition of significant extreme points is given as follows.

**Definition 4: (*Significant Extreme Points*)** A univariate time series $T = t_1,...,t_N$ has a *significant minimum* at position $m$ with $1 < m < N$, if a subsequence $(t_i, \ldots, t_j)$ with $1 \leq i < j \leq N$ in $T$ exists, such that $t_m$ is the minimum of all points of this subsequence and $t_i \geq R \times t_m$, $t_j \geq R \times t_m$ with user-defined $R \geq 1$.

Similarly, a *significant maximum* is existent at position $m$ with $1 < m < N$, if a subsequence $(t_i, \ldots, t_j)$ with $1 \leq i < j \leq N$ in $T$ exists, such that $t_m$ is the maximum of all points of this subsequence and $t_i \leq t_m/R$, $t_j \leq t_m/R$ with user-defined $R \geq 1$.

Notice that in the above definition, the parameter $R$ is called *compression rate* which is greater than one and an increase of $R$ leads to selection of fewer significant extreme points. Figure 1 illustrates the definition of significant minima (a) and maxima (b).

Given a time series $T$, starting at the beginning of the time series, all significant minima and maxima of the time series are computed by using the procedure given in Pratt and Fink [19]. This procedure has linear time and constant memory. It can process new points as they arrive, without storing the original time series.

The details of the segmentation step for extracting pattern candidates are given as follows:

(i)  We extract all significant extreme points of the time series $T$. The result of this step is a sequence of extreme points $EP = (ep_1,.., ep_l)$

(ii)  We compute all the pattern candidates iteratively. A pattern candidate $PC_i(T)$, $i = 1,..., l - 2$ is the subsequence of $T$ that is bounded by the two extreme points $ep_i$ and $ep_{i+2}$. Pattern candidates are the subsequences that may have different lengths.

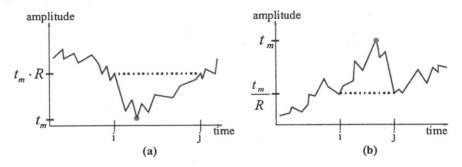

**Fig. 1.** Illustration of significant extreme points: (a) Minimum, (b) Maximum ([19])

## 3.2   Homothetic Transformation

To ensure the effectiveness of our proposed method, in Step 2 of our FindCBD algorithm, we have to apply some interpolation technique for transforming the pattern candidates of different lengths to those of the same length. Spline interpolation can be selected for this task as suggested in by Gruber et al. [7]. However, spline interpolation is not only complicated in computation, but also can modify undesirably the shapes of the motif candidates. In this work, we apply homothetic transformation, a simpler and more effective technique which also can transform the subsequences with different lengths to those of the same length. Due to the limit of space, we can not explain the use of homothetic transformation here, interested readers can refer to our previous work [20] for more details.

## 3.3   SAX Discretization

In our discord discovery method, we use Squeezer algorithm to cluster the pattern candidates (i.e. subsequences). But Squeezer algorithm operates on categorical dataset. Therefore, we need some discretization method to convert the subsequences to symbolic strings. Here we select to use Symbolic Aggregate Approximation (SAX) method ([16]) to transform the subsequences to symbolic strings. The SAX representation that is used in Step 2 of our FindCBD algorithm can be explained briefly as follows.

A time series $C = c_1...c_N$ of length $N$ can be represented in a reduced $w$-dimensional-space as another time series $D = d_1...d_w$ by segmenting $C$ into $w$ equally-sized segments and then replacing each segment by its mean value $d_i$. This dimensionality reduction technique is called Piecewise Aggregate Approximation (PAA) [12]. After this step, the time series $D$ is transformed into a symbolic sequence $A = a_1 \ldots a_w$ in which each real value $d_i$ is mapped to a symbol $a_i$ through a table look-up. The lookup table contains the *breakpoints* that divide a Gaussian distribution in an arbitrary number (e.g. from 3 to 10) of equi-probable regions. This discretization is based on the assumption that the reduced time series have a Gaussian distribution.

Notice that since pattern candidates extracted in Step 1 are always short time series, after being transformed by PAA and SAX, the dimensionality of the pattern candidates becomes sufficiently small and Squeezer can cluster efficiently these objects with low dimensionality.

## 3.4 How to Compute CBLOF of Each Object

**Definition 5:** Let $A_1$, ..., $A_m$ be a set of categorical attributes with domains $D_1$, ..., $D_m$ respectively. Let the dataset $D$ be the set of tuples where each tuple $t$: $t \in D_1 \times \ldots \times D_m$. The results of a clustering algorithm executed on $D$ is denoted as: $C = \{C_1, C_2, \ldots, C_k\}$ where $C_i \cap C_j = \varnothing$ and $C_1 \cup C_2 \ldots \cup C_k = D$. The number of clusters is $k$.

**Definition 6:** (*Large and Small Cluster*) Suppose $C = \{C_1, C_2, \ldots, C_k\}$ is the set of clusters in the sequence that $|C_1| \geq |C_2| \geq \ldots \geq |C_k|$. Given two numeric parameters $\alpha$ and $\beta$, we define $b$ the boundary of large and small if one of the following formulas holds:

$$(|C_1| + |C_2| + \ldots + |C_b|) \geq |D| * \alpha \tag{1}$$

$$|C_b|/|C_{b+1}| \geq \beta \tag{2}$$

The set of large clusters is defined as $LC = \{C_i \mid i \leq b\}$ and the set of small cluster is defined as: $SC = \{C_j \mid j > b\}$.

Definition 6 gives a measure to distinguish large and small clusters. Formula (1) considers the fact that most data points in the dataset are not outliers. Therefore, clusters that contain a large portion of data points should be taken as large clusters. For example, if $\alpha$ is set to 90 %, we intend to regard clusters contain 90 % of data points as large clusters. Formula (2) considers the fact that large and small clusters should have significant differences in size. For instance, if we set $\beta$ to 5, the size of any cluster in $LC$ is at least five times of the size of the cluster in $SC$.

**Definition 7:** (*Cluster-Based Local Outlier Factor*) Suppose $C = \{C_1, C_2, \ldots, C_k\}$ is the set of clusters in the sequence that $|C_1| \geq |C_2| \geq \ldots \geq |C_k|$ and the meanings of $\alpha$, $\beta$, $b$, $LC$ and $SC$ are the same as they are formalized in Definition 4. For any records $t$, the cluster-based local outlier factor of $t$ is defined as:

$$CBLOF(t) = |C_i| * \min(distance(t, C_j)) \quad \text{if } t \in C_i, C_i \in SC \text{ and } C_j \in LC(j : 1 \to b)$$
$$= |C_i| * (distance(t, C_i)) \quad \text{if } t \in C_i, C_i \in LC$$

From Definition 7, the CBLOF of an object is determined by the size of its cluster, and the distance between the object and its closest large cluster (if this object lies in small cluster) or the distance between the object and the cluster it belongs to (if this object belongs to a large cluster).

### 3.5   The Squeezer Algorithm

Let $A_1$, ..., $A_m$ be a set of categorical attributes with domains $D_1$, ..., $D_m$. respectively. Let the dataset $D$ be the set of tuples where each tuple $t$: $t \in D_1 \times ... \times D_m$. Let $TID$ be the set of unique identifiers of every tuple. For each $tid \in TID$, the attribute value for $A_i$ of corresponding tuple is represented as $tid. A_i$.

**Definition 8: (Cluster)** $Cluster \subseteq TID$ is a subset of $TID$.

**Definition 9:** Given a cluster $C$, the set of different attribute values on $A_i$ with respect to $C$ is defined as: $VAL_i(C) = \{tid . A_i \mid tid \in C\}$ where $1 \le i \le m$.

**Definition 10:** Given a cluster $C$, let $a_i \in D_i$, the support of $a_i$ in $C$ with respect to $A_i$ is defined as: $Sup(a_i) = |\{tid \mid tid . A_i = a_i, tid \in C\}|$.

**Definition 11: (Similarity)** Given a cluster $C$ and a tuple $t$ with $tid \in TID$, the similarity between $C$ and $tid$ is defined as:

$$Sim(C, tid) = \sum_{i=1}^{m} \left( \frac{Sup(a_i)}{\sum_{a_j \in VAL_i(C)} Sup(a_j)} \right)$$

where $a_i = tid. A_i$

To compute CBLOF for object $t$, He et al. need a background clustering algorithm and the clustering algorithm used is the Squeezer algorithm (He et al. [8]). The Squeezer algorithm has some advantageous features. First, it achieves both high quality of clustering results and scalability. Second, it does not require the number of desired clusters as an input parameter. Third, it can handle high dimensional datasets effectively. However, Squeezer is for clustering categorical data.

From Definition 11, it is clear that the similarity used here is statistics based. That means if the similarity between a tuple and an existed cluster is large enough, it means that the probability of the tuple belongs to this cluster is larger.

The Squeezer algorithm has $n$ tuples as input, similarity threshold $s$ as a parameter and produces clusters as final results. Initially, the first tuple in the database is read in and the first cluster is constructed to contain the first tuple, i.e. $C = \{1\}$. Then, the consequence tuples are read iteratively. The outline of the Squeezer algorithm is described as follows.

```
Algorithm Squeezer (D, s)
begin
    while (D has unread tuple) {
        tuple = getCurrentTuple (D)
        if (tuple.tid = = 1) {
                addNewClusterStructure (tuple.tid)}
        else {
                for each existed cluster C
                        simComputation (C, tuple)
                get the max value of similarity: sim_max
                get the corresponding Cluster Index: index
                if sim_max >= s
                        addTupleToCluster (tuple, index)
                else
                        addNewClusterStructure (tuple.tid)}
                    }
    }
    outputClusteringResult ()
end
```

Note: In the formula to compute the CBLOF of a tuple, the distance from a tuple to a given cluster can be computed using the similarity between that tuple to the cluster. That means

$$distance(t, C) = 1/(1 + Sim(C, t))$$

## 3.6    The Parameters of the FindCBD Algorithm

Due to the combination of segmentation, homothetic transform and cluster-based outlier detection, our FindCBD algorithm requires eight parameters which are defined as follows.

$R$: compression ratio for extracting important extreme points from a time series. If $R$ is larger, fewer extreme points are selected, otherwise, more extreme points selected.

$l\_max$: the maximum length of pattern candidates.

$l\_min$: the minimum length of the pattern candidates. If a pattern candidate with length less than $l\_min$, it will be ignored.

$a$: alphabet size, $w$: window size for SAX discretization.

$s$: similarity threshold. This threshold is used by the Squeezer algorithm to determine which cluster a pattern candidate belongs to.

Parameter $\alpha$ indicates the percentage of pattern candidates in the candidate set that belongs to large clusters. Parameter $\beta$ determines the difference in size between a large cluster and a small cluster. The parameters $\alpha$ and $\beta$ are used in computing the outlier factors of each pattern candidates.

Note that FindCBD does not require user to determine the discord length, but the user has to estimate the maximum and the minimum values for the discord length through the two parameters *l_max* and *l_min*.

## 4  Experimental Evaluation

We implemented the comparative methods with Microsoft Visual C# and conducted the experiments on an Intel(R) Core(TM) 2 Duo CPU T6400 @ 2.00 GHz, 2 GB RAM PC.

In this experiment, we compare the proposed algorithm to the HOT SAX algorithm. The HOT SAX is selected for comparison due to its popularity. It is the most cited algorithm for detecting time series discords up to date and was applied in many applications. The comparison is in terms of time efficiency and discord detection accuracy.

**Table 1.** Parameter settings of the two discord discovery algorithms on the five datasets

| Dataset | FindCBD | HOT SAX |
|---|---|---|
| ECG | $R = 1.2$, $l\_max = 250$, $l\_min = 40$ $w = 20$, $a = 8$, $s = 12$, $\alpha = 0.9$, $\beta = 5$ | $w = 20$, $a = 8$, $m = 100$ |
| AEM | $R = 1.4$, $l\_max = 250$, $l\_min = 40$ $w = 20$, $a = 8$, $s = 12$, $\alpha = 0.9$, $\beta = 5$ | $w = 20$, $a = 8$, $m = 200$ |
| ERP | $R = 1.35$, $l\_max = 350$, $l\_min = 30$ $w = 20$, $a = 20$, $s = 12$, $\alpha = 0.9$, $\beta = 5$ | $w = 20$, $a = 20$, $m = 1200$ |
| STOCK | $R = 1.03$, $l\_max = 500$, $l\_min = 50$ $w = 20$, $a = 20$, $s = 15$, $\alpha = 0.9$, $\beta = 5$ | $w = 20$, $a = 20$, $m = 600$ |
| POWER | $R = 1.15$, $l\_max = 200$, $l\_min = 50$ $w = 20$, $a = 20$, $s = 12$, $\alpha = 0.9$, $\beta = 5$ | $w = 20$, $a = 20$, $m = 800$ |

We conducted the experiment on five datasets: ECG (20000 data points), AEM (20000 data points), ERP (25000 data points), STOCK (20000 data points) and POWER (25000 data points). All the datasets are obtained from the UCR Time Series Data Mining Archive (Keogh et al. [15]).

The parameter settings for two algorithms: FindCBD and HOT SAX over each dataset are given in Table 1. For the HOT SAX algorithm, we have the three following parameters: SAX alphabet size $a$, the length of a SAX word $w$ and the length of the discord $m$. For the FindCBD, we have eight parameters: the compression ratio $R$, the maximum length of pattern candidates, $l\_max$, the minimum length of pattern candidates $l\_min$, SAX alphabet size $a$, the length of a SAX word $w$, the similarity threshold $s$, the parameter $\alpha$, and the parameter $\beta$ (for distinguishing small clusters and large clusters).

Notice that with all five datasets, we choose the window size $w = 20$. Due to that after PAA and SAX transformation, the dimensionality of pattern candidates is 20. With this dimensionality, the Squeezer algorithm can work effectively. For all the

**Table 2.** Experimental results on the run times of the two discord discovery algorithms.

| Dataset | Length | Method | Run time (s) | Speedup |
|---|---|---|---|---|
| ECG | 20000 | FindCBD | 0.041 | 2390 |
| | | HOT SAX | 98 | |
| AEM | 20000 | FindCBD | 0.016 | 16250 |
| | | HOT SAX | 260 | |
| ERP | 25000 | FindCBD | 0.027 | 21629 |
| | | HOT SAX | 584 | |
| STOCK | 20000 | FindCBD | 0.024 | 6250 |
| | | HOT SAX | 150 | |
| POWER | 20000 | FindCBD | 0.052 | 3192 |
| | | HOT SAX | 166 | |
| Average | | | | 9942.2 |

experiments, the two parameters $\alpha$, $\beta$ needed when computing anomaly scores are set to 90 % and 5 separately.

The experimental results on the run times of the two algorithms on the five datasets are shown in Table 2.

From the experimental results, we can see that for all the datasets our FindCBD is remarkably faster than HOT SAX. In average, FindCBD is faster than HOT SAX about 10,000 times. Efficiency is achieved because of two reasons. First, sliding over the set of segments extracted from a time series in FindCBD is much faster than sliding the window over the time series one data point at a time in HOTSAX. Segment-based sliding window, which does not incur any information loss, has been supported by several previous works in time series anomaly detection as well as motif discovery

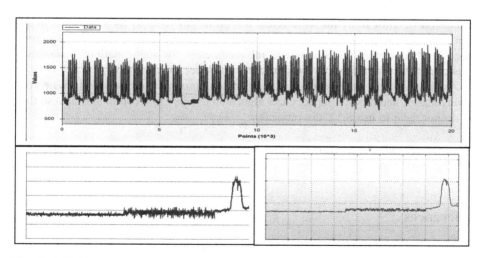

**Fig. 2.** POWER dataset (top). The top discord discovered in the dataset by HOT SAX (bottom-left). The top discord discovered in the dataset by FindCBD (bottom-right).

([2, 7, 20]). Second, both the segmentation basing on significant extreme points and the Squeezer algorithm for clustering can work very fast.

Now we turn our discussion to the accuracy of the proposed discord discovery algorithm. Following the tradition established in previous works, such as [1, 2, 13, 14], the accuracy of a given discord discovery algorithms is basically based on human analysis of the discords discovered by that algorithm. That means through human inspection we can check if the discords identified by a proposed algorithm on a given time series dataset are almost the same as those identified by the baseline discord discovery algorithm (here we select HOT SAX as the baseline algorithm). If the check result is positive in most of the test datasets, we can conclude that the proposed discord discovery algorithm brings out the same accuracy as the baseline algorithm.

Due to space limit, Fig. 2 shows only one example of the top discord discovered in the POWER dataset by the FindCBD and HOT SAX algorithm. From Fig. 2, we can see that the top discord discovered by our proposed algorithm is exactly the same as that discovered by HOT SAX algorithm. In fact, over all five datasets, the discords discovered by FindCBD are almost the same as those discovered by HOT SAX.

## 5   Conclusions

This work is the first of our attempt to apply outlier detection techniques in discord discovery for time series data. The main idea of our proposed method is to combine segmentation and cluster-based outlier detection in one framework. The segmentation is based on significant extreme points ([19]) and the cluster-based outlier detection is based on the method proposed by He et al. [8].

We experimented our proposed method for time series discord discovery on five real world datasets. The experimental results show that our approach is much faster than the HOTSAX algorithm in detecting time series discords while the anomalous patterns discovered by the two methods perfectly match with each other. One major conclusion we draw from this work is that it is promising to apply the techniques in the field of outlier detection to time series discord discovery. One limitation of our proposed method is that it requires several parameters for segmentation, homothetic transform, SAX discretization and clustering by Squeezer algorithm.

As future work, we intend to experiment our proposed method with more real world datasets and modify the Squeezer algorithm to adapt it to continuous data so that we do not have to use SAX discretization.

**Acknowledgement.** We are grateful to Prof. Eamonn Keogh for his kindly providing all the test datasets used in this work.

## References

1. Bu, Y., Leung, T.W., Fu, A., Keogh, E., Pei, J., Meshkin, S.: WAT: finding Top-K discords in time series database. In: Proceedings of the 2007 SIAM International Conference on Data Mining (SDM 2007), Minneapolis, MN, USA (26–28 April 2007)

2. Chuah, M.C., Fu, F.: ECG anomaly detection via time series analysis. In: Thulasiraman, P., He, X., Xu, T.L., Denko, M.K., Thulasiram, R.K., Yang, L.T. (eds.) ISPA Workshops 2007. LNCS, vol. 4743, pp. 123–135. Springer, Heidelberg (2007)
3. Duan, L.D., Xu, L., Guo, F., Lee, J., Yan, B.: A local density based spatial clustering with noise. Inf. Syst. **32**(7), 978–986 (2007)
4. Duan, L.D., Xu, L., Liu, Y., Lee, J.: Cluster-based outlier detection. Ann. Oper. Res. **168**, 151–168 (2009)
5. Ester, M., Kriegel, H., Sander, J., Xu, X.: A density-based algorithm for discovering clusters in large spatial databases with noises. In: Proceedings of 2nd International Conference on Knowledge Discovery and Data Mining, pp. 226–231. AAAI Press, Portland (1996)
6. Guha, S., Rastogi, R., Shim, K.: CURE: an efficient clustering algorithm for large databases. In: Tiwary, A., Franklin, M. (eds.) Proceedings of 1998 ACM SIGMOD International Conference on Management of Data, Seattle, Washington, USA, pp. 73–84 (01–04 June 1998)
7. Gruber, C., Coduro, M., Sick, B.: Signature verification with dynamic RBF network and time series motifs. In: Proceedings of 10th International Workshop on Frontiers in Handwriting Recognition (2006)
8. He, Z., Xu, X., Deng, S.: Squeezer: an efficient algorithm for clustering categorical data. J. Comput. Sci. Technol. **17**(5), 611–624 (2002)
9. He, Z., Xu, X., Deng, S.: Discovering cluster-based local outliers. Pattern Recogn. Lett. **24**(9–10), 1641–1650 (2003)
10. Hawkins, D.: Identification of Outliers. Chapman and Hall, London (1980)
11. Jiang, M.F., Tseng, S.S., Su, C.M.: Two phase clustering process for outlier detection. Pattern Recogn. Lett. **22**(6–7), 691–700 (2001)
12. Keogh, E., Chakrabarti, K., Pazzani, M., Mehrotra, S.: Dimensionality deduction for fast similarity search in large time series database. J. Knowl. Inf. Syst. **3**(3), 263–286 (2001)
13. Keogh, E., Lonardi, S., Chiu, B.: Finding surprising patterns in a time series database in linear time and space. In: KDD 2002: Proceedings of 8th ACM SIGKDD International Conference on Knowledge Discovery and Data Mining, New York, NY, USA, pp. 550–556 (2002)
14. Keogh, E., Lin, J. and Fu, A.: HOT SAX: efficiently finding the most unusual time series subsequence. In: Proceedings of 5th IEEE International Conference on Data Mining (ICDM), pp. 226–233 (2005)
15. Keogh E., Xi X., Wei L., Ratanamahatana C.A.: The UCR time series classification/clustering homepage (2013). www.cs.ucr.edu/~eamonn/time_series_data
16. Lin, J., Keogh, E., Lonardi, S., Chiu, B.: A symbolic representation of time series, with implications for streaming algorithms. In: Proceedings of 8th ACM SIGMOD Workshop on Research Issues in Data Mining and Knowledge Discover (DMKD 2003), pp. 2–11 (13 June 2003)
17. Ma, J., Perkins, S.: Online novelty detection on temporal sequences. In: Proceedings of the 9th ACM SIGKDD International Conference on Knowledge Discovery and Data Mining, NY, USA, pp. 614–618. ACM Press (2003)
18. Oliveira, A.L.I., Neto, F.B.L., Meira, S.R.L.: A method based on RBF-DAA neural network for improving novelty detection in time series. In: Proceedings of 17th International FLAIRS Conference, AAAI Press, Miami Beach, Florida, USA (2004)
19. Pratt, K.B., Fink, E.: Search for pattern in compressed time series. Int. J. Image Graph. **2**(1), 89–106 (2002)

20. Truong, C.D., Anh, D.T.: An efficient method for discovering motifs in large time series. In: Selamat, A., Nguyen, N.T., Haron, H. (eds.) ACIIDS 2013, Part I. LNCS, vol. 7802, pp. 135–145. Springer, Heidelberg (2013)
21. Zhang, T., Ramakrishnan, R., Livny, M.: BIRCH: an efficient data clustering method for very large databases. In: Proceedings of the 1996 ACM SIGMOD International Conference on Management of Data, Montreal, Quebec, Canada, pp. 103–114 (04–06 June 1996)

# Web Site Audience Segmentation Using Hybrid Alignment Techniques

Vinh-Trung Luu[✉], Germain Forestier, Frédéric Fondement,
and Pierre-Alain Muller

MIPS, Université de Haute Alsace, 12, rue des frères Lumière,
68093 Mulhouse Cedex, France
{trung.luu-vinh,germain.forestier,
frederic.fondement,pierre-alain.muller}@uha.fr

**Abstract.** We are working on behavioral marketing in the Internet. On one hand we observe the behavior of visitors, and on the other hand we trigger (in real-time) stimulations intended to alter this behavior. Real-time and mass-customization are the two challenges that we have to address. In this paper, we present a hybrid approach for clustering visitor sessions, based on a combination of global and local sequence alignments, such as Needleman-Wunsch and Smith-Waterman. Our goal is to define very simple approaches able to address about 80 % of visitor sessions to be segmented, and which can be easily turned into small pieces of program, to be run in parallel in thousands of web browsers.

**Keywords:** Web mining · Sequential pattern mining · Clustering

## 1 Introduction

Behavioral marketing in the Internet includes adapting web sites to the interests of the visitors in real-time, while they are browsing. Web usage mining has been widely used to transform low-level browsing data (such as page- and click-stream) into actionable knowledge, which makes sense in the business arena. This calls for operators able to compute a measure of similarity between any two sessions, in order to define groups of similar sessions, and further to segment the audience. In our case, as we want to act in real-time, we also have to provide similarity operators which can be executed quickly (in a time which is compatible with the browsing speed of visitors). Sessions can be considered as sequences of events. The granularity of these events can be fine-tuned, from pages-loads down to low-level JavaScript events. In this paper, for the sake of simplicity, we will talk of sequences of symbols, such as A-B-C-D-E-F. Luckily, we have access daily to hundred thousands of such sequences, which are recorded by our industrial partner (BeamPulse). These sequences originate mainly from e-commerce applications.

There is a large amount experience in sequence analysis in the field of DNA sequences comparison. Sequence alignment has been widely used to identify regions of similarity of DNA, RNA or protein sequences in bioinformatics.

© Springer International Publishing Switzerland 2015
X.-L. Li et al. (Eds.): PAKDD 2015, LNCS 9441, pp. 29–40, 2015.
DOI: 10.1007/978-3-319-25660-3_3

Two main approaches - global and local alignment of sequences - have been proposed, respectively by Needleman-Wunsch [1] (NW) and Smith-Waterman [2] (SW). Weinan Wang et al. [3] labeled sitemaps as tree structures and compared pairs of sessions using sequences comparison by applying global sequence alignment. In another research, LI Chaofeng et al. [4] introduced a scoring method by combination of visiting time and URLs similar to [3]. However, according to Poornalatha Ga et al. [5], the optimal similarity between two sequences or clustering outliers can be found by an algorithm based on Smith-Waterman local alignment method only. An approach to cluster web sessions was proposed by Bhupendra S. Chordia et al. [6] where the clusters are initialized using the longest and most dissimilar sequences. Then, a combination of local and global alignment is used to update the clusters. Alternatively, Costantinos Dimopoulos et al. [7] modeled users navigation history and web page content using weighted suffix trees. Their system was then used for the prediction of web page usage. Dynamic Time Warping (DTW), another widely used sequence alignment, has been frequently used to cluster time series [8]. For example, Warissara Meesrikamolkul et al. [9] proposed a method to combine DTW and K-Means to cluster time-series efficiently. They significantly improved the execution time and improved the accuracy of the clusters. Meanwhile, Atsuyoshi Nakamura et al. [10] studied a method named packing alignment to study sequences of various length. This method is partly similar to DTW but allows gaps and limits consecutive events. DTW approach has also been the basis or reference to propose new algorithms, such as [11] by Alice Marascu et.al taking distance measure LCSS having similar distance matrix like DTW into consideration to detect similarity matching in data streams.

This paper aim at introducing a new approach for clustering sessions, by defining a combination of local and global sequence alignments for computing similarity between two pages visit sequences. As we do not target 100 % applicability, issues such as impreciseness of sequence glocal (hybrid) metric, caused by the somewhat ignorance of sequences dissimilarity when lengths are uneven, can be overcome.

The remainder of this paper is organized as follows: Sect. 2 details our approach and provides illustrative examples. Experimental result is described in Sect. 3. In Sect. 4, we present related works and explain how our approach compares to theses earlier techniques. Finally, Sect. 5 concludes our paper and suggests some future research directions.

## 2   Proposed Method

As introduced previously, the Needleman-Wunsch [1] (NW) algorithm creates a global alignment of two sequences. This algorithm aims at detecting the optimal alignment over the entire length of two sequences. Thus, this algorithm is appropriate to align pair of sequences of similar length. Meanwhile, the Smith-Waterman [2] (SW) algorithm is dedicated to local sequence alignment and is then suitable when comparing two sequences with significant difference in lengths. In this paper, we used the NW scoring scheme of +1 for matching and

−1 for non-matching pair of items in sequences, and the SW scoring scheme of +2 for matching and −1 for non-matching inside matching, ignore non-matching outside. We selected these two algorithms for their simple and efficient alignment scoring scheme. To detect the best alignment of sequences pair, these two algorithms use a matrix with a number of rows and columns corresponding to the sequences lengths. This matrix is filled by aligning score between these two sequences, and finally a trace back is performed [1,2].

NW and SW, by their featured alignments, measure similarity of sequence pairs in different evaluations. For instance, SW score of Fig. 1 and NW scores of Figs. 2 and 3 are equal. However, if we take the rate of similarity lengths over sequence lengths into consideration, the similarity of Fig. 1 is not as much as Figs. 2 and 3.

**A**BCDEFGHIJK

**A**

**Fig. 1.** Sequence alignment on two sequences having a common subsequence but different lengths

**AB**

**AB**

**Fig. 2.** Sequence alignment on two identical sequences

**ABC**D

**ABC**E

**Fig. 3.** Sequence alignment on two sequences having a common subsequence and similar lengths

In the comparison of web access sequences, the pairs of sequences in Figs. 2 and 3 are more likely to be similar than the sequences of Fig. 1 as they contains the same number of items. However, their similarity scores are mostly same. Alternatively, Figs. 4 and 5 show cases of pairs of sequences that have the same length and the same NW score. However, the first pair in Fig. 4 is more consecutive than the one in Fig. 5. In other words, SW score of the first pair is higher than the second. This consecution, in our opinion, makes the first pair more similar in web access sequence comparison.

A**BC**D

X**BC**Y

**Fig. 4.** Sequence alignment on two sequences having a common subsequence and similar lengths

A**B**D**C**

X**B**Y**C**

**Fig. 5.** Sequence alignment on two sequences having common subsequences and similar lengths

Since the clustering of web sessions is based on the alignment scores, these scores have to reflect the real similarity of the sequences. In our opinion, the *real* similarity of web sessions pair should not only consider a specific rate of common pages but should also take into account the consecution in those common pages. This consecution plays an important role in web usage mining, where the same set of pages but in different order represents dissimilar accessing behaviors. Accordingly, we propose a method to compute what is expected of similar pairs of sequences. As mentioned previously, a global view in sequence alignment is NW strong advantage. Its scoring scheme takes both similarity and dissimilarity into account but does not really reflect the consecution of similar items. Therefore, another algorithm focusing on this consecution should be employed to process the result provided by NW. SW is a good candidate as it focuses on local similarity in sequence alignment. Thus, the method proposed in this paper takes the advantages of NW and SW and reduce their disadvantages in web access sequence alignment.

We selected five pairs of sequences: (ABCDEFG, BCDEFG), (ABCDEFGH, ABXDYFGH), (ABCDEFG, CDEFG) (DEFG, DEFG) and (ABCDEF, CDEF) that have specific properties to illustrate the method. We proposed a set of rules that combine NW and SW alignment scores. We expect that similar pairs of sequences match the rules for both alignments. Furthermore, the order of the rules should not affect the final result. We recommend to first check the rules using NW alignment score and then the rules using SW alignment. Using this process, we start by considering a global alignment of the sequences and then a local alignment. In other words, SW alignment works on NWs result. We define rule matching (✓) and rule non-matching (✗) pairs through checking as result in Table 1.

**Table 1.** Rule matching and non-matching pairs in sequence alignments result

|          | NW score > 2 | NW score > 2 and SW score > 10 |
|----------|:---:|:---:|
| ABCDEFG BCDEFG | ✓ | ✓ |
| ABCDEFGH ABXDYFGH | ✓ | ✗ |
| ABCDEFG CDEFG | ✓ | ✗ |
| DEFG DEFG | ✓ | ✗ |
| ABCDEF CDEF | ✗ | ✗ |

The values 2 and 10 have been chosen as initial thresholds based on the average lengths of sequence pairs. As one can see, by defining these thresholds the similar pairs match the NW rule. However, some others pairs such as (ABCDEF,

CDEF) does not. If we want sequence pairs to have a similarity score higher than half of the sequence length, the longer sequences length has to be used within the rule. Integrating this length also allows overcoming another drawback of NW similarity metric as NW scoring scheme counts correlation between similarity and dissimilarity but ignores the ratio of similarity/dissimilarity over sequence lengths. Thus, we enhanced the rule to make NW score value dependent of the longer sequence length as described in Table 2, with the corresponding coefficient equals to 1/4 then all pairs match:

**Table 2.** Rule matching and non-matching pairs in sequence alignments result after taking longer sequence length into account through its coefficient

|  | NW score > longer sequence length/4 | NW score > longer sequence length/4 and SW score > 10 |
|---|---|---|
| ABCDEFG BCDEFG | ✓ | ✓ |
| ABCDEFGH ABXDYFGH | ✓ | ✗ |
| ABCDEFG CDEFG | ✓ | ✗ |
| DEFG DEFG | ✓ | ✗ |
| ABCDEF CDEF | ✓ | ✗ |

However, by applying SW rule as threshold for the expected consecution, many pairs in NWs result are non-matching with this rule. We analyze the non-matching pairs as following:

- ABCDEFGH/ABXDYFGH: Resulting SW score = 10 when aligning with ABCDEFGH or other sequences because of its inner dissimilarity comparing to the other ones. This web access sequence is not similar to the other one in pair because the consecution is not matching SW rule
- CDEFG/DEFG: Resulting SW score = 8 when aligning with the other sequence or itself because of one disadvantages of this approach: SW score set in rule affects the sequence lengths in result, because these lengths have to be equal or greater than the threshold. Nevertheless, this can be improved by setting the SW score in the rule dependent of the shorter sequence of the set. For example, in order to select pairs that shorter sequence are sub sequence of longer one, similarity length aligned by SW must equal to the shorter sequence length.

With the above given matching score of SW aligning is 2, we change the rule condition from "> 10" to "=shorter sequence length x 2". Corresponding result is in Table 3, which shows the final result of proposed combination of NW and SW:

**Table 3.** Rule matching and non-matching pairs in sequence alignment result after taking longer and shorter sequence length into account through their coefficients

|  | NW score > longer sequence length/4 | NW score > longer sequence length/4 and SW score = shorter sequence length x 2 |
|---|---|---|
| ABCDEFG BCDEFG | ✓ | ✓ |
| ABCDEFGH ABXDYFGH | ✓ | ✗ |
| ABCDEFG CDEFG | ✓ | ✓ |
| DEFG DEFG | ✓ | ✓ |
| ABCDEF CDEF | ✓ | ✓ |

Another possible approach is binary Dynamic Time Warping (DTW). Back to sequence pair examples from Figs. 1 to 5, the application of DTW results are close to NW. If the rule is, for example, DTW score $\leq 2$, pairs in Figs. 2 to 5 are similar and pair in Fig. 1 is not. The combination of DTW and SW returns a similar result than NW and SW when sequences pair in Fig. 5 eliminated from similarity set of pairs. In DTW, conditional value in rule can depend on sequence length too, since the sequences pair considered similar if the dissimilarity not greater than some threshold.

For instance, (AAAA,A) is a case that could not be considered similar in web usage mining context because there might be a reason why a web visitor stayed longer on a page. Nevertheless, DTW does not align with gaps as NW; hence it treats sequence of identical symbols not as a kind of user accessing behavior but as duplication. Therefore, DTW scores is 0 for this example, no matter how long is the duplication in the longer sequence. This limitation makes NW more suitable than DTW in page visit sequence alignment.

*Time and Space Complexity:* According to Alexander Chan in [12], time and space complexity of NW and SW are the same, $O(mn)$, given by $m$ and $n$ are sequence lengths. In our proposed method, each sequence pair is aligned by both of algorithms, thus the total time and complexity processing each pair should be $O(mn)$.

## 3    Experimental Result

The dataset used for the experiments was collected from a University campus website. This website has more than 20,000 visits monthly. A deployed service has taken part in preparation phase [13, 14] of the clustering process. Written in Javascript and Java, these services allow us to extract information from University campus data like cookies and other associated information such as page visit order, activity time or duration of page visit. In addition, the output format is optional which is convenient to work with variety of mining tool if needed. The extracted information is then checked and validated before applying algorithms to mine them.

Building web access sequences is the next phase. As mentioned earlier and in related works [3–7], sequence of visits plays an important role in user behaviors analyzing. In order to improve the performance of sequence alignment, URLs have to be shortened optimally by the presentation of symbols set like numbers. Similar to [5–7], session contains ordered URLs like, for example:

1 = http://www.campus-fonderie.uha.fr/fr/droit/
2 = http://www.campus-fonderie.uha.fr/fr/economie-et-societe/
3 = http://www.campus-fonderie.uha.fr/fr/management/
4 = http://www.campus-fonderie.uha.fr/fr/management-interculturel/

will be represented by symbol set $\{1, 2, 3, 4\}$, and turn to be page visit sequence like S = 1_2_3_4. In this sequence, page access order is respected and each symbol represents only a unique page. Pairwise alignments are made through all pairs of page visit sequence to score their similarity. As proposed in [3], similarity matrix of web sessions is then computed from this pairwise alignment results.

In the first experiment, we show results on 32 sample sessions that have been selected according to their length, duplication and order of visits as representative of the whole dataset. The goal of this experiment is to highlight specific features of the method. We focus this experiment on three rules: "NW score > longer sequence length/4" (NW), "SW score = shorter sequence length x 2" (named SW), and the combition "NW & SW" (the rule in the last column of Table 3). We applied independently the three rules on the similarty matrix obtained by comparing the 32 sequences. We then computed single linkage clustering using the three matrices using $R^1$. The clustering results are displayed using dendrograms on Fig. 6 for NW, Fig. 7 for SW and Fig. 8 for NW & SW.

As we can see on Figs. 6, 7 and 8, there are respectively 26, 32 and 23 sessions after the applications of the rules. Applying NW rule results (Fig. 6) leads to more similar sessions with higher global similar, but sequences like 10_8_1_9_2_4 or 1_2_3_4_5 are not locally similar to others by SW rule. In contrary, applying only SW rule (Fig. 7) leads to the existence of sequences such as 10_1_12_13_4_9_14 9_3_4 11_11_11,10_8_15_10, 10_8_1_9_2_4, etc. that are not globally similar to others by NW rule.

A noticeable sequence 9_3_4 exists in single rule cases because it is matching either but not both. Finally, the combination of NW and SW (Fig. 8) rules extracts less but satisfied sequences of global and local similarity.

---

[1] https://stat.ethz.ch/R-manual/R-patched/library/stats/html/dendrogram.html.

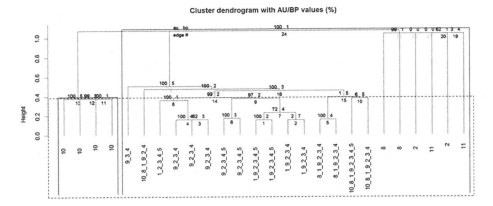

**Fig. 6.** Dendrogram of NW score > longer sequence length/4 (NW)

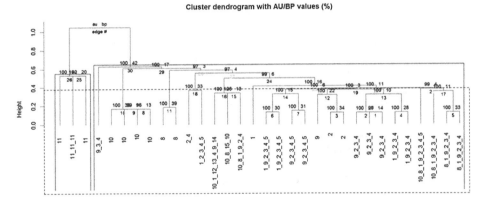

**Fig. 7.** R2: Dendrogram of SW score = shorter sequence length x 2 (SW)

Consequently, the first top-down pair of Fig. 8 is different from the others on global and local similarity. Considering clusters at a specific height, for instance 0.4, by looking inside dashed frame, some following features can be seen:

- The number of clusters produced using NW, SW and NW&SW rules are respectively 11, 10 and 13 ;
- The NW&SW similarity inside the clusters is the best, most of the clusters are 100 % similar inside, except one. Meanwhile, there are two and three of such clusters in NW and SW. The rate of clusters with 100 % inside similarity over number of cluster are respectively 92 %, 81 % and 70 % in NW, SW and NW&SW ;
- Clusters with dissimilarity inside of NW&SW are smaller than NW, and such clusters in NW are generally smaller than them in SW, considering the cluster size by number of sequence ;

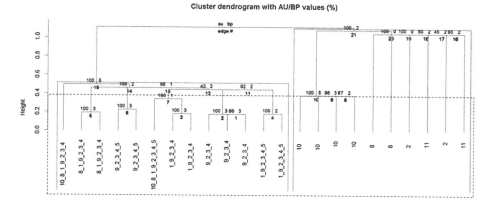

**Fig. 8.** Dendrogram of NW score > longer sequence length/4 and SW score = shorter sequence length x 2 (NW&SW)

- Clusters with dissimilarity inside of NW&SW are more similar than NW, and such clusters in NW are generally more similar than them in SW, considering the rate of similar sequences over number of sequences ;
- The necessary hierarchical level number by NW, SW and NW&SW rules are respectively 24, 30 and 21.

Experiments performed in the sample of 32 sessions show that the combination of NW and SW rules eliminates dissimilar sequence pairs from the similarity matrix compared to single NW and SW rules. As described previously, the combination of NW and SW rules generates more clusters from less sequence, more clusters 100 % similar inside, even smaller and better similarity inside of dissimilar clusters, requires less hierarchical level than single NW and SW rules.

We also performed a similar experiment on another dataset containing 1128 page visit records of 282 sessions. We used the implementation proposed in[2], agglomerative hierarchical clustering algorithm in[3], and implement an algorithm to get clusters by optional level on tree. We also include the "no rule" when working on similarity matrix, to compare the number of clusters and execution times among rules application as in Tables 4, 5 and 6, that present result after one of about fifty performing times of this experiment. Thus, Table 4 shows the number of clusters at some specific hierarchical levels by applying no rule and rule of "NW score > longer sequence length/4". Correspondingly, Table 5 is about cluster number by applying rules of "SW score = shorter sequence length x 2" and "NW score > longer sequence length/4 and SW score = shorter sequence length x 2" at same levels. Finally, in Table 6 we present execution times after running on corresponding rules. This result presents all mentioned advantages of NW and SW rules combination, as in the previous experiment with 32 sample

---

[2] https://code.google.com/p/himmele/source/browse/trunk/Bioinformatics/.
[3] https://github.com/lbehnke/hierarchical-clustering-java/tree/master/src.

sessions. Additionally, the execution times are also in the same order of "No rule" > "SW rule" > "NW+SW rule" > "NW rule" like Table 6. Therefore, the rules combination of NW and SW is better than others in clustering exactness, with some difference in execution time.

**Table 4.** Number of clusters on hierarchical tree at some specific levels, by no rule and NW rule.

|  | No rule | NW score > longer sequence length/4 |
|---|---|---|
| Hierarchical level 5 | 8 | 17 |
| Hierarchical level 7 | 11 | 34 |
| Hierarchical level 9 | 20 | 49 |
| Hierarchical level 11 | 33 | 63 |

**Table 5.** Number of clusters on hierarchical tree at some specific levels, by SW rule and rule combination of NW and SW

|  | SW score = shorter sequence length x 2 | NW score > longer sequence length/4 and SW score = shorter sequence length x 2 |
|---|---|---|
| Hierarchical level 5 | 12 | 18 |
| Hierarchical level 7 | 21 | 37 |
| Hierarchical level 9 | 29 | 49 |
| Hierarchical level 11 | 33 | 67 |

**Table 6.** Clustering execution time by no rule, NW rule, SW rule and rule combination of NW and SW

|  | Execution Time (in second) |
|---|---|
| No rule | 692.7 |
| NW score > longer sequence length/4 | 558.9 |
| SW score = shorter sequence length x 2 | 578.0 |
| NW score > longer sequence length/4 and SW score = shorter sequence length x 2 | 561.3 |

## 4   Related Work

Our approach focuses on sequence alignment and ignores URL structural similarity suggested in some previous approaches [3,4]. The reason is, without content mining, the use of website tree structure to represent the similarity of user interest may practically encounter some shortcomings such as:

- URLs are not always in any fixed structure form. Nowadays, they tend to be shorten by some unstructured presentation string
- The similarity of URL structure does not completely reflect the common interest of visitors. Two pages like `math.html` and `art.html` probably explored by two separated visitors groups and maybe shown in different categories on website, though they got the same prefix

In another approach [5], SW might be more global by counting the longer sequence length in pairwise alignment but our paper focuses on the combination of primitives. Proposed sequence alignment methods in [6,7], using a hybrid metric by incorporation global into local alignment of 2 sequences. According to the formula, the more different in sequences length, the more local alignment should be taken into account, and vice versa. Because it turns to be global for the shorter sequence and local for the longer sequence, this metric is meaningful in some contexts. Nevertheless, it is not really in ours, because a local alignment scoring scheme like SW not counting the rest different length of sequences, although the longer these parts length is, the more important it will be in similarity metric when sequence lengths are significantly different.

Using similar pairwise alignment implemented by dynamic programming, DTW optimally minimizes the cost function [9,10] i.e. distance between pair of sequences whereas NW optimally maximizes similarity score. As a result, DTW measures the dissimilarity between sequences. In our context of web usage mining, two sessions with less dissimilarity in page visits are more similar, then DTW can be taken into account in considering proposed methods of sequence alignment. As our DTW analysis result above, DTW is appropriate for time series stretching or compressing but not for strings like our approach.

## 5   Conclusion

Sequence alignment techniques have been used widely in DNA sequences comparison, and have also been applied to segmentation of Web sessions. However, these techniques were not originally dedicated to web usage clustering, and there is room for optimization in order to adapt these alignments techniques to the specificities of real-time Web marketing, which is our field of application.

We have made the choice of a simple threshold-driven combination of the well-known Needleman-Wunsch and Smith-Waterman global and local alignment techniques. Values of these thresholds can be considered parameters of a given Web site, and we follow currently some simple heuristics to define them.

Our experiences show that our pairwise distance metric, based on the successive alignment of NW and SW in sequence pair, is a simple and realistic way to combine global and local approaches.

With the raise of mobile devices and tablets, there is now a significant difference in terms of low-level events that can observed between those devices and traditional computers (with a mouse). We need to better understand how the granularity of the events included in the sequences affects these thresholds. Therefore, future work is needed to fine-tune our heuristics for setting thresholds.

# References

1. Needleman, S.B., Wunsch, C.D.: A general method applicable to the search for similarities in the amino acid sequence of two proteins. J. Mol. Biol. **48**(3), 443–453 (1970)
2. Smith, T.F., Waterman, M.S.: Identification of common molecular subsequences. J. Mol. Biol. **147**(1), 195–197 (1981)
3. Wang, W., Zaïane, O.R.: Clustering web sessions by sequence alignment. In: Proceedings of 13th International Workshop on Database and Expert Systems Applications, 2002, pp. 394–398. IEEE (2002)
4. Li, C., Lu, Y.: Similarity measurement of web sessions based on sequence alignment. Wuhan Univ. J. Nat. Sci. **12**(5), 814–818 (2007)
5. Poornalatha, G., Raghavendra, P.: Alignment based similarity distance measure for better web sessions clustering. Procedia Comput. Sci. **5**, 450–457 (2011)
6. Chordia, B.S., Adhiya, K.P.: Grouping web access sequences using sequence alignment method. Indian J. Comput. Sci. Eng. (IJCSE) **2**(3), 308–314 (2011)
7. Dimopoulos, C., Makris, C., Panagis, Y., Theodoridis, E., Tsakalidis, A.: A web page usage prediction scheme using sequence indexing and clustering techniques. Data Knowl. Eng. **69**(4), 371–382 (2010)
8. Petitjean, F., Forestier, G., Webb, G., Nicholson, A., Chen, Y., Keogh, E.: Dynamic time warping averaging of time series allows faster and more accurate classification. In: IEEE International Conference on Data Mining (2014)
9. Meesrikamolkul, W., Niennattrakul, V., Ratanamahatana, C.A.: Shape-based clustering for time series data. In: Tan, P.-N., Chawla, S., Ho, C.K., Bailey, J. (eds.) PAKDD 2012, Part I. LNCS, vol. 7301, pp. 530–541. Springer, Heidelberg (2012)
10. Nakamura, A., Kudo, M.: Packing alignment: alignment for sequences of various length events. In: Huang, J.Z., Cao, L., Srivastava, J. (eds.) PAKDD 2011, Part II. LNCS, vol. 6635, pp. 234–245. Springer, Heidelberg (2011)
11. Marascu, A., Khan, S.A., Palpanas, T.: Scalable similarity matching in streaming time series. In: Tan, P.-N., Chawla, S., Ho, C.K., Bailey, J. (eds.) PAKDD 2012, Part II. LNCS, vol. 7302, pp. 218–230. Springer, Heidelberg (2012)
12. Chan, A.: An analysis of pairwise sequence alignment algorithm complexities: needleman-wunsch, smith-waterman, fasta, blast and gapped blast (2013)
13. Cooley, R., Mobasher, B., Srivastava, J.: Grouping web page references into transactions for mining world wide web browsing patterns. In: Proceedings of Knowledge and Data Engineering Exchange Workshop, 1997, pp. 2–9. IEEE (1997)
14. Cooley, R., Mobasher, B., Srivastava, J.: Data preparation for mining world wide web browsing patterns. Knowl. Inf. Syst. **1**(1), 5–32 (1999)

# Mining Massive-Scale Spatiotemporal Trajectories in Parallel: A Survey

Pengtao Huang$^{(\boxtimes)}$ and Bo Yuan

Intelligent Computing Lab, Division of Informatics, Graduate School at Shenzhen,
Tsinghua University, Shenzhen 518055, People's Republic of China
hpt13@mails.tsinghua.edu.cn, yuanb@sz.tsinghua.edu.cn

**Abstract.** With the popularization of positioning devices such as GPS navigators and smart phones, large volumes of spatiotemporal trajectory data have been produced at unprecedented speed. For many trajectory mining problems, a number of computationally efficient approaches have been proposed. However, to more effectively tackle the challenge of big data, it is important to exploit various advanced parallel computing paradigms. In this paper, we present a comprehensive survey of the state-of-the-art techniques for mining massive-scale spatiotemporal trajectory data based on parallel computing platforms such as Graphics Processing Unit (GPU), MapReduce and Field Programmable Gate Array (FPGA). This survey covers essential topics including trajectory indexing and query, clustering, join, classification, pattern mining and applications. We also give an in-depth analysis of the related techniques and compare them according to their principles and performance.

**Keywords:** Spatiotemporal · Trajectory mining · Parallel computing

## 1 Introduction

In the past decade, positioning technologies have received tremendous development and location-aware sensors such as GPS devices and smart phones have become ubiquitous, collecting large volumes of trajectory data continuously. Although a variety of technologies have been proposed to analyze these data for different applications, they are facing more and more difficulties when handling massive-scale spatiotemporal trajectories due to prohibitive computational cost. In recent years, parallel data mining approaches have emerged with convincing performance in dealing with big data.

In general, a spatiotemporal trajectory can be represented as a sequence of points $(x_1, y_1, t_1)$, $(x_2, y_2, t_2)$, ..., $(x_n, y_n, t_n)$, where $(x_i, y_i)$ is the spatial location consisting of longitude and latitude (sometimes altitude), and $t_i$ is the time when the spatial location $(x_i, y_i)$ is recorded [17].

The paradigm of trajectory mining can be stated as "trajectory preprocessing (prior databases) → trajectory indexing and retrieval (in databases) → advanced topics (above databases)" [45]. Among them the in-database phase and above-database phase are more challenging and worth detailed study, and the advanced

© Springer International Publishing Switzerland 2015
X.-L. Li et al. (Eds.): PAKDD 2015, LNCS 9441, pp. 41–52, 2015.
DOI: 10.1007/978-3-319-25660-3_4

topics can be broadly classified into trajectory mining techniques, trajectory patterns and practical applications. The main topics of trajectory mining are illustrated in Fig. 1.

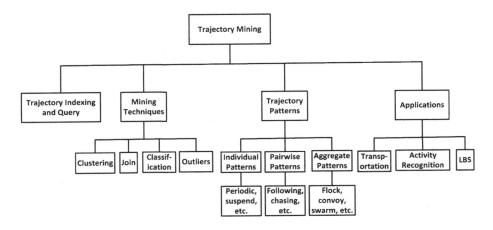

**Fig. 1.** Main topics of trajectory mining

The trajectory mining techniques extend traditional data mining techniques to trajectory data, including clustering [16], join [3], classification [15] and so on, which can be used to further discover trajectory patterns. It should be noted that clustering aims at discovering groups of similar objects from a single trajectory collection while join is a specific operation that computes pairs of similar objects from two trajectory collections [45].

Trajectory pattern (T-pattern) was introduced by Giannotti et al. [7] as concise descriptions of frequent behaviours in terms of both space and time and later extended to other motion patterns and behaviour patterns. Trajectory patterns can be classified according to different standards. In terms of the number of moving objects, they can be divided into individual patterns, pairwise patterns and aggregate patterns. Individual patterns include periodic patterns [20], suspension [27] etc. Pairwise patterns include following pattern [21], attraction or avoidance [19] etc. The aggregate patterns include flock [9], convoy [12], swarm [18] etc. Furthermore, more complex aggregate patterns can be found in many real-world applications including urban transportation, animal protection, human activity recognition and location-based services.

The main contribution of this paper is a novel and comprehensive survey of parallel trajectory mining algorithms based on GPU, MapReduce and FPGA. In Sect. 2, we review several parallel trajectory indexing and query algorithms. Existing parallel trajectory mining techniques and trajectory pattern mining algorithms are introduced in Sects. 3 and 4, respectively. In Sect. 5, we present the survey of some classical applications of trajectory mining. This paper is concluded in Sect. 6 with a summary of challenges and future work.

## 2    Trajectory Indexing and Query

Trajectory databases that support effective trajectory indexing and query are the basis of trajectory mining. Trajectory queries aim to evaluate spatiotemporal relationships among spatial data objects, which can be classified into three types: trajectories and points (P-Query), trajectories and regions (R-Query), trajectories and trajectories (T-Query). Trajectory indexing techniques can accelerate query processing, which can also be classified into three types [45]. The first is to extend existing methods such as R-tree with augmentation in temporal dimensions (e.g., 3DR-tree or STR-tree). The second approach uses multiversion structures and builds a separate R-tree for each time stamp and shares common parts between two consecutive R-trees (e.g., MR-tree, HR-tree, HR+-tree, and MV3R-tree). The third approach divides the spatial dimension into grids, and then builds a separate temporal index for each grid (e.g., SETI, and MTSB-tree).

You et al. [40] presented a GPU-based approach to index and query large-scale geospatial data using R-Trees. GPUs were mainly used to accelerate both R-Tree bulk loading and spatial window query processing, making the data layout schema very efficient. The GPU-based approach achieved around 10x speedups on average over 8-core CPU parallel implementations. The GPU-based approach (NVIDIA Quadro 6000 GPU) achieved around 10x speedups on average over the 8-core CPU parallel implementations (two Intel E5405 processors) for query processing on synthetic datasets. Furthermore, on two large scale real-world datasets, the GPU implementation achieved around 4x speedup on the R-Tree bulk loading task compared to the CPU parallel implementation. The advantage of GPU increased to around 10x speedup on the query processing task.

Gowanlock and Casanova [8] focused on a trajectory similarity search, the distance threshold query, which finds all trajectories within a given distance $d$ of a query trajectory over a time interval. They provided a GPU-friendly indexing method which achieved a speedup of 15.2 over the sequential CPU implementation and a speedup of 3.3 over the OpenMP parallel CPU implementation.

Ma et al. [24] presented a paradigm called PRADASE (Query Processing of Massive TRAjectory DAta baSEd on MapReduce) for query processing over massive trajectory data based on MapReduce, relying on a GFS (Google File System) -style storage, which only supports appending data and two strategies by which a large historical trajectory data set is partitioned into data chunks. Traditional trajectory data partitioning, indexing, and query processing technologies were extended to fully utilize the highly parallel processing power of large-scale clusters. The framework scales well in terms of the size of trajectory data but is not efficient for real time queries due to frequent communications among computers.

Sun et al. [33] proposed a spatiotemporal index algorithm named Layer-by-layer Index Based on Grid Partition (LIBGP) running on MapReduce. Navigation and location services data and six kinds of retrieval patterns were formally defined and several index algorithms of different dimensions suitable for the LBS data were put forward. LIBGP avoids the problem of low trajectory recognition rate based on grid. Besides, it can retrieve gigabytes of data efficiently and shows good scalability in terms of data dimension and size.

You's and Gowanlock's algorithms are both based on R-Trees or improved versions running on GPUs, and their speedup rates are very close. PRADASE and LIBGP are both partition-based query methods working on MapReduce platforms. In addition to the above algorithms, some frameworks have been proposed to integrate several operations and techniques, such as SpatialHadoop and Parallel SECONDO.

Eldawy and Mokbel [4] presented SpatialHadoop as the first full-fledged MapReduce framework for spatial data, which employs a simple spatial high level language, a two-level spatial index structure, basic spatial components built inside the MapReduce layer, and three basic spatial operations: range queries, k-NN queries, and spatial join. SpatialHadoop can achieve order(s) of magnitude better performance than Hadoop for spatial data. Besides, it is open source and allows researchers to further extend its functionality.

Lu and Gting [22] extended SECONDO [11] to a cluster of computers to improve the efficiency of processing large-scale queries so that users can convert large-scale sequential queries to parallel queries without learning the MapReduce programming details. Usually Parallel SECONDO needs more queries for the same step than sequential processing, but it achieves an impressive speedup on all steps, especially for large-scale problems. Compared with SpatialHadoop [4], which extends the capability of spatial data processing inside the core functionality of Hadoop, Parallel SECONDO applies existing SECONDO technologies directly without implementing them again according to the MapReduce paradigm.

The comparison of the above trajectory indexing and query algorithms or frameworks is shown in Table 1.

## 3   Trajectory Mining Techniques

Trajectory mining techniques including clustering, join, classification, outlier detection and so on create the foundation for further discovering detailed trajectory patterns, which extend the data types in traditional data mining techniques to spatiotemporal trajectory data. In the following, we will introduce some typical parallel trajectory mining techniques proposed in recent years, which are summarized in Table 2.

Sart et al. [30] investigated both GPU and FPGA based acceleration of subsequence similarity search under the Dynamic Time Warping (DTW) measure. By exploiting the massive computing power of parallel hardware accelerators, the algorithms achieved two orders of magnitude speedup with GPUs and four orders of magnitude speedup with FPGAs, which makes it possible to test DTW for all possible alignments/shifts and bring the accuracies to a higher new level.

Wang et al. [39] proposed a novel stream-oriented framework for FPGA based subsequence similarity search and a novel PE-ring structure for DTW calculation. The framework guarantees accuracy with a two-phase precision reduction

**Table 1.** Comparison of trajectory indexing and query algorithms

| Algorithm | Domain | Related techniques | Platform | Feature |
|---|---|---|---|---|
| You et al. [40] | Large-scale geospatial data indexing and query | R-Trees | GPU | 10x speedups on average |
| Gowanlock and Casanova [8] | Distance threshold query | A GPU-friendly indexing method | GPU | 15.2x speedup |
| Ma et al. [24] (PRADASE) | Trajectory data query | Extended partitio-ning, indexing, and query processing | Map-Reduce | Scalable but not efficient for real time queries |
| Sun et al. [33] (LIBGP) | Navigation and location services data index | Layer-by-layer Index Based on Grid Partition | Map-Reduce | Real time and good scalability |
| Eldawy and Mokbel [4] (Spatial-Hadoop) | A framework for spatial data | Language, storage, MapReduce and operations layers | Map-Reduce | Order(s) of magnitude |
| Lu and Gting [23] (Parallel SECONDO) | Large-scale parallel queries for moving objects | Parallel SECONDO databases | Map-Reduce | Needs more quer-ies but achieves an impressive speed-up |

**Table 2.** Comparison of trajectory mining techniques

| Algorithm | Domain | Related techniques | Platform | Feature |
|---|---|---|---|---|
| Sart et al. [30] | Subsequence similarity search | Dynamic Time Warping measure | GPU FPGA | GPU: two orders; FPGA: four orders |
| Wang et al. [39] | Subsequence similarity search | A FPGA frame-work and a PE-ring structure | FPGA | Several orders of magnitude over [30] |
| Zhao et al. [44] | Clustering mol-ecular simula-tion trajectories | k-centers algori-thm utilizing tri-angle inequality | GPU | Two orders of magnitude |
| Gudmundsson et al. [10] | Clustering sub-trajectories | Continuous Fréchet distance | GPU | 11x faster |
| Fang et al. [5] | Trajectory joins | K-NN and (h,k)-NN | Map-Reduce | Twice faster, not efficient for complex join queries |

while achieving several orders of magnitude speedup over the best software and GPU/FPGA implementations [30] by exploiting the fine-grained parallelism of DTW. Furthermore, the PE-ring structure supports the on-line updating of patterns of arbitrary lengths.

Zhao et al. [44] implemented a GPU-based parallel k-centers algorithm that utilizes triangle inequality to cluster molecular simulation trajectories. The algorithm behaves well with the increase of cluster number and can achieve up to two orders of magnitude faster than the CPU implementation. Besides, it can faithfully recover the underlying density of the dataset but the triangle inequality becomes less effective in higher dimensions.

Gudmundsson and Cereceda [10] implemented a subtrajectory clustering algorithm to report all subtrajectory clusters of a trajectory based on GPUs. Continuous Fréchet distance is used to measure the similarity between curves which allows applying compressing/simplification techniques to the input data without loosing much information. The GPU-based approach can be 11x faster than the original serial algorithm in [2].

Fang et al. [5] presented an efficient framework for answering k-NN join queries using MapReduce. It partitions the trajectories using spatial grids, and then computes a time-dependent upper bound (TDB), allowing trajectories to be pruned in parallel. Besides, k-NN join was extended to (h, k)-NN join and a new tight TDB was proposed to improve efficiency.

In summary, Zhao's and Gudmundsson's algorithms are both for trajectory clustering, which aim at discovering groups of similar objects from a single trajectory collection with very high efficiency. Fang's algorithm focuses on trajectory join, which is used to compute pairs of similar objects from two trajectory collections, but it is not very efficient to answer very complex join queries and there is still room for improvement.

## 4   Trajectory Patterns

Trajectory pattern mining aims at discovering groups of trajectories based on their proximity in a spatial or spatiotemporal sense, which is an emerging and rapidly developing topic in spatiotemporal data mining and query processing. This section will present some recent parallel trajectory pattern mining algorithms and the comparison of them is shown in Table 3.

Qiao et al. [28] proposed a parallel sequential pattern mining (plute) algorithm for massive trajectory data, which includes three essential techniques: prefix projection, data parallel formulation and task parallel formulation. MapReduce is employed in the third technique in a scalable and easy-to-use fashion. The algorithm shows good performance on parallel computing time and communication cost among processors, outperforming PartSpan [29] in many aspects.

Jinno et al. [13,32] proposed a hierarchical grid-based approach with quadtree search to discover frequent movement patterns from the trajectories of moving objects. The algorithm is naturally parallelized and implemented on MapReduce, which is able to identify complex patterns that cannot be identified by a single grid approach with a fixed resolution and requires less memory and processing time. However, when the minimum support becomes lower, significantly more memory is required.

Moussalli et al. [25,26] presented FPGA- and GPU-based solutions for parallel matching of variable-enhanced complex patterns by stream-mode (single pass) filtering. Both implementations are able to process the trajectory data in a single pass when handing pattern queries with no more than one variable or no

**Table 3.** Comparison of trajectory pattern mining algorithms

| Algorithm | Domain | Related techniques | Platform | Feature |
|---|---|---|---|---|
| Qiao et al. [28] (plut) | Mining sequential trajectory patterns | Prefix projection, data parallel formulation and task parallel formulation | Map-Reduce | Less than two times faster; less communication cost |
| Jinno et al. [13,32] | Discovering frequent movement patterns | A hierarchical grid-based approach with quadtree search | Map-Reduce | At most tens of times smaller memory usage; processing time increasing marginally |
| Moussalli et al. [25,26] | Complex pattern matching over spatio-temporal streams | FlexTrack system and hardware based architectures | FPGA GPU | GPU: up to two orders; FPGA: over three orders |
| Sun et al. [34] ($uPST_{MR}^{+}$) | Mining patterns from uncertain sequence data | Probabilistic Suffix Trees; NodeArray | Map-Reduce | A little extra memory, but much faster |
| Valladares [37] | Finding extremal sets | Discarding the non maximal or minimal sets | GPU | 6 times faster |
| Valladares [37] | Detecting intersection sets | Input domain reduction; empty and duplicated sets removal | GPU | Saving much computation and memory |
| Fort et al. [6] | Reporting flock patterns | Variants discussion and complexity analysis | GPU | On average 23 and maximally $10^3$ times faster |

wildcards with two or more variables, but result in false positive matches when two or more variable occur in a pattern query alongside wildcards. The parallel solutions can outperform the current state-of-the-art CPU-based approaches by two or three orders of magnitude at certain circumstances and shows very good scalability with regard to pattern complexity.

Tsai et al. [36] proposed an algorithm to mine movement pattern from uncertain trajectory data based on MapReduce, and Sun et al. [34] proposed two MapReduce algorithms named $uPST_{MR}$ and $uPST_{MR}^{+}$ to discover the hidden patterns from a large amount of uncertain sequence data. Probabilistic Suffix Trees (PST) are constructed in a progressive, multi-layered and iterative manner for huge data with uncertainties. A NodeArray data structure is used to reduce disk I/O and reduce execution time requiring a little extra memory. $uPST_{MR}^{+}$ shows excellent performance with good scalability and stability.

As to finding flock patterns in large trajectory databases, Valladares [37] presented a GPU-based approach for finding extremal sets within a family $\mathcal{F}$ of $k$ finite sets, which has no restrictions on the input family and runs up to 6 times faster than the algorithm by Bayardo and Panda [1]. He also presented another parallel approach for computing the intersection between two families of sets, which is the first implementation of the problem. The approach shows good efficiency and scalability and saves much computation and memory with the input domain reduction and the empty and duplicated sets removal. Both the algorithms are necessary for finding the flock patterns in [6].

Fort et al. [6] studied the problem of finding flock patterns in trajectory databases and presented some parallel algorithms based on GPU for reporting all maximal flocks, the largest flock and the longest flock. The number of maximal potential flocks was reduced by half and the GPU algorithm was on average 23 and maximally $10^3$ times faster than the best known sequential algorithm [38] with more robust and scalable response.

## 5    Applications of Trajectory Mining

Nowadays, the capability of analyzing large volumes of trajectory data is in increasing demand in many applications, including transportation optimization, trajectory planning, popular place discovery, crowd analysis and so on. Some recent practical applications of trajectory mining are summarized as follows (in Table 4).

Kondekar et al. [14] provided a MapReduce-based solution to the large scale Time Dependent Vehicle Routing Problem with Time Window (TDVRPTW) in dynamic network with fluctuant link travel time. The dynamic traffic conditions of the road network are considered, which make the problem more difficult to solve but the results are also more reliable. The island approach to the genetic algorithm can be easily modeled on MapReduce and the inherent parallel nature

**Table 4.** Comparison of applied trajectory mining algorithms

| Algorithm | Domain | Related techniques | Platform | Feature |
|---|---|---|---|---|
| Kondekar et al. [14] | Time Dependent Vehicle Routing Problem with Time Window | Hybrid genetic solution using island approach | Map-Reduce | A tremendous improvement both on time and efficiency |
| Thakur et al. [35] | USV trajectory palnning | State transition models and Markov Decision Process | GPU | A factor of 43.4 |
| Li et al. [19] | Calibrating bus trajectory data | K-NN | Map-Reduce | At lease a factor of two |
| Cereceda [37] | Computing popular places | Popular regions visualization and schematization; popularity map | GPU | Good efficiency and scalability |
| Scheepens et al. [31] | Visualizing vessel movement predictions | Similarity to historical trajectories; Monte Carlo simulation | GPU | Can be stored and visualized in real-time |
| Zhang et al. [41–43] | Online spatial, temporal and spatiotemporal aggregations | Timestamp compression; simple linear data structures | GPU | Dozens of times faster |

of genetic algorithms are exploited to improve efficiency, making it easy to solve large scale VRP with minimal time and full resource utilization.

Thakur et al. [35] described GPU-based algorithms to compute state transition models for Unmanned Surface Vehicle (USV) trajectory planning problem. GPU is used to accelerate the computation of state-transition probabilities which is subsequently used to solve the Markov Decision Process (MDP) to obtain trajectory plan, so that dynamically feasible trajectories for USVs can be generated. The GPU-based methods gain dozens of times of speedup but introduce some simulation error. The approach is flexible and is capable of handling any USV geometry, dynamics parameters and sea-state, but not suitable for fast moving boats or dynamic environmental disturbances with dynamic obstacles.

Li et al. [19] used MapReduce to calibrate massive bus trajectory data, correcting the direction correcting and projecting the bus GPS point to the road link. Both the map matching problem and the direction calibrating problem are very suitable to run on MapReduce because of the characteristics of traffic data. Besides, K-Nearest Neighbour algorithm (K-NN) is utilized to evaluate the final result of travelling direction and improves the accuracy significantly.

Valladares [37] studied the problem of computing popular places, regions that are visited by at least a given number of entities and proposed two practical models to solve the problem for the first time. The GPU-based implementation shows very good efficiency and scalability which allows constraints to be added on both the input and output paths.

Scheepens et al. [31] presented two models to predict positions of moving objects and visualize them in an interactive mode. One is based on comparing the current state of the reference vessel with a large set of historical trajectories and building a PDF from these trajectories, and the other on Monte Carlo simulations of a large number of trajectories based on movement statistics derived from vessels similar to the reference in a large set of historical trajectories. GPU is used to compute and visualize PDFs efficiently. The methods can be used in maritime domain like avoiding collision, and detecting piracy or smuggling as well as other domains like urban law enforcement domain for pedestrian movements. However, the current methods do not apply to domains with more uncertainty such as animal movement or more than two vessels.

Zhang et al. [41–43] developed some data management frameworks including $U^2$STRA and $U^2$SOD-DB to efficiently manage large-scale trajectory data, and a set of parallel techniques based on multi-core CPUs and many-core GPUs to associate taxi pickup location points with their nearest street segments and then reduce online spatial, temporal and spatiotemporal aggregations to relational aggregations, which play an important role in understanding urban dynamics and facilitating decision making. The GPU-based implementations can be dozens of times faster than serial CPU implementations and several times faster than multi-core CPU implementations for spatial, temporal and spatiotemporal aggregations. However, for relational aggregations, the GPU implementations just perform slightly better than the multi-core implementations using dynamic arrays because of the Thrust library overheads.

# 6    Conclusions and Future Work

In this paper, we present the first comprehensive survey of the state-of-the-art algorithms for massive-scale spatiotemporal trajectory mining based on parallel computing platforms including GPU, MapReduce and FPGA. It is evident that these hardware-accelerated algorithms can often achieve orders of magnitude speedup compared to traditional sequential algorithms without compromising the quality of solutions. Note that the many-core architecture GPUs are more engergy/space efficient and cost effective compared to CPU-based distributed systems. As a result, it is preferable to deploy GPU-based techniques for applications where the size of data is up to the GB level while Hadoop/MapReduce-based techniques are more suitable for handling data at TB or above level.

In the future, more advanced high-performance computing platforms can be applied to trajectory mining, such as Mars, Spark and so on. It is also worth considering real-time trajectory streams and more complex scenarios (e.g., road networks and rough terrain).

# References

1. Bayardo, R., Panda, B.: Fast Algorithms for Finding Extremal Sets. In: Proceedings of the 2011 SIAM International Conference on Data Mining, pp. 25–34 (2011)
2. Löffler, M., et al. Detecting commuting patterns by clustering subtrajectories. In: Hong, S.-H., Hong, S.-H., Fukunaga, T., Fukunaga, T., Nagamochi, H., Nagamochi, H. (eds.) ISAAC 2008. LNCS, vol. 5369, pp. 644–655. Springer, Heidelberg (2008)
3. Ding, H., Trajcevski, G., Scheuermann, P.: Efficient similarity join of large sets of moving object trajectories. In: The 15th International Symposium on Temporal Representation and Reasoning, pp. 79–87. IEEE (2008)
4. Eldawy, A., Mokbel, M.F.: A demonstration of spatialhadoop: an efficient MapReduce framework for spatial data. Proc. VLDB Endowment **6**(12), 1230–1233 (2013)
5. Fang, Y., Cheng, R., Tang, W., Maniu, S., Yang, X.: Evaluating Nearest-Neighbor Joins on Big Trajectory Data. Technical report (2014)
6. Fort, M., Sellarès, J.A., Valladares, N.: A parallel GPU-based approach for reporting flock patterns. Int. J. Geogr. Inf. Sci. **28**(9), 1877–1903 (2014)
7. Giannotti, F., Nanni, M.: Trajectory pattern mining. In: Proceedings of the 13th ACM SIGKDD International Conference on Knowledge Discovery and Data Mining, pp. 330–339. New York (2007)
8. Gowanlock, M.G., Casanova, H.: Parallel Distance Threshold Query Processing for Spatiotemporal Trajectory Databases on the GPU. Technical report (2014)
9. Gudmundsson, J., van Kreveld, M.: Computing longest duration flocks in trajectory data. In: Proceedings of the 14th Annual ACM International Symposium on Advances in Geographic Iinformation Systems, pp. 35–42. ACM Press, New York (2006)
10. Gudmundsson, J., Valladares, N.: A GPU approach to subtrajectory clustering using the Fréchet distance. IEEE Trans. Parallel Distrib. Sys. **PP**(99), 1–16 (2014)
11. Güting, R.H., Behr, T., Düntgen, C.: SECONDO : a platform for moving objects database research and for publishing and integrating research implementations. Bull. IEEE Comput. Soc. Tech. Committee Data Eng. **33**(2), 56–63 (2010)

12. Jeung, H., Yiu, M.L., Zhou, X., Jensen, C.S., Shen, H.T.: Discovery of convoys in trajectory databases. Proc. VLDB Endowment **1**(1), 1068–1080 (2008)
13. Jinno, R., Seki, K., Uehara, K.: Parallel distributed trajectory pattern mining using MapReduce. In: 2012 IEEE 4th International Conference on Cloud Computing Technology and Science, pp. 269–274 (2012)
14. Kondekar, R., Gupta, A., Saluja, G.: A MapReduce based hybrid genetic algorithm using island approach for solving time dependent vehicle routing problem. In: International Conference on Computer&Information Science (ICCIS), pp. 263–269. No. 2003 (2012)
15. Lee, J., Han, J., Li, X., Gonzalez, H.: TraClass: trajectory classification using hierarchical region-based and trajectory-based clustering. Proc. VLDB Endowment **1**(2), 1081–1094 (2008)
16. Lee, J., Han, J., Whang, K.: Trajectory Clustering : A partition-and-group framework. In: Proceedings of the 2007 ACM SIGMOD International Conference on Management of Data, pp. 593–604. New York (2007)
17. Li, Z.: Spatiotemporal pattern mining: algorithms and applications. In: Aggarwal, C.C., Han, J. (eds.) Frequent Pattern Mining, pp. 283–306. Springer International Publishing, Heidelberg (2014)
18. Li, Z., Ding, B., Han, J., Kays, R.: Swarm: mining relaxed ttemporal moving object clusters. Proc. VLDB Endowment **3**(1–2), 723–734 (2010)
19. Li, Z., Ding, B., Wu, F., Lei, T.: Attraction and avoidance detection from movements. Proc. VLDB Endowment **7**(3), 157–168 (2013)
20. Li, Z., Ding, B., Han, J., Kays, R., Nye, P.: Mining periodic behaviors for moving objects. In: Proceedings of the 16th ACM SIGKDD International Conference on Knowledge Discovery and Data Mining, pp. 1099–1108. ACM Press, New York (2010)
21. Li, Z., Wu, F., Crofoot, M.C.: Mining following relationships in movement data. In: IEEE 13th International Conference on Data Mining, pp. 458–467. IEEE (2013)
22. Lu, J., Guting, R.H.: Parallel secondo: boosting database engines with hadoop. In: 2012 IEEE 18th International Conference on Parallel and Distributed Systems, pp. 738–743. IEEE, Los Alamitos (2012)
23. Lu, J., Guting, R.H.: Parallel SECONDO: a practical system for large-scale processing of moving objects. In: 2014 IEEE 30th International Conference on Data Engineering, pp. 1190–1193. IEEE (2014)
24. Ma, Q., Yang, B., Qian, W., Zhou, A.: Query processing of massive trajectory data based on MapReduce. In: Proceeding of the First International Workshop on Cloud Data Management - CloudDB 2009, pp. 9–16. ACM Press, Hong Kong (2009)
25. Moussalli, R., Absalyamov, I., Vieira, M.R., Najjar, W., Tsotras, V.J.: High performance FPGA and GPU complex pattern matching over spatio-temporal streams. GeoInformatica **19**(2), 405–434 (2014)
26. Moussalli, R., Moussalli, R., Vieira, M.R., Vieira, M.R., Najjar, W., Najjar, W., Tsotras, V.J., Tsotras, V.J.: Stream-mode FPGA acceleration of complex pattern trajectory querying. In: Sellis, T., et al. (eds.) SSTD 2013. LNCS, vol. 8098, pp. 201–222. Springer, Heidelberg (2013)
27. Orellana, D., Wachowicz, M.: Exploring patterns of movement suspension in pedestrian mobility. Geogr. Anal. **43**(3), 241–260 (2011)
28. Qiao, S., Li, T., Peng, J., Qiu, J.: Parallel sequential pattern mining of massive trajectory data. Int. J. Comput. Intell. Sys. **3**(3), 343–356 (2010)
29. Qiao, S., Tang, C., Dai, S., Zhu, M., Peng, J., Li, H., Ku, Y.: PartSpan: Parallel Sequence mining of trajectory patterns. In: 2008 Fifth International Conference on Fuzzy Systems and Knowledge Discovery, pp. 363–367. No. 2006, IEEE (2008)

30. Sart, D., Mueen, A., Najjar, W., Keogh, E., Niennattrakul, V.: Accelerating dynamic time warping subsequence search with GPUs and FPGAs. In: 2010 IEEE International Conference on Data Mining, pp. 1001–1006. IEEE (2010)
31. Scheepens, R., van de Wetering, H., van Wijk, J.J.: Contour based visualization of vessel movement predictions. Int. J. Geogr. Inf. Sci. **28**(5), 891–909 (2014)
32. Seki, K., Jinno, R., Uehara, K.: Parallel distributed trajectory pattern mining using hierarchical grid with MapReduce. Int. J. Grid High Perform. Comput. **5**(4), 79–96 (2013)
33. Sun, F., Wang, W., Zhou, B., Chen, F.: The design and application of navigation and location services data index. In: 2013 International Conference on Computational and Information Sciences, pp. 774–777. IEEE (2013)
34. Sun, Z.-Y., Sun, Z.-Y., Tsai, M.-C., Tsai, M.-C., Tsai, H.-P., Tsai, H.-P.: Mining Uncertain Sequence Data on Hadoop Platform. In: Peng, W.-C., et al. (eds.) PAKDD 2014 Workshops. LNCS, vol. 8643, pp. 204–216. Springer, Heidelberg (2014)
35. Thakur, A., Svec, P., Gupta, S.K.: GPU based generation of state transition models using simulations for unmanned surface vehicle trajectory planning. Robot. Auton. Sys. **60**(12), 1457–1471 (2012)
36. Tsai, H.P.: Mining Movement Pattern from Uncertain Trajectory Data with MapReduce (2011). http://nchuir.lib.nchu.edu.tw/handle/309270000/89680
37. Valladares, N.: GPU Parallel Algorithms For Reporting Movement Behaviour Patterns in Spatio-temporal Databases. Ph.D. thesis, University of Girona (2013)
38. Vieira, M.R., Bakalov, P., Tsotras, V.J.: On-line discovery of flock patterns in spatio-temporal data. In: Proceedings of the 17th ACM SIGSPATIAL International Conference on Advances in Geographic Information Systems - GIS 2009, pp. 286–295. ACM Press, New York (2009)
39. Wang, Z., Huang, S., Wang, L., Li, H., Wang, Y., Yang, H.: Accelerating subsequence similarity search based on ddynamic time warping Ddistance with FPGA. In: Proceedings of the ACM/SIGDA International Symposium on Field Programmable Gate Arrays - FPGA 2013, pp. 53–62. ACM Press, New York(2013)
40. You, S., Zhang, J., Gruenwald, L.: Parallel spatial query processing on GPUs using R-trees. In: Proceedings of the 2nd ACM SIGSPATIAL International Workshop on Analytics for Big Geospatial Data - BigSpatial 2013, pp. 23–31 (2013)
41. Zhang, J., You, S., Gruenwald, L.: High-performance online spatial and temporal aggregations on multi-core CPUs and many-core GPUs. In: Proceedings of the Fifteenth International Workshop on Data Warehousing and OLAP (DOLAP 2012), pp. 89–96. ACM, Maui (2012)
42. Zhang, J., You, S., Gruenwald, L.: U2STRA : High-performance data management of ubiquitous urban sensing trajectories on GPGPUs. In: Proceedings of the 2012 ACM Workshop on City Data Management Workshop -CDMW 2012. pp. 5–12 (2012)
43. Zhang, J., You, S., Gruenwald, L.: parallel online spatial and temporal aggregations on multi-core CPUs and many-core GPUs. Inf. Sys. **44**, 134–154 (2014)
44. Zhao, Y., Sheong, F.K., Sun, J., Sander, P., Huang, X.: A fast parallel clustering algorithm for molecular simulation trajectories. J. Comput. Chem. **34**(2), 95–104 (2013)
45. Zheng, Y., Zhou, X.: Computing with Spatial Trajectories. Springer New York Dordrecht Heidelberg London, New York (2011)

# Manifold Regularized Symmetric Joint Link Model for Overlapping Community Detection

Hao Chen, Xianchao Zhang, Wenxin Liang$^{(\boxtimes)}$, and Feng Ding

Dalian University of Technology, Dalian 116620, China
chenhaoac@gmail.com, {xczhang,wxliang,dingfeng}@dlut.edu.cn

**Abstract.** Overlapping community detection is an important research topic in analyzing real-world networks. Among existing algorithms for detecting overlapping communities, generative models have shown their superiorities. However, previous generative models do not consider the intrinsic geometry of probability distribution manifold. To tackle this problem, we propose a Manifold Regularized Symmetric Joint Link Model (MSJL), which utilizes the local geometrical structure of manifold to improve the performance of overlapping community detection. MSJL assumes that the community probability distribution lives on a submanifold, and adopts the manifold assumption which specifically requires two close nodes in an intrinsic geometry to have similar community distribution. The structure of the intrinsic manifold is modeled by a nearest neighbor graph, and MSJL incorporates the graph Laplacian as a manifold regularization into the maximum likelihood function of the standard SJL model. Experiments on synthetic benchmarks and real-world networks demonstrate that MSJL can significantly improve the performance compared with the state-of-the-art methods.

**Keywords:** Overlapping community detection · Generative model · Manifold regularization · Graph laplacian

## 1 Introduction

Overlapping community detection is an important research topic in analyzing and understanding real-world networks such as social networks, citation networks and biological networks. In real-world networks, it is intuitive that each node belongs to multiple groups. For instance, a person may be connected to family, friends and fellow colleagues in a social network. Based on this intuition, a number of approaches have been developed to find overlapping communities.

Recently, some probabilistic generative models [2,15,17,20] have been proposed for overlapping community detection. Compared to heuristic methods [1,7,8,11,12], generative models are able to give a strict mathematical significance and offer natural probabilistic interpretations to overlapping belongings of each node. However, previous generative models assume that the community probability distribution generates data in the Euclidean space, without considering the case of manifold structure.

© Springer International Publishing Switzerland 2015
X.-L. Li et al. (Eds.): PAKDD 2015, LNCS 9441, pp. 53–65, 2015.
DOI: 10.1007/978-3-319-25660-3_5

From the studies of manifold learning, many researchers [3,4,18,19] have pointed out that the data is usually sampled from a low-dimensional *submanifold* [13] embedded in a high-dimensional ambient space, and the learning performance will be greatly improved by considering the geometrical structure.

In this paper, we propose a Manifold Regularized Symmetric Joint Link Model (MSJL), which explicitly incorporates local manifold structure into the standard SJL model for community detection. We assume the community probability distribution lives on a submanifold, and adopts the manifold assumption which specifically requires two close nodes in an intrinsic geometry to have similar community distribution. To model the structure of intrinsic manifold, we construct the nearest neighbor graph using the cosine similarity matrix exacted from the original network. We employ the Generialized Expectation Maximization (GEM) algorithm and the Newton-Raphson method for maximizing the objective function, which combines the manifold regularization term with the network generating likelihood. Experiments on synthetic benchmarks and real-world networks have showed that MSJL can significantly improve the performance compared with the state-of-the-art methods, suggesting the necessity of combining geometrical structure of manifold in community detection.

In the following sections, we first review the methods in overlapping communities and manifold learning in Sect. 2. Section 3 introduces the proposed MSJL model and the parameter estimation processes. In Sect. 4, we detail the experiments setting and present the results on synthetic benchmarks and real-world networks. Section 5 concludes this paper.

## 2    Related Work

### 2.1    Overlapping Community Detection

An early algorithm for overlapping community detection was the Clique Percolation Method (CPM) proposed by Palla [7], which takes communities as unions of adjacent complete subgraphs and searches all cliques of size $k$ in a network. Later Ahn et al. [1] partitioned link communities via hierarchical clustering with a similarity metric of edges. Since each node inherits all memberships of its links, it can belong to multiple overlapping communities. Lancichinetti et al. [11,12] tried to expand communities from random seeds based on the local optimization of a fitness function. Gregory et al. [8] extended the label propagation algorithm to find overlapping communities by allowing one node belonging to multiple communities. Although these methods give some reasonable results in practice, they lack a strict mathematical significance and the ability to generate new links, which can be used for problems like connections predicting.

In contrast, probabilistic generative models give rigorous generative process and the ability to generate new data. The basic idea is to design a generative process based on model parameters to describe the probability of generating a network. The soft community memberships of nodes are inferred by fitting the model to the observed real network. Newman et al. [15] proposed a mixture model for network structure, in which nodes with a similar connection preference rather than the highly connected nodes will be classified into the same group. Ball, et al. [2] developed a Poisson community model for detecting link communities. In Ball's method, edges have $K$ different colors to represent the communities assignments and model is parameterized by a set of parameters $\theta_{iz}$, where $\theta_{iz}$ denotes the propensity of node $i$ to have edges of color $z$. However, they assumed the number of edge between two nodes follows Poisson distribution, which allows more than one edge between a pair of nodes and is unrealistic in most real-world networks. Symmetric Joint Link (SJL) model [17,20] adopts the idea of topic models and generates links with a mixture model with $K$ topics by the joint link probability $P(e_{ij})$. More generally, SJL does not require multiple edges between two nodes.

## 2.2 Manifold Learning

In mathematics, a manifold is a topological space in which each point has a neighborhood that is homeomorphic to the Euclidean space. In recent years, many researchers [3,4,18,19] have considered that data is drawn from sampling a probability distribution that lives on a low-dimensional submanifold embedded in a high-dimensional ambient space.

Since data generated from submanifold cannot "fill up" the high dimensional Euclidean space uniformly, the intrinsic manifold structure needs to be considered while learning from examples. In order to exploit the geometrical manifold structure, many manifold learning algorithms have been proposed, such as Isomap [19], Locally Linear Embedding (LLE) [18], and Laplacian Eigenmap (LE) [3]. Those algorithms adopt the locally invariant idea, such as requiring two close points in the intrinsic geometry have similar embeddings. Besides the nonlinear dimensionality reduction algorithms [18,19] and semi-supervised learning algorithms [4], Cai et al. have also showed the learning performance can be greatly improved when incorporating the geometric knowledge of manifold into NMF [5], document clustering [6], Gaussian mixture model (GMM) [9].

# 3  Manifold Regularized Symmetric Joint Link Model

## 3.1  Background

Suppose there is a network $G = (V, E)$. The core of Symmetric Joint Link (SJL) model [17,20] is a latent variable model for co-occurrence data which associates an unobserved community indicator $z_k \in \{z_1, \cdots, z_K\}$ with the $e_{i,j} \in E$. The SJL model follows this generate process:

1. For each edge $e_{i,j} \in E$:
    (a) Select the edge's community indicator $z_k$ with probability $\omega_k$.
    (b) generate one end $i$ with probability $\theta_{ik}$, which indicates the intensity of the relationship between the node $i$ to the community $k$.
    (c) generate the other end $j$ with probability $\theta_{jk}$.

Translating the generation process of the whole graph $G$ into a joint probability results in the expression

$$P(G) = P(A|\boldsymbol{\omega}, \boldsymbol{\theta}) = \prod_{ij}(\sum_k \omega_k \theta_{ik} \theta_{jk})^{A_{ij}}, \tag{1}$$

where $A$ is the adjacency matrix and $\sum_k \omega_k = 1, \sum_i \theta_{ik} = 1$. The parameters can be estimated by maximizing the log-likelihood

$$\mathcal{L} = \ln P(A|\boldsymbol{\omega}, \boldsymbol{\theta}) = \sum_{ij} A_{ij} \ln P(e_{ij}|\boldsymbol{\omega}, \boldsymbol{\theta}) = \sum_{ij} A_{ij} \ln(\sum_k \omega_k \theta_{ik} \theta_{jk}) . \tag{2}$$

For each node $i$, its community membership can be calculated by conditional probability $\frac{\omega_k \theta_{ik}}{\sum_k \omega_k \theta_{ik}}$. To get overlapping communities, we can sort the conditional probability in descending order and retain the first $n$ communities in condition that the gap between the $n$-th and $(n+1)$-th communities is the largest.

The SJL model only assumes that the community probability distribution generates data in Euclidean space. Now we want to make use of the local geometrical structure of community probability manifold to improve the performance of community detection.

## 3.2   The MSJL Model

According to the standard learning framework, we have data $X$ and there is a probability distribution $P$ on $X \times \mathbb{R}$ to generate examples. For clustering problem, examples are simply drawn according to the marginal distribution $\mathcal{P}_X$ of $P$. As [4] shows, we can exploit the knowledge of marginal $\mathcal{P}_X$ to get better function learning because of some identifiable relation between $\mathcal{P}_X$ and the condition $P(y|x)$, where $y$ is the community label. Belkin, et al. [4] proposes the manifold assumption that if two points $x_1, x_2 \in X$ are close in the intrinsic geometry of $\mathcal{P}_X$, then the conditional probabilities $P(y|x_1)$ and $P(y|x_2)$ are similar. This assumption is nature when applied to our case: two nodes share a lot of neighbors in common should have similar probability distribution over different communities.

Although the data manifold is usually unknown, the local geometric structure can be modeled effectively by the *graph Laplacian*, which requires a nearest neighbor graph according to the spectral graph theory and manifold learning theory [3]. From the adjacency matrix $A$ we can observe $m$ data points $\{c_1, c_2, \cdots, c_m\} \subset \mathbb{R}^n$, which are coordinates mapped from data points $X$ in manifold space to Euclidean space. We calculate the cosine similarity matrix between nodes and construct the nearest neighbor graph. The equation is written as follows:

$$S_{ij} = \begin{cases} \dfrac{c_i^T c_j}{\sqrt{|c_i||c_j|}} & c_i \in N_p(c_j) \text{ or } c_j \in N_p(c_i) \\ 0 & \text{others} \end{cases} , \tag{3}$$

where $c_i$ is the $i$-th vector of $A$ and $N_p(c_i)$ denotes the set of $p$ nearest neighbors of $c_i$. Since $A_{ij} \in \{0, 1\}$, the dot product of vector $c_i$ and $c_j$ is equal to the number of common neighbors between these two nodes.

Thus, the manifold regularization term can be defined as

$$R(G) = \frac{1}{2}\sum_{k=1}^{K}\sum_{i,j=1}^{N}(\theta_{ik} - \theta_{jk})^2 S_{ij} = \sum_{k=1}^{K}(\sum_{i=1}^{N}\theta_{ik}^2 D_{ii} - \sum_{i,j=1}^{N}\theta_{ik}\theta_{jk}S_{ij})$$
$$= \sum_{k=1}^{K}(\boldsymbol{\theta}_k^T D\boldsymbol{\theta}_k - \boldsymbol{\theta}_k^T S\boldsymbol{\theta}_k) = \sum_{k}^{K}\boldsymbol{\theta}_k^T L\boldsymbol{\theta}_k \ , \tag{4}$$

where $D$ is diagonal matrix whose entries are row sums of $S$, $D_{ii} = \sum_j S_{ij}$, and $L = D - S$ is the Laplacian matrix [3]. The smaller of $R(G)$, the smoother of $P(y|c)$ over the graph and consequently along the geodesics in the intrinsic geometry of data.

Now we define the MSJL model by incorporating the regularization term into the likelihood of original SJL as follows.

$$\overline{\mathcal{L}} = \mathcal{L} - \lambda R(G) = \sum_{ij} A_{ij} \ln(\sum_k \omega_k \theta_{ik}\theta_{jk}) - \frac{\lambda}{2}\sum_{k=1}^{K}\sum_{i,j=1}^{N}(\theta_{ik} - \theta_{jk})^2 S_{ij} \ . \tag{5}$$

In Eq. (5), our goal is to maximize likelihood $\mathcal{L}$ and minimize $R(G)$ simultaneously, and $\lambda$ is the weight parameter used to control the balance between the likelihood and the smoothness of the community distribution among the neighbors. It is obvious that the SJL model is the special case of the MSJL model when $\lambda = 0$.

### 3.3  Parameter Estimation

Since MSJL model involves unobserved latent variables and the object function is difficult to optimize, we use the Expectation Maximization (EM) algorithm to estimate them. The EM algorithm iterates in two steps to compute a local maximum of $\overline{\mathcal{L}}$. Specifically, in the **E-step** we compute the posterior probabilities as

$$q_{ijk} = P(z_k|e_{ij}, \boldsymbol{\omega}, \boldsymbol{\theta}) = \frac{\omega_k\theta_{ik}\theta_{jk}}{\sum_{ijk}A_{ij}\omega_k\theta_{ik}\theta_{jk}}, \tag{6}$$

and the regularized expectation of complete log-likelihood as

$$\mathcal{Q}(\Psi;\Psi_n) = Q(\Psi;\Psi_n) - \lambda R(G)$$
$$= \sum_{ij} A_{ij}\sum_k q_{ijk}[\ln(\omega_k\theta_{ik}\theta_{jk})] - \frac{\lambda}{2}\sum_{k=1}^{K}\sum_{i,j=1}^{N}(\theta_{ik} - \theta_{jk})^2 S_{ij}, \tag{7}$$

where $\Psi = (\boldsymbol{\omega}, \boldsymbol{\theta})$, $\Psi_n$ denotes the value of $\Psi$ in the previous $n$-th iteration and $Q(\Psi;\Psi_n)$ is the expectation of complete log-likelihood.

In the **M-step**, the goal is to maximize $\mathcal{Q}(\Psi;\Psi_n)$ with respect to the parameters $\boldsymbol{\theta}$ and $\boldsymbol{\omega}$. Since the manifold regularization $\mathcal{R}(G)$ only relates to $\boldsymbol{\theta}$, we can easily maximize $\mathcal{Q}(\Psi; \Psi_n)$ with respect to $\boldsymbol{\omega}$ by the method of Lagrange multipliers and get the equation as follows.

$$\omega_k = \frac{\sum_{ij} A_{ij} q_{ijk}}{\sum_{ijk} A_{ij} q_{ijk}} \;. \tag{8}$$

Next we keep $\boldsymbol{\omega}$ fixed, then the relevant part of $\mathcal{Q}(\Psi; \Psi_n)$ to $\boldsymbol{\theta}$ becomes

$$\mathcal{Q}(\boldsymbol{\theta}; \boldsymbol{\theta}_n) = Q(\boldsymbol{\theta}; \boldsymbol{\theta}_n) - \lambda R(G) \;. \tag{9}$$

Unfortunately, it is difficult to maximize $\mathcal{Q}(\boldsymbol{\theta}; \boldsymbol{\theta}_n)$ directly through a closed-form solution of $\boldsymbol{\theta}$. Thus we solve this problem with the generalized EM algorithm (GEM) [14] to maximize the regularized log-likelihood. The difference between GEM and EM is that GEM only needs to find a "better" $\boldsymbol{\theta}_{n+1}$ to make sure $\mathcal{Q}(\boldsymbol{\theta}_{n+1}; \boldsymbol{\theta}_n) \geq \mathcal{Q}(\boldsymbol{\theta}_n; \boldsymbol{\theta}_n)$ rather than maximizing $\mathcal{Q}(\boldsymbol{\theta}; \boldsymbol{\theta}_n)$ in the M-step.

To satisfy the condition $\mathcal{Q}(\boldsymbol{\theta}_{n+1}; \boldsymbol{\theta}_n) \geq \mathcal{Q}(\boldsymbol{\theta}_n; \boldsymbol{\theta}_n)$, we first choose the initial value $\boldsymbol{\theta}_{n+1}^{(0)}$ which maximizes $Q(\boldsymbol{\theta}; \boldsymbol{\theta}_n)$ as follows.

$$\theta_{ik} = \frac{\sum_{jk} A_{ij} q_{ijk}}{\sum_{ijk} A_{ij} q_{ijk}} \;. \tag{10}$$

Then we use the Newton-Raphson method [6] to decrease $R(G)$ using update formula $x_{t+1} = x_t - \gamma \frac{f'(x)}{f''(x)}$, where $0 \leq \gamma \leq 1$ is the step parameter. Since we can get $R(G) \geq 0$ in Eq. (4), the Newton-Raphson method will decrease $R(G)$ and likely increase $\mathcal{Q}(\boldsymbol{\theta}; \boldsymbol{\theta}_n)$ in each step by updating $\boldsymbol{\theta}$ in the following equation as

$$(\theta_{ik})_{n+1}^{t+1} = (1 - \gamma)(\theta_{ik})_{n+1}^t + \gamma \frac{\sum_{j=1}^N S_{ij} (\theta_{ik})_{n+1}^t}{\sum_{j=1}^N S_{ij}} \;. \tag{11}$$

We repeatedly update $\theta$ using Eq. (11) until $\mathcal{Q}(\boldsymbol{\theta}_{n+1}^{(t+1)}, \boldsymbol{\theta}_n) \leq \mathcal{Q}(\boldsymbol{\theta}_{n+1}^{(t)}, \boldsymbol{\theta}_n)$ or max number of iteration $T$ reached. Then we compare whether $\mathcal{Q}(\boldsymbol{\theta}_{n+1}^{(t)}, \boldsymbol{\theta}_n) \geq \mathcal{Q}(\boldsymbol{\theta}_{n+1}^{(0)}, \boldsymbol{\theta}_n)$: if it is true, $\boldsymbol{\theta}_{n+1}^{(0)}$ is replaced by $\boldsymbol{\theta}_{n+1}^{(t)}$; else we keep current $\boldsymbol{\theta}_{n+1}^{(0)}$ and continue the next E-step. The pseudo-code of the MSJL algorithm is showed in Algorithm 1.

### 3.4   Complexity Analysis

In each E-step of MSJL, it takes $\mathcal{O}(|E|K)$ operations to compute $q_{ijk}$ with Eq. (6), where $|E|$ is the number of links in the network and $K$ is number of communities. In each M-step, computing $\omega_k$ and $\theta_{ik}$ need $\mathcal{O}(NK)$ operations and the Newton-Raphson method takes $\mathcal{O}(T(NK+Np))$ operations to maximize problem in Eq. (9), where $N$ is the number of nodes in the network, $p$ is the number of nearest neighbor and $T$ is the number of max iteration number in the Newton-Raphson method. Thus the MSJL algorithm has a time complexity of $\mathcal{O}(M(|E|K + NK + T(NK + Np)))$, where $M$ is the number of iterations. Compared to SJL model, MSJL has addtional steps to optimize $\boldsymbol{\theta}$ in Newton-Raphson method.

---

**Algorithm 1.** Generialized EM for MSJL

---

1: Compute the $p$-nearest neighbor graph matrix S as in Eq. (3)
2: Random initialize the parameters $\boldsymbol{\omega} = (\omega_k)_{k=1}^K$ and $\boldsymbol{\theta} = ((\theta_{ik})_{n=1}^N)_{k=1}^K$ respectively.
3: $n \leftarrow 0$
4: **repeat**
5:    **E-step**:
6:    Compute $P(z_k|e_{ij}, \boldsymbol{\omega}, \boldsymbol{\theta})$ as in Eq. (6)
7:    **M-step**:
8:    Compute $\boldsymbol{\omega}$ as in Eq. (8)
9:    Compute $\boldsymbol{\theta}_{n+1}$ as in Eq. (10)
10:    $t \leftarrow 0$
11:    $\boldsymbol{\theta}_{n+1}^{(0)} \leftarrow \boldsymbol{\theta}_{n+1}$
12:    Compute $\boldsymbol{\theta}_{n+1}^{(1)}$
13:    **while** $\mathcal{Q}(\boldsymbol{\theta}_{n+1}^{(t+1)}, \boldsymbol{\theta}_n) > \mathcal{Q}(\boldsymbol{\theta}_{n+1}^{(t)}, \boldsymbol{\theta}_n)$ and $t <$ maxstep $T$ **do**
14:      $\mathcal{Q}(\boldsymbol{\theta}_{n+1}^{(t)}) \leftarrow \mathcal{Q}(\boldsymbol{\theta}_{n+1}^{(t+1)})$
15:      Compute $\mathcal{Q}(\boldsymbol{\theta}_{n+1}^{(t+1)})$ as in Eq. (11)
16:    **end while**
17:    **if** $\mathcal{Q}(\boldsymbol{\theta}_{n+1}^{(t)}, \boldsymbol{\theta}_n) \geq \mathcal{Q}(\boldsymbol{\theta}_{n+1}, \boldsymbol{\theta}_n)$ **then**
18:      $\boldsymbol{\theta}_{n+1} \leftarrow \boldsymbol{\theta}_{n+1}^{(t)}$
19:    **else**
20:      Keep $\boldsymbol{\theta}_{n+1}$
21:    **end if**
22:    $n \leftarrow n + 1$
23: **until** convergence or maxiter

---

## 4 Experiments

In this section, we compare the proposed MSJL model with other overlapping community detection algorithms in synthetic benchmark and real-world networks. The baseline algorithms are as follows.

- **SJL** [17]: The Symmetric Joint Link model.
- **Possion** [2]: The Poisson community model fit with EM.
- **COPRA** [8]: The Community Overlap PRopagation Algorithm based on label propagation.
- **CPM** [7]: The Clique Percolation Method.
- **OSLOM** [12]: The Order Statistics Local Optimization Method for finding statistically significant local communities.

For CPM and OSLOM, we use their default parameters. For COPRA, the community number $\upsilon$ varies from 2 to 10. For MSJL, we empirically set the number of nearest neighbors $p$ to 5, Newton step parameter $\gamma$ to 0.1, Newton max iteration number $T$ to 5 and regularization parameter $\lambda$ to 100. Since SJL, MSJL and Possion need certain community number $K$, we adopt the Bayes Information Criterion (BIC) to find the number of communities for networks without ground truth. We use $K$ that achieves the smallest value of BIC:

$$BIC(K) = -2\mathcal{L} + NK \log |E|. \tag{12}$$

## 4.1   Evaluation Metrics

In these experiments, we use the extended Normalized Mutual Information (NMI) [11] and the average F1-score to evaluate the quality of communities detection results with ground truth. For communities without ground truth, we use overlapping modularity $Q_{ov}$ [16]. The value of these metrics is between 0 and 1. For a detected cover of overlapping communities, the values closer to 1 indicate a better matching to the real cover.

- **Normalized Mutual Information** (NMI). NMI adopts the criterion used in information theory to compare the detected communities and the ground-truth communities. Lacncichinetti [11] extended NMI to measure overlapping covers.
- **Average F1-score.** Suppose we have a set of ground truth communities $C^*$ and a set of detected communities $\hat{C}$. We define F1-score to be the average F1-score of the best matching ground-truth community to each detected community and the F1-score of the best-matching detected community to each ground-truth community.
- **Overlapping Modularity** $(Q_{ov})$. Overlapping modularity $Q_{ov}$ [16] is an extension of the Newman-Girvan modularity to deal with overlapping communities. To calculate $Q_{ov}$, a linear function $f(x) = 60x - 30$ is adopted according to the suggestion in [16].

## 4.2   Results on Synthetic Networks

In this section, we use the Lancichinetti-Fortunato-Radicchi (LFR) benchmark [10] to generate networks in size $N = 1000$ and test different parameters including mixing parameter $\mu^1$, the number of overlapping nodes $O_n$, and the number of communities $O_m$ to which each overlapping node belongs. The average degree $k$ is set to 10, which approaches the most real-world social networks case according to [21]. For other parameters, the maximum degree is set to 50 and community sizes vary in the range $[20, 50]$. We run each algorithm 10 times and the adopt average values.

Figure 1(a) and (b) show the NMI and F1-score values of the detected communities with $O_m$ ranging from 2 to 8, which indicates the diversity of overlapping nodes; Fig. 1(c) and (d) show the NMI and F1-score values of the detected communities with the mixture parameter $\mu$ ranging in $[0, 0.45]$. We can see that the detection performance decays since the connections inside communities become weaker for larger $\mu$; Fig. 1(e) and (f) show the NMI and F1-score values of the detected communities as a function of $O_n$ ranging in $[50, 500]$. From the results it can be seen that the proposed MSJL model outperforms other algorithms over different kinds of networks structures. The NMI and F1-score values of all the algorithms decrease with the three parameters increasing. However, the values of MSJL model decrease much slower than the other algorithms, showing the effectiveness and robustness of manifold regularization.

---

[1] Mixing parameter $\mu$ is the fraction of links of a node that connect to other nodes outside its community.

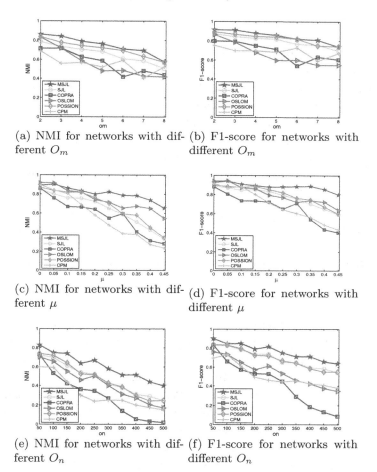

(a) NMI for networks with different $O_m$

(b) F1-score for networks with different $O_m$

(c) NMI for networks with different $\mu$

(d) F1-score for networks with different $\mu$

(e) NMI for networks with different $O_n$

(f) F1-score for networks with different $O_n$

**Fig. 1.** Comparison of MSJL with other methods on LFR benchmark networks

## 4.3   Results on Real Networks

We further analyze MSJL model on several real-world networks[2] which are commonly employed in community detection literature (Table 1). All these networks are treated as unweighted and undirected. For networks with ground truth, NMI and F1-score are applied for evaluation. For networks without ground truth, we used $Q_{ov}$ to evaluate the results.

As shown in Tables 2 and 3, MSJL achieves the best results on nine networks and the second best on the blogs dataset. MSJL has gained 22.7 % relative improvement in NMI and 5.6 % relative improvement in $Q_{ov}$ over SJL on average.

To further observe the effectiveness of manifold regularization, we visualize the community detection results of SJL and MSJL on the dolphins network in

---

[2] Networks data are download from http://www-personal.umich.edu/~mejn/netdata/.

**Table 1.** Real-world networks with community structure

| Network | Description | Vertices | Edges |
|---------|-------------|----------|-------|
| karate | Zacharys karate club | 34 | 78 |
| dolphins | Dolphin social network | 62 | 159 |
| polbooks | Books about US politics | 105 | 441 |
| football | American college football | 115 | 613 |
| blogs | Political blogs | 1224 | 9250 |
| lemis | Les miserables co-appearance characters | 34 | 78 |
| jazz | Jazz musicians networks | 198 | 5484 |
| email | Univeristy e-mail interchanges | 1133 | 5451 |
| neural | C. elegans neural network | 297 | 2345 |
| power | US. power grid | 4941 | 6594 |

**Table 2.** The NMI's and F1-score's on real-world networks with ground truth

| Metric | Network | MSJL | SJL | COPRA | OSLOM | POSSION | CPM |
|--------|---------|------|-----|-------|-------|---------|-----|
| NMI | karate | **1** | 0.8322 | 0.2922 | 0.6388 | 0.8429 | 0.2219 |
| | dolphins | **0.8144** | 0.5456 | 0.4775 | 0.5942 | 0.5759 | 0.3306 |
| | polbooks | **0.4132** | 0.3352 | 0.3824 | 0.2994 | 0.3199 | 0.3234 |
| | football | **0.7522** | 0.7 | 0.7166 | 0.6762 | 0.7128 | 0.7471 |
| | blogs | 0.7091 | 0.7013 | 0.4741 | 0.1324 | **0.7197** | 0.113 |
| F1-score | karate | **1** | 0.9405 | 0.4564 | 0.7447 | 0.9490 | 0.3765 |
| | dolphins | **0.9640** | 0.8640 | 0.7173 | 0.7846 | 0.8654 | 0.6327 |
| | polbooks | **0.7298** | 0.6851 | 0.7192 | 0.6327 | 0.6944 | 0.6238 |
| | football | **0.8503** | 0.8127 | 0.8339 | 0.7875 | 0.8080 | 0.8452 |
| | blogs | 0.9459 | 0.9418 | 0.6010 | 0.2031 | **0.9501** | 0.1793 |

Fig. 2. From Fig. 2(a) it can be seen that SJL fails to preserve the local geometry structure and gives some unreasonable partitions. Conversely, from Fig. 2(b) it can be seen that MSJL smooths the community probability along the manifold intrinsic geometry, where nearby nodes get the same community assignments.

## 4.4 Parameter Sensitiveness

MSJL model contains two major parameters, the number of nearest neighbors $p$ and the regularization parameter $\lambda$. In order to analyze the influence of these parameters, we run MSJL with different $p$ and $\lambda$ respectively on the LFR benchmark network with $\mu = 0.2$, $O_m = 2$ and $O_n = 100$. As can be seen in Fig. 3, the average NMI of MSJL is quite stable with both two parameters. The performance decrease slightly as $p$ increase. This is reasonable because the similarity between

**Table 3.** The $Q_{ov}$'s on real-world networks without ground truth

| Network | MSJL | SJL | COPRA | OSLOM | POSSION | CPM |
|---------|------|-----|-------|-------|---------|-----|
| lemis | **0.7654** | 0.7338 | 0.7173 | 0.7095 | 0.7336 | 0.634 |
| jazz | **0.7542** | 0.7256 | 0.7047 | 0.4455 | 0.7439 | 0.5959 |
| email | **0.6681** | 0.6273 | 0.3891 | 0.499 | 0.6074 | 0.4626 |
| neural | **0.7016** | 0.6799 | 0.1841 | 0.4242 | 0.6692 | 0.3939 |
| power | **0.8866** | 0.8040 | 0.2846 | 0.4568 | 0.7916 | 0.1525 |

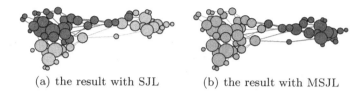

(a) the result with SJL          (b) the result with MSJL

**Fig. 2.** The result of SJL and MSJL on the dolphins dataset

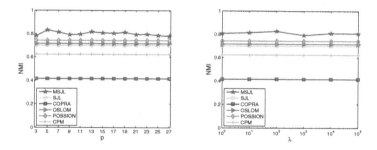

**Fig. 3.** Perfomance of MSJL under different parameter $p$ and $\lambda$

a node and its neighbor decreases when we choose latter nodes, which does not help to hold the manifold assumption.

## 5 Conclusion

In this paper, we have presented a Manifold Regularized Symmetric Joint Link Model (MSJL), which incorporates local manifold structure into the standard SJL model for overlapping community detection. To utilize the local geometrical structure, MSJL assumes the community probability distribution lives on a manifold, and the structure of the intrinsic manifold is modeled by a nearest neighbor graph. MSJL uses the graph Laplacian to smooth the community probability along the manifold intrinsic geometry. Experiments have showed that MSJL can significantly improve the performance compared with existing algorithms, showing the effectiveness combining geometrical structure of manifold in community detection. However, MSJL is not perfect because the additional Newton-Raphsion procedure costs more running times. We hope to develop more effective methods to reduce running time in the future.

**Acknowledgments.** This work was supported by National Science Foundation of China (No. 61272374 and No. 61300190), Specialized Research Fund for the Doctoral Program of Higher Education (No. 20120041110046) and Key Project of Chinese Ministry of Education (No. 313011).

# References

1. Ahn, Y.Y., Bagrow, J.P., Lehmann, S.: Link communities reveal multiscale complexity in networks. Nature **466**(7307), 761–764 (2010)
2. Ball, B., Karrer, B., Newman, M.: Efficient and principled method for detecting communities in networks. Phys. Rev. E **84**(3), 036103 (2011)
3. Belkin, M., Niyogi, P.: Laplacian eigenmaps and spectral techniques for embedding and clustering. NIPS **14**, 585–591 (2001)
4. Belkin, M., Niyogi, P., Sindhwani, V.: Manifold regularization: a geometric framework for learning from labeled and unlabeled examples. J. Mach. Learn. Res. **7**, 2399–2434 (2006)
5. Cai, D., He, X., Han, J., Huang, T.S.: Graph regularized nonnegative matrix factorization for data representation. IEEE Trans. Pattern Anal. Mach. Intell. **33**(8), 1548–1560 (2011)
6. Cai, D., Mei, Q., Han, J., Zhai, C.: Modeling hidden topics on document manifold. In: CIKM, pp. 911–920. ACM (2008)
7. Dernyi, I., Palla, G., Vicsek, T.: Clique percolation in random networks. Phys. Rev. Lett. **94**(16), 160202 (2005)
8. Gregory, S.: Finding overlapping communities in networks by label propagation. New J. Phys. **12**(10), 103018 (2010)
9. He, X., Cai, D., Shao, Y., Bao, H., Han, J.: Laplacian regularized gaussian mixture model for data clustering. IEEE Trans. Knowl. Data Eng. **23**(9), 1406–1418 (2011)
10. Lancichinetti, A., Fortunato, S.: Benchmarks for testing community detection algorithms on directed and weighted graphs with overlapping communities. Phys. Rev. E **80**(1), 016118 (2009)
11. Lancichinetti, A., Fortunato, S., Kertsz, J.: Detecting the overlapping and hierarchical community structure in complex networks. New J. Phys. **11**(3), 033015 (2009)
12. Lancichinetti, A., Radicchi, F., Ramasco, J.J., Fortunato, S.: Finding statistically significant communities in networks. PloS One **6**(4), e18961 (2011)
13. Lee, J.: Introduction to Smooth Manifolds, vol. 218. Springer, New York (2012)
14. Neal, R.M., Hinton, G.E.: A view of the EM algorithm that justifies incremental, sparse, and other variants. In: Jordan, M.I. (ed.) Learning in Graphical Models, pp. 355–368. Springer, Netherlands (1998)
15. Newman, M.E., Leicht, E.A.: Mixture models and exploratory analysis in networks. Proceedings of the National Academy of Sciences **104**(23), 9564–9569 (2007)
16. Nicosia, V., Mangioni, G., Carchiolo, V., Malgeri, M.: Extending the definition of modularity to directed graphs with overlapping communities. J. Stat. Mech. Theor. Exp. **2009**(03), P03024 (2009)

17. Ren, W., Yan, G., Liao, X., Xiao, L.: Simple probabilistic algorithm for detecting community structure. Phys. Rev. E **79**(3), 036111 (2009)
18. Roweis, S.T., Saul, L.K.: Nonlinear dimensionality reduction by locally linear embedding. Science **290**(5500), 2323–2326 (2000)
19. Tenenbaum, J.B., De Silva, V., Langford, J.C.: A global geometric framework for nonlinear dimensionality reduction. Science **290**(5500), 2319–2323 (2000)
20. Wang, Z., Hu, Y., Xiao, W., Ge, B.: Overlapping community detection using a generative model for networks. Physica A: Stat. Mech. Appl. **392**(20), 5218–5230 (2013)
21. Xie, J., Kelley, S., Szymanski, B.K.: Overlapping community detection in networks: the state-of-the-art and comparative study. ACM Comput. Surv. (CSUR) **45**(4), 43 (2013)

# High Dimensional Explicit Feature Biased Matrix Factorization Recommendation

Weibin Sun, Xianchao Zhang, Wenxin Liang$^{(\boxtimes)}$, and Zengyou He

Dalian University of Technology, Dalian, China
swb0802@126.com, {xczhang,wxliang,zyhe}@dlut.edu.cn

**Abstract.** Collaborative Filtering method using latent factor model is one of the most popular approaches in personal recommending system. It is famous for its good performance by using only user-item rating matrix. The latent progress intelligently factorizes users' preference on different items through the rating matrix. However, the factorization progress is completely implicit. Thus, it is difficult to integrate new observed features, and it becomes more complicated when one feature has multiple values. In this paper, we propose a new algorithm based on Matrix Factorization to model explicit features besides rating values by adding high dimensional factors, which makes the factorized presentation explainable. The algorithm is generally applicable for such discrete features as type, genres, age and so on. Experimental results show that our approach outperforms the state-of-the-art methods using latent factor model.

## 1 Introduction

Recommending system plays an important role in solving information overloading problems. It helps to filter information and benefits not only the information consumers, but also information providers as online shops and social networks.

Matrix Factorization approach, hereinafter referred to as MF approach, becomes famous for its efficiency and simplicity since the Netflix Prize [1]. It only utilizes user-item rating matrix to get user and item feature matrices in which each row represents one user/item. The feature matrices are then used to predict unknown rating values.

The main advantage of MF approaches is that it needs only rating matrix to make the prediction. However, one of the limitation of MF is that its factorization progress is completely implicit. Even though the latent factor model is solved, whether the key features are contained and which vector represents which feature remain unknown.

Some efforts have been made to add additional information to MF method. In [16] considers social relations, [3] concerns time factor, and [12] integrates

This work was supported by National Science Foundation of China (No. 61272374, 61300190), Specialized Research Fund for the Doctoral Program of Higher Education (No. 20120041110046) and Key Project of Chinese Ministry of Education (No. 313011).

© Springer International Publishing Switzerland 2015
X.-L. Li et al. (Eds.): PAKDD 2015, LNCS 9441, pp. 66–77, 2015.
DOI: 10.1007/978-3-319-25660-3_6

ingredients information for recipe recommendation. However, the problem mentioned above still remains. Besides, these methods fail when one feature contains multiple values.

Considering these limitations, in this paper we propose a novel MF method. The main contributions of this paper are summarized as follows.

- The proposed model is applicable when one feature contains multiple values.
- Instead of increasing the dimensions of user and item feature vectors which is unexplainable and increases the over fitting problem, we add an additional dimension which represents the key feature. It is proved to be effective through experiments.
- Experimental results demonstrate that our approach outperforms the state-of-the-art methods using latent factor model.

The rest of the paper is organized as follows. Section 2 introduces previous works of Collaborative Filtering, especially MF based work. Section 3 describes details about MF methods. Section 4 brings up our method. The experiment and results analysis are shown in Sect. 5, followed by the conclusion in Sect. 6.

## 2   Related Work

### 2.1   Traditional Recommender Algorithms

Collaborative Filtering (CF) [19,21] is the most popular algorithm in recommending system which is based on user-item rating matrix. Taking the advantages of crowds makes it different from traditional Content-based algorithms, which focus on analyzing user and item features of history records. There are two types of CF algorithms: memory-based methods and model-based methods; Memory-based methods explicitly figure out the user and item similarity [4,7] and make the prediction directly basing on the target user's history behavior. Person correlation and cosine similarity are the common methods to determine similar users and items which are called "nearest neighbors".

The model-based approaches use the observed ratings to train a predefined learning model. The ratings are then predicted via the trained model instead of directly manipulating the original rating database as the memory-based approaches do. Common algorithms in this category include Ranking based model [14] and Clustering model. In the ranking model, they measure the similarity between users based on the correlation between their rankings of items rather than the rating values and propose new collaborative filtering algorithms for ranking items based on preferences of similar users [14]. Various matrix clustering techniques have been investigated in an attempt to address the problems of efficiency, scalability and sparsity [26]. User clustering and item clustering methods [18] cluster user or item vectors first, and nearest neighbors of a user or item are restricted to its cluster. Co-clustering method views the contingency table as an empirical joint probability distribution of two discrete random variables and poses the co-clustering problem as an optimization problem in information theory the optimal co-clustering maximizes the mutual information between the clustered random variables subject to constraints on the number of row and column clusters [5,6,11]. Clustering based model usually greatly increase the scalability problem and each user or item can only fall into one cluster, which is not always true in the real world.

## 2.2 Matrix Factorization Algorithms

Matrix factorization methods in recommender systems normally seek to factorize the user-item rating matrix into two low rank user-specific and item-specific matrices, and then utilize the factorized matrices to make further predictions [15]. Singular Value Decomposition (SVD) is the basic method to minimize sum square errors based MF problems [2,22,23].

In [24], Expectation Maximization (EM) algorithm was used to find the local optimal solution. Besides, Non-Negative Matrix Factorization (NMF) [10,13] is another method to solve similar problem which constrains that all the values in matrix are non-negative. In [25], they focus on using "low-norm" factorizations for collaborative prediction instead of dimensionality. But SVD and NMF are still not efficient enough because the effects of small updates to the rating matrix are not localized [26].

Probabilistic Matrix Factorization (PMF) models can be viewed as graphical models in which hidden factor variables have directed connections to variables that represent user rating. Ruslan Salakhutdinov et al. presented the Probabilistic Matrix Factorization (PMF) model which scales linearly with the number of observations and performs well on the large, sparse, and very imbalanced Netflix dataset [17]. In their following work [20], they have presented a fully Bayesian treatment of Probabilistic Matrix Factorization by placing hyperpriors over the hyperparameters and using Markov Chain Monte Carlo methods to perform approximate inference.

Hu Liang et al. [8] proposed a generalized Cross Domain Triadic Factorization (CDTF) model over the triadic relation user-item-domain, which can better capture the interactions between domain-specific user factors and item factors. However, in this paper, our algorithm is different from Hu Liang's work. We consider this situation that some features may have multiple values which is true in the real world.

## 3   Matrix Factorization for Recommending Systems

The basic form of Matrix Factorization objective function is shown as follow:

$$\min_{p_u, q_i} \frac{1}{2} \sum_{(u,i) \in K} (r_{ui} - p_u^T q_i)^2 + \frac{\lambda_u}{2} \|P\|^2 + \frac{\lambda_i}{2} \|Q\|^2 \tag{1}$$

where $p_u$ and $q_i$ correspond to feature vectors, $r_{ui}$ is the observed value and $p_u^T q_i$ is predicted values. The last two terms are used to prevent over fitting. The algorithm aims at solving the unknown matrix $P$ and $Q$ using rating data set $K$.

For this kind of problems, we have stochastic gradient descent method to achieve the local optimal solution, and the main iteration process is shown as follows.

$$p_u \leftarrow p_u + lr((r_{ui} - p_u^T q_i)q_i - \lambda_u p_u) \tag{2}$$

$$q_i \leftarrow q_i + lr((r_{ui} - p_u^T q_i)q_i - \lambda_i q_i) \tag{3}$$

A biased version of MF method is proved to be more effective [9] which takes the following estimate form:

$$\hat{r}_{ui} = a + b_u + b_i + p_u^T q_i \tag{4}$$

where $a$ is the average rating for all items, $b_u$ is the rating bias for user $u$, and $b_i$ for item $i$.

## 4 High Dimensional Explicit Feature Biased MF

In this section, we will propose an improved algorithm of Baseline MF by adding explicit factors.

As we mentioned before, MF algorithm only utilizes rating information. Moreover, the factors in $P$, $Q$ matrix representing user preference and item information is latent, which cannot be explained. Although these factors greatly simplify the MF algorithm, there is still improvement that can be made.

In the following sections, movies rating progress is used to illustrate the high dimensional MF method and movies type (also known as genres) information is viewed as explicit feature to correct the latent factors in the model.

### 4.1 Bias Adjustment for Multiple Feature Values

Each user has different preference on different item of a particular feature. It is reasonable to add biases on different types rather than one bias for each user. Take movie for instance. As shown in Fig. 1, David prefers Horror movie most and does not like Action movie. Obviously, if we take David's average rating 6.46 as baseline to predict, the type preference information will be lost. It is the same to item. Bias setting could not be the same between popular items and unpopular ones. Thus, we add another dimension to user bias $b_u$ and item bias $b_i$. Moreover, we modified the average variable $a$ over all items to the average of each feature type to make the bias adjustment more specific.

Item's feature values may be multiple. For example, movie Interstellar have type value Fantasy and Adventure and one music may multiple artists. We calculate the bias of each feature value separately, and then average them one rating bias. The formula is shown as follows.

$$bias = \frac{\sum_{c \in C(i)} a_c + b_{uc} + b_{ic}}{|Ci|}, \tag{5}$$

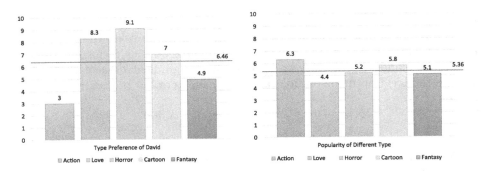

**Fig. 1.** Type preference of different users and items

where $a_c$ is the average rating for type value $c$, $b_u c$ is the bias rating that user $u$ prefers type $c$, $b_i c$ is the popularity bias of item $i$ on type $c$, $C(i)$ is the type value set that $i$ belongs to, and $|C(i)|$ represents the elements count.

### 4.2 Explicit Feature Factorization with High Dimensional Solution

As items contain type information, each rating of a specific user not only represents his explicit preference on this item, but also preference on the type that the item belongs to. As shown in Fig. 2(a)(b), traditional MF uses latent factor model, which factorizes the rating matrix into user and item feature matrices with k-dimension. Thus, there are k latent factors for each user and item. They perhaps contain the type factor or probably not because the factorizing progress is totally latent and is not controllable to us.

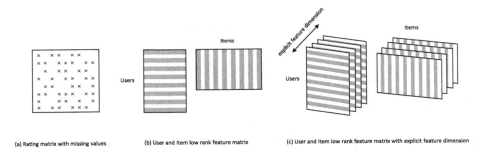

**Fig. 2.** Matrix factorization models

However, in our approach as shown in Fig. 2(c), we convert the type information from latent factor to explicit one. Each user and item has t-dimension factor matrix and each matrix represents its type specific feature. In other words, instead of increasing user and item feature vector dimensions, we convert them from flat to three-dimensional.

As the same is with the bias settings, we also add type dimension to user factor matrix $p_u$ and item factor matrix $q_i$, converting them from flat to three-dimension. The explicit feature type is definitely contained in the model. The user and item factor interaction is finally shown as follows.

$$\frac{\sum_{c \in C(i)} p_{uc}^T q_{ic}}{|Ci|}, \tag{6}$$

where $p_{uc}^T q_{ic}$ converts factorization procession from user-item to user-type-item. Type features are presented as new dimension explicitly.

## 4.3  Model Integration and Evaluation

From previous Sects. 4.1 and 4.2, we demonstrated how to modify explicit feature bias as well as user and item factors interaction utilizing type information. Now finally designed the objective function as follow.

$$\min_{b*, p_{uc}, q_{ic}} \frac{1}{2} \sum_{(u,i) \in K} (r_{ui} - \frac{\sum_{c \in C(i)} a_c + b_{uc} + b_{ic} + p_{uc}^T q_{ic}}{|C(i)|})^2$$
$$+ \frac{1}{2} \sum_{c \in C(i)} (\lambda_{u1}(b_{uc})^2 + \lambda_{i1}(b_{ic})^2 + \lambda_{u2}\|p_{uc}\|^2 + \lambda_{i2}(q_{ic})^2), \tag{7}$$

where $a_c$, $b_{uc}$, $b_{ic}$ are scalars. $p_{uc}$ and $q_{ic}$ are vectors. We add all the unknown variables into regularization term to prevent overfitting. In Eq. (13), type dimension is added to the bias part, in Eq. (14) to the user-item interaction part and in Eq. (7) to both.

We adopt the stochastic gradient descent approach to update each parameters. Take Eq. (7) for instance, the iteration process is as follows.

$$b_{uc} \leftarrow b_{uc} + lr(\nabla r - \lambda_{u1} b_{uc}) \tag{8}$$

$$b_{ic} \leftarrow b_{ic} + lr(\nabla r - \lambda_{i1} b_{ic}) \tag{9}$$

$$p_{uc} \leftarrow p_{uc} + lr(\nabla r q_{ic} - \lambda_{u2} p_{uc}) \tag{10}$$

$$q_{ic} \leftarrow q_{ic} + lr(\nabla r b_{uc} - \lambda_{i2} q_{ic}), \tag{11}$$

where $lr$ is the learning rate, and

$$\nabla r = r_{ui} - \frac{\sum_{c \in C(i)} a_c + b_{uc} + b_{ic} + p_{uc}^T q_{ic}}{|C(i)|}. \tag{12}$$

In order to see the impact of different partitions in the objective function, we designed another two estimating formula which are shown as follows.

$$\hat{r}_{ui} = (r_{ui} - (a + b_u + b_i + \frac{\sum_{c \in C(i)} p_{uc}^T q_{ic}}{|C(i)|}))^2 \tag{13}$$

$$\hat{r}_{ui} = (r_{ui} - (\frac{\sum_{c \in C(i)} a_c + b_{uc} + b_{ic}}{|C(i)|} + p_u^T q_i))^2 \tag{14}$$

We use Mean Absolute Error (MAE) and Root Mean Square Error (RMSE) metrics to measure the models. MAE is defined as follows.

$$MAE = \frac{\sum_{(u,i) \in T} |r_{ui} - \hat{r}_{ui}|}{|T|} \tag{15}$$

where $r_{ui}$ represents the actual rating score that user $u$ rated on item $i$. $\hat{r}_{ui}$ is the predicted score. Similarly, RMSE is defined as follows.

$$RMSE = \sqrt{\frac{\sum_{(u,i) \in T} (r_{ui} - \hat{r}_{ui})^2}{|T|}}, \tag{16}$$

## 5 Experiments

### 5.1 Dataset

We use two movie rating datasets in our experiment. Each dataset contains movie ratings of 1 to 5 scale. Each movie belongs to several types.

The first dataset is the popular MovieLens10M dataset, which contains 10,000,054 ratings from 69,878 users and 10,677 movies. Each movie has at least one type information and there are 20 different movie types.

The second dataset is crawled from Douban, which is a famous Chinese Web 2.0 web site providing user ratings and reviews for books, movies, music and so on. We spend several months to get 11,229,246 ratings from 34,145 users and 23,502 movies, including type information for each movie.

### 5.2 Methods for Comparison

We compare some relative models using MF algorithm. The details of each model are listed as follows.

**User Mean (UMean)**: The mean rating score of each user is used as prediction for unknown rating of this user.

**Item Mean (IMean)**: The mean rating score of each movie is used as prediction for unknown rating of this movie.

**NMF**: This method is proposed in [10]. It uses Non-negative Matrix Factorization with only user-item rating matrix for recommendation which is widely used in collaborative filtering.

**BLMF**: Baseline MF, which is mentioned in [9]. The estimate equation is shown as Eq. (4). It is the base algorithm of our methods.

**BPMF**: This algorithm uses Markov Chain Monte Carlo to train Bayesian Probabilistic Matrix Factorization [20].

**HEMF1**: This method is the improved Baseline MF which adds explicit feature dimension to bias part. The objective function is shown as Eq. (13).

**HEMF2**: This method is the improved Baseline MF which adds explicit feature dimension to user-item interaction part. The objective function is shown as Eq. (14).

**HEMF3**: This method is the improved Baseline MF which adds explicit feature dimension to both bias and user-item interaction part. The objective function is shown as Eq. (7).

## 5.3   Data Preparation

For each of this two dataset, we randomly selected 90 % of the ratings as training set and the remaining as the testing set. During the splitting process, we make sure that for each user and item appearing in the testing set, there are at least one rating in the training set. In another word, there are no brand new users or items in the testing set.

## 5.4   Parameter Settings

In order to perform a convictive comparison, we employ similar parameter settings among different algorithms. We conducted all the algorithms under both 10 dimension and 30 dimension. For all the regularization term, we set them to 0.1. The learning rate is set to 0.05 and all the algorithms are iterated until the training RMSE or MAE begin to increase.

**Table 1.** Performance comparisons on MovieLens dataset

| Dataset | D | Matrix | UMean | IMean | NMF | BLMF | BPMF | HEMF1 | HEMF2 | HEMF3 |
|---------|---|--------|-------|-------|-----|------|------|-------|-------|-------|
| MovieL | 10 | MAE | 0.7683 | 0.7384 | 0.7151 | 0.7081 | 0.6809 | 0.6974 | 0.6680 | 0.6645 |
| | | Improve | 13.51 % | 10.01 % | 7.08 % | 6.61 % | 2.41 % | | | |
| | | MAE | 0.9779 | 0.9442 | 0.9208 | 0.8965 | 0.8647 | 0.8794 | 0.8516 | 0.8423 |
| | | Improve | 13.87 % | 10.79 % | 8.53 % | 6.05 % | 2.59 % | | | |
| | 30 | MAE | 0.7683 | 0.7384 | 0.7363 | 0.7012 | 0.6860 | 0.6968 | 0.6540 | 0.6510 |
| | | Improve | 14.88 % | 11.43 % | 11.18 % | 6.75 % | 5.10 % | | | |
| | | MAE | 0.9779 | 0.9442 | 0.9557 | 0.8958 | 0.8781 | 0.8567 | 0.8570 | 0.8480 |
| | | Improve | 13.28 % | 10.19 % | 11.27 % | 5.35 % | 3.43 % | | | |

## 5.5   Result Analysis

The results on MovieLens and Douban are shown in Tables 2 and 3. The percentages in the tables are improvements that our methods outperform others. Figures (3) and (4) show the iteration process of each method. The rest algorithms converge within 40 iteration. We summarized some key conclusions as follows.

**Table 2.** Performance comparisons on douban dataset

| Dataset | D | Matrix | UMean | IMean | NMF | BLMF | BPMF | HEMF1 | HEMF2 | HEMF3 |
|---------|---|--------|-------|-------|-----|------|------|-------|-------|-------|
| Douban | 10 | MAE | 0.6923 | 0.6017 | 0.5957 | 0.5887 | 0.5399 | 0.6344 | 0.5631 | 0.5734 |
| | | Improve | 18.92 % | 6.71 % | 5.77 % | 4.65 % | -3.69 % | | | |
| | | MAE | 0.8633 | 0.7539 | 0.7550 | 0.7365 | 0.6866 | 0.8358 | 0.7166 | 0.7235 |
| | | Improve | 16.99 % | 4.95 % | 5.09 % | 2.70 % | -4.37 % | | | |
| | 30 | MAE | 0.6923 | 0.6018 | 0.6136 | 0.6268 | 0.5463 | 0.6351 | 0.5617 | 0.5729 |
| | | Improve | 18.87 % | 6.67 % | 8.46 % | 10.39 % | -2.82 % | | | |
| | | MAE | 0.8633 | 0.7539 | 0.7899 | 0.7888 | 0.6956 | 0.8360 | 0.7177 | 0.7230 |
| | | Improve | 16.87 % | 4.80 % | 9.14 % | 9.01 % | -3.20 % | | | |

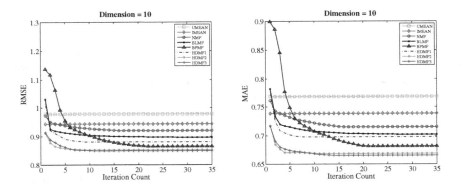

**Fig. 3.** Performance comparison of different alg. on MovieLens

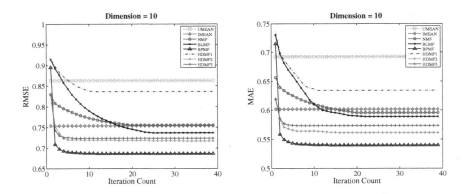

**Fig. 4.** Performance comparison of different alg. on Douban

1. Our High Dimensional Explicit Feature biased MF methods (HEMF1, HEMF2 and HEMF3) outperform most of the algorithms (except BPMF on the Douban dataset). This proved that the explicit feature with high dimension factors information will improve the performance. While there is still some interesting phenomena in these two datasets. On one hand, the Item Mean algorithm outperforms the User Mean in both datasets, which indicates that user ratings are more fluctuant while movie tends to receive relative consistent rating scores. This is reasonable because one user may watch movies of different qualities while for each movie, its quality determines relative concentrated rating scores. On the other hand, the difference between these two algorithms in Douban dataset is larger than that in MovieLens, which may indicate that the users on Douban Website are easier to be influenced by movie's previous ratings or their tastes are more concentrated. This difference may be the reason that BPMF outperforms our algorithm in Douban dataset while not in MovieLens.

2. The difference between BLMF and HEMF1 is that HEMF1 adds type dimension to user-item interaction in objective function Eq. (13). HEMF1 performs better than BLMF on the MovieLens dataset, but worse on the Douban dataset. We can see from Table 1 that these two dataset have similar data sparsity, but Douban have more item types than MovieLens, which means that Douban received less training probability on each type in the PQ matrix than MovieLens. This data feature may lead to the bad performance in user-item interaction. The same result also appears in HEMF2 and HEMF3. This indicates that user-item interaction with explicit feature dimension method is more applicable when feature count is not too large.

3. The difference between BLMF and HEMF2 is that HEMF2 adds type dimension to bias part in objective function Eq. (14). Explicit feature bias method is more accurate than that using overall bias discarding type distinction.

4. From the dimension perspective, not all the algorithm will perform better when dimension increase from 10 to 30. Almost all the algorithm suffer from the over-fitting problem. On the other hand, when characteristic matrix dimension increase from two-dimension to three-dimension (i.e. from $n \times k$, corresponding to BLMF, to $n \times t \times k$, corresponding to HEMF), the performance increases remarkably. This result confirms that increase dimension by converting implicit characters into explicit ones outperforms simply increase explicit characters, which will relieve the over-fitting problem.

## 6   Conclusion

In this paper, we proposed a variation of bias based baseline MF algorithm using explicit feature information. Converting observed features from implicit factorization, which is uncontrollable, to explicit ones helps to improve the performance. It increases the dimension of user and item features from another perspective which relieves the over fitting problem. It is applicable when the item have to multiple values and is more effective when the number of feature values is not too large.

# References

1. Bennett, J., Lanning, S.: The netflix prize. In: Proceedings of KDD Cup and Workshop, vol. 2007, p. 35 (2007)
2. Brand, M.: Fast online SVD revisions for lightweight recommender systems. In: SDM, pp. 37–46. SIAM (2003)
3. Chen, T., Zheng, Z., Lu, Q., Jiang, X., Chen, Y., Zhang, W., Chen, K., Yu, Y., Liu, N., Cao, B., et al.: Informative ensemble of multi-resolution dynamic factorization models. In: KDD-Cup Workshop (2011)
4. Deshpande, M., Karypis, G.: Item-based top-n recommendation algorithms. ACM Trans. Inf. Syst. (TOIS) 22(1), 143–177 (2004)
5. Dhillon, I.S., Mallela, S., Modha, D.S.: Information-theoretic co-clustering. In: Proceedings of the Ninth ACM SIGKDD International Conference on Knowledge Discovery and Data mining, pp. 89–98. ACM (2003)
6. George, T., Merugu, S.: A scalable collaborative filtering framework based on co-clustering. In: Fifth IEEE International Conference on Data Mining, p. 4. IEEE (2005)
7. Herlocker, J.L., Konstan, J.A., Borchers, A., Riedl, J.: An algorithmic framework for performing collaborative filtering. In: Proceedings of the 22nd Annual International ACM SIGIR Conference on Research and Development in Information Retrieval, pp. 230–237. ACM (1999)
8. Hu, L., Cao, J., Xu, G., Cao, L., Gu, Z., Zhu, C.: Personalized recommendation via cross-domain triadic factorization. In: Proceedings of the 22nd International Conference on World Wide Web, pp. 595–606. International World Wide Web Conferences Steering Committee (2013)
9. Koren, Y., Bell, R., Volinsky, C.: Matrix factorization techniques for recommender systems. Computer 42(8), 30–37 (2009)
10. Lee, D.D., Seung, H.S.: Algorithms for non-negative matrix factorization. In: Advances in Neural Information Processing Systems, pp. 556–562 (2001)
11. Leung, K.W.T., Lee, D.L., Lee, W.C.: CLR: a collaborative location recommendation framework based on co-clustering. In: Proceedings of the 34th International ACM SIGIR Conference on Research and Development in Information Retrieval, pp. 305–314. ACM (2011)
12. Lin, C.-J., Lin, C.-J., Kuo, T.-T., Kuo, T.-T., Lin, S.-D., Lin, S.-D.: A content-based matrix factorization model for recipe recommendation. In: Tseng, V.S., Tseng, V.S., Ho, T.B., Ho, T.B., Zhou, Z.-H., Zhou, Z.-H., Chen, A.L.P., Chen, A.L.P., Kao, H.-Y., Kao, H.-Y. (eds.) PAKDD 2014, Part II. LNCS, vol. 8444, pp. 560–571. Springer, Heidelberg (2014)
13. Liu, C., Yang, H.c., Fan, J., He, L.W., Wang, Y.M.: Distributed nonnegative matrix factorization for web-scale dyadic data analysis on mapreduce. In: Proceedings of the 19th International Conference on World Wide Web, pp. 681–690. ACM (2010)
14. Liu, N.N., Yang, Q.: Eigenrank: a ranking-oriented approach to collaborative filtering. In: Proceedings of the 31st Annual International ACM SIGIR Conference on Research and Development in Information Retrieval, pp. 83–90. ACM (2008)
15. Ma, H.: An experimental study on implicit social recommendation. In: Proceedings of the 36th International ACM SIGIR Conference on Research and Development in Information Retrieval, pp. 73–82. ACM (2013)
16. Ma, H., Zhou, D., Liu, C., Lyu, M.R., King, I.: Recommender systems with social regularization. In: Proceedings of the Fourth ACM International Conference on Web Search and Data mining, pp. 287–296. ACM (2011)

17. Mnih, A., Salakhutdinov, R.: Probabilistic matrix factorization. In: Advances in Neural Information Processing Systems, pp. 1257–1264 (2007)
18. O'Connor, M., Herlocker, J.: Clustering items for collaborative filtering. In: Proceedings of the ACM SIGIR Workshop on Recommender Systems, vol. 128. Citeseer (1999)
19. Resnick, P., Varian, H.R.: Recommender systems. Commun. ACM **40**(3), 56–58 (1997)
20. Salakhutdinov, R., Mnih, A.: Bayesian probabilistic matrix factorization using markov chain monte carlo. In: Proceedings of the 25th International Conference on Machine Learning, pp. 880–887. ACM (2008)
21. Sarwar, B., Karypis, G., Konstan, J., Riedl, J.: Analysis of recommendation algorithms for e-commerce. In: Proceedings of the 2nd ACM Conference on Electronic Commerce, pp. 158–167. ACM (2000)
22. Sarwar, B., Karypis, G., Konstan, J., Riedl, J.: Application of dimensionality reduction in recommender system-a case study. Technical report, DTIC Document (2000)
23. Sarwar, B., Karypis, G., Konstan, J., Riedl, J.: Incremental singular value decomposition algorithms for highly scalable recommender systems. In: Fifth International Conference on Computer and Information Science, pp. 27–28. Citeseer (2002)
24. Srebro, N., Jaakkola, T., et al.: Weighted low-rank approximations. In: ICML, vol. 3, pp. 720–727 (2003)
25. Srebro, N., Rennie, J., Jaakkola, T.S.: Maximum-margin matrix factorization. In: Advances in Neural Information Processing Systems, pp. 1329–1336 (2004)
26. Zhang, W., Wang, J., Chen, B., Zhao, X.: To personalize or not: a risk management perspective. In: Proceedings of the 7th ACM Conference on Recommender Systems, pp. 229–236. ACM (2013)

# A Simhash-Based Generalized Framework
# for Citation Matching in MapReduce

Pengsen Wang$^{(\boxtimes)}$, Bin Wu, Xiaoming Li, Lin Wang, and Bai Wang

Beijing Key Laboratory of Intelligent Telecommunications Software
and Multimedia, Beijing University of Posts and Telecommunications,
Beijing 100876, China
{wps1992,xiaomingli007,chestnutwl}@gmail.com,
{wubin,wangbai}@bupt.edu.cn

**Abstract.** Citation matching is to find the cited papers according to only a small amount of information. There have been some works on citation matching. Most of the solutions require expensive model processing to achieve good results. However, when dealing with millions of citations in large digital libraries, these solutions may not be efficient enough. To address this problem, we propose a simhash-based generalized framework in MapReduce for citation matching. In the framework, we use title exact matching and distance-based short text similarity metrics to implement citation matching. Moreover, customizing citation fields, citation field weights and word segmentation weights are used for improving the accuracy. We also design a heuristic algorithm which can automatically calculate the weights of each citation field. For disposing the large-scale datasets, we implement the framework in Hadoop, a popular parallel computation platform. We do our experiments with real datasets from a Chinese Medicine Digital Library, and a comparative experiment with Cora corpus (McCallum's citation matching test set). The results of experiments confirm the efficiency and effectiveness of our framework.

**Keywords:** Citation matching · Parallelization · Short text similarity · MapReduce

## 1 Introduction

Citations in research publications represent an important knowledge source regarding the context of scientific work [1]. For a digital library, building the link between the citations and the cited papers is significant. It will provide better user-friendly interface to get the cited papers by citations. Moreover, it can also build citation network more accurately and completely which can be analyzed for paper identification of related research, importance, research trend prediction and so on.

Citation matching is the problem to find the cited literatures according to only a small amount of information. In reality, some citation records are incomplete, inaccurate, or lacking of DOI (Digital Object Unique Identifier). So we cannot decide whether two records describe the same article directly. With the rapid growth of the number of the publications, matching large-scale citations with incomplete and inaccurate information effectively and efficiently is a big challenge.

© Springer International Publishing Switzerland 2015
X.-L. Li et al. (Eds.): PAKDD 2015, LNCS 9441, pp. 78–90, 2015.
DOI: 10.1007/978-3-319-25660-3_7

Since Hitchcock et al. [4] demonstrated a proof-of-concept system that performed autonomous linking within Cognitive Science Open Journal, the problem of citation matching problem has been of interest to researchers [1, 2, 4–7, 9]. However, most of them require expensive model processing and are just suitable for specific language. The time-consuming methods are not the solutions for large scale citation matching.

In this paper, we propose a simhash-based generalized framework for citation matching in MapReduce. Because of spelling errors and incompletion, mere title exact matching is not enough for all matching situations. We combine title exact matching with short text similarity metrics in order to propose a generalized framework for citation matching. And we implement our framework in MapReduce to make it more effective. The experimental evaluation shows efficiency and effectiveness of the framework. Our contributions can be summarized as follows:

- We show that Charikar's simhash [3] is practically useful for large scale citation matching. We modify simhash method and experimentally validate that the framework can get the best performance with hamming distance k = 7.
- We design a heuristic algorithm which can automatically calculate the weights of each filed of the citation, and we develop a generalized framework for citation matching with high accuracy, efficiency and stability in different languages.
- We implement the framework in MapReduce. Experiments on huge real datasets verify the efficiency and scalability of our framework.

The rest of the paper is organized as follows. Related work is given in Sect. 2. In Sect. 3, we introduce problem definition. We describe our framework in Sect. 4 and citation matching in MapReduce in Sect. 5. Section 6 presents our experiments and the results. We end with conclusions and future work in Sect. 7.

## 2 Related Work

As a standardized part of a scientific article, citations have great values to be explored, and there have been numerous works on parsing and analyzing citations for different purposes [1]. Blocking methods are proposed to efficiently process multi-dimensional citation records [1, 6, 13]. It uses several citation fields to split the dataset into blocks. But citation record pairs can be compared in the same block with relatively high computation cost.

The approach Pasula et al. [2] proposed is based on the use of a relational probability model to define a generative model for the domain, including models of author and title corruption and a probabilistic citation grammar. Bilenko [12] presented a framework for improving duplicate detection using trainable measures of textual similarity. Machine learning methods can be utilized to improve citation matching performance, but the computational complexity of the algorithm is high and it cannot be able to dispose large-scale data in practical applications. Liao et al. [5] proposed an alternative joint inference approach–Generalized Joint Segmentation. It can effectively deal with the situation when the dataset type is unknown. But it focused on different types of citation data instead of a specific method. Koo et al. [6] study the best combination of citation record fields that helps increase citation matching performance and is applicable regardless of which research framework one may adopt. But this article mainly works on the effects of citation fields in citation matching performance. They don't have their own method to do citation matching. Fedoryszak et al. [9] use appropriate indexing and MapReduce to do citation matching. Their method performance good in small dataset, but they don't valid the effectiveness for large scale data with indexing.

In our work, we propose a simhash-based generalized framework for citation matching in MapReduce. The experiments show that this framework is effective and efficient. The framework can be used to do citation matching to construct large-scale digital library with less manual identification and labeling.

# 3 Problem Definition

Our aim is to develop a generalized framework which can be efficiently applied in citation matching cases. To describe the problem more succinctly, we introduce some definitions related to our framework.

***Definition 1.*** *A* ***citation dataset*** *CSet is a set of tuples <id, C>, where C is a set of fields and id is a local identifier for the citation in the dataset.*

A tuple of the citation data always consists of some fixed fields such as id, title ($T$), author ($A$), year ($Y$), month ($M$), volume ($V$) and page ($P_a$). And we denote fields except id as $C$.

***Definition 2.*** *A* ***cited paper dataset*** *QSet is a set of tuples <id, Q>, where Q is a set of fields extract from a paper and id is a local identifier for the paper.*

A tuple of the cited paper data always consists of some fixed fields, such as that in citation. And we denote fields except id as $Q$.

***Definition 3.*** *The* ***citation matching*** *is that for a tuple <id, C> in the citation dataset, we find a unique tuple <id, Q> in the cited paper dataset with the common fields (title ($T$), author($A$), year($Y$), month($M$), volume($V$) and page($Pa$)) in C and Q.*

To match these two datasets, we develop a framework for citation matching.

In order to describe succinctly, we define some symbols as follows:

| | |
|---|---|
| $CSet$: The citation dataset. | $P_i$: The $i_{th}$ word of the publisher of citation($P_i$) obtained by segmentation. |
| $QSet$: The cited paper dataset. | |
| $C$: A citation tuple in the $CSet$. | $W_T$: the weight of $T$. |
| $T$: The title of the citation. | $W_{Ti}$ : The weight of $Ti$ . |
| $A$: The author of the citation. | $W_A$: The weight of $A$. |
| $P$: The source of the citation. | $W_{Ai}$:The weight of $Ai$. |
| $Y$: The publishing year of the citation. | $W_P$ : The weight of $P$. |
| $M$: The publishing month of the citation. | $W_{Pi}$ : The weight of $Pi$. |
| $V$: The volume (volume, issue). | $Vector^T$ : Vector with the same dimension consisting of 0 and 1. 1 representing including the part of citations and 0 being opposite. |
| $P_a$: The publishing pages of the citation. | |
| $T_i$: The $i_{th}$ word in title by segmentation | |
| $A_i$: The $i_{th}$ author of the citation | |

## 4     Framework for Citation Matching

Citation data records usually consist of some fixed parts, e.g. citation title, citation author, publisher, citation publishing year, citation volume (volume, issue) etc. We can also extract the data from cited paper data. Thus, we can get the common fields of citations and cited paper datasets, e.g. title, author, publisher and year.

The structure of the framework is shown in the following Fig. 1.

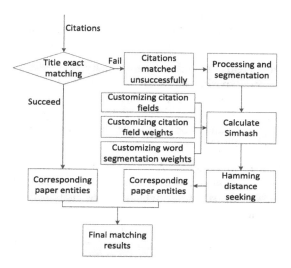

**Fig. 1.** The structure of framework

### 4.1     Title Exact Matching

The citation is a reference giving the source of the cited article and has a variety of forms. Different citations of one cited paper written by different people vary a lot. The title field of the citation is errorless most of the time. Due to the significance of the title field, people always pay more attention to it. In this paper, we use title exact matching to process the citation data first. Then we can get a smaller dataset to do more complex processing. The experiments in Sect. 6 show that the title exact matching provides a high accuracy.

### 4.2     Citation Match Based on Simhash

With regard to the citations which failed to be matched exactly by title, we need to use the textual similarity method to match them. Simhash algorithm transforms the text message into n-bit binary string, which can distinguish text message more effectively [3]. We use simhash to do citation matching in this paper. First, remove the punctuations and specific symbols in the citation and paper records. Then select the proper fields and give them weights. Third, segment the fields and calculate the simhash value of the citation and paper records.

Each field of citation, including citation title, citation author, publisher, year, citation volume (volume, issue), etc., has its own format, and each field embodies different information of the citation. Among them, citation title, citation author and publisher ought to be segmented further, and the basic formula for the simhash of citation is:

$$simhash(C) = simhash(T, A, P, Y, M, V, P_a) \tag{1}$$

The formula is displayed in terms of simhash calculation. There are some improvements in our algorithm on the basis of traditional simhash algorithm. The modified algorithm improves the effectiveness, efficiency, and generality.

**Customizing Citation Fields.** Different from ordinary short text, citations and paper records consist of several specific fields, of which every field is limited to a fixed format. Thus we can select some fields of citation for citation matching. A simple method is giving the weights of every field and determining whether it is selected according to the trend of F1 value. For large-scale citation matching, we can sample the whole dataset for a small amount of data to figure out the optimal setting of weights.

**Customizing Citation Field Weights.** As mentioned above, citation is different from normal short message. Citation consists of many specific fields, each of which has its own role. Therefore, we can set the weight of every citation field according to the characteristics of the dataset.

In this paper, we design a heuristic algorithm (Algorithm 1) for seeking the optimal parameter setting of weights. First, we give the initial weights according to the selected citation fields. If the field is selected, its initial weight is 1 and if not, the weight is 0. Second, we compute the F1 value of experiment results with the set weights. (In this paper, we use F1 value to judge the setting of weights. Precision and recall can be used as the criteria as well.) After that, we increase the weight of every field respectively by a 'step value' and compute the F1 value. If the F1 value is the largest ever, continue to increase the weight until the computed F1 value is not larger than the largest one. After computing all weights of fields successively, repeat the procedure of increasing weights until the largest F1 value is fixed. Finally we can get an optimal setting of weights.

The complexity of heuristic algorithm is relatively high. Therefore we sample it as well to figure out the optimal setting of weights and apply it to large-scale citation data.

**Customizing Word Segmentation Weights.** When calculating simhash value, word segmentation weights are needed. This framework can change word segmentation weights (W) as needed. Therefore we can use different segment weights according to the dataset to improve the performance of the framework. Then we have:

$$
\begin{aligned}
simhash(C) &= simhash(T, A, P, Y, M, V, P_a, W) \\
&= \text{sign} \left( \begin{array}{c} sim(T, W_T) + sim(A, W_A) + sim(P, W_P) + hashCode(Y) \\ + hashCode(M) + hashCode(V) + hashCode(P_a) \end{array} \right) \tag{2}
\end{aligned}
$$

Where:

$$sim(T, W_T) = \sum W_{Ti} \cdot hashCode(T_i) \tag{3}$$

$$sim(A, W_A) = \sum W_{Ai} \cdot hashCode(A_i) \tag{4}$$

$$sim(P, W_P) = \sum W_{Pi} \cdot hashCode(P_i) \tag{5}$$

*hashCode()* can calculate the hash code vector.
*sign()* can replace 0, 1 with −1, 1 respectively in hash code vector.

In this paper, most of the words are characteristics with high level of differentiation after segmentation. So, we set all words with the same weight. The final formula is:

$$
\begin{aligned}
&simhash(C) \\
&= sign\left( \begin{array}{l} \alpha \cdot sim(T, W) + \beta \cdot sim(A, W) + \gamma \cdot sim(P, W) + \delta \cdot hashCode(Y) \\ + \varepsilon \cdot hashCode(M) + \lambda \cdot hashCode(V) + \mu \cdot hashCode(P_a) \end{array} \right) Vector^T
\end{aligned}
\tag{6}
$$

Where α, β, γ, δ, ε, λ, μ are the weight of each part of the citation.

### 4.3 Distance-Based Similarity Metrics

Rather than learning-based techniques, we use Hamming Distance similarity metrics. In our framework, we define a threshold k for the simhash similarity metrics. When the Hamming Distance between two simhash strings is less than or equal to k, the two simhash strings match, otherwise they don't. What we should do is to ascertain an appropriate value of the threshold. In Sect. 6, we experimentally validate that the framework can get the best performance with hamming distance k = 7.

| Alg 1: | Heuristic algorithm for citation field weights |
|---|---|
| **Input:** | $W$: Initial weights according to the selected of citation fields |
| **Output:** | $W$: Weights after optimizing |
| 1 | Inaitially, $W'$ are all -1, $F1_{max}$ is 0 |
| 2 | $F1_{current} \leftarrow F1\_Fun(W)$ |
| 3 | **while** $W' != W$ |
| 4 | **foreach** $W_i \in W$ |
| 5 | **while** $F1_{current} > F1_{max}$ |
| 6 | $F1_{max} \leftarrow F1_{current}$ |
| 7 | $W' = W$ |
| 8 | $W_i = W_i + step$ |
| 9 | $F1_{current} \leftarrow F1\_Fun(W)$ |
| 10 | $W_i = W_i - step$ |
| 11 | **return** $W$ |

| Alg 2: Citation Matching in MapReduce | |
|---|---|
| **Input:** | CitationData and Cited Data |
| **Output:** | CitationData with matched cited paper label |
| 1 | **Function Map()** |
| 2 | A = simHash(Citation Record) |
| 3 | **for** i ∈ {1, ..., (d' + 1)} |
| 4 | $(A_i, B_i)$ = Trans(A, i) |
| 5 | //The Second Dividing |
| 6 | **for** j ∈ {1, ..., (d' + 1)} |
| 7 | $(B_{ij}, C_{ij})$ = Trans1($B_i$, i) |
| 8 | emit($A_i + B_{ij}, C_{ij}$) |
| 9 | |
| 10 | **Function Reduce(k, $values[n]$)** |
| 11 | **for** v ∈ values[n] |
| 12 | make Citation List and Paper List |
| 13 | **for** c ∈ Citation List |
| 14 | **if** c matched records in Paper List |
| 15 | **emit**(c, matched records) |

## 5    Citation Matching in MapReduce

There is a huge collection of papers in a digital library. With respect to it, parallel computation is a valid solution for matching massive citations effectively. In general, the matching ($m$ to $n$) needs to match every target with every existing record, so the algorithmic complexity is O($m * n$). It is definitely time consuming to do the similarity matching of mass data with this algorithmic complexity.

In this paper, we get the simhash value by extracting valid citation fields, segmenting the fields and customizing word segmentation weights. It is the Hamming Distance of the simhash value that determines whether the citation is matched successfully. In order to reduce the searching space of similarity matching and accomplish the simhash similarity matching of mass data, we divide the $n$-bit fingerprint into fields on the basis of Pigeonhole Principle and a certain Hamming Distance.

Supposing that there are $n$ records in a dataset, the number of bits of simhash value is $d$ and the Hamming Distance is $d'$. If a $d$-bit simhash value is divided equally into $(d' + 1)$ parts, according to Pigeonhole Principle, for the matched record, the different bit of the simhash value of which the Hamming Distance is no more than $d'$ is in at most $d'$ parts. Namely, at least one part is identical to the counterpart of the other record. With this dividing method, the number of index bits is $d/(d' + 1)$ and one record increases to $2^{d'}$ records. But, the searching space is likely to be reduced to $1/(2^{d/(d'+1)-d'})$ of the former one under ideal conditions by index bits.

This dividing method converts the original simhash value into key-value pairs, adjusting the structure to parallel computing framework MapReduce. In this paper we implemented simhash citation matching in a parallel way based on MapReduce.

We select 64 as the length of simhash bits. As for the Hamming Distance $d'$, we select a reasonable number 7 through Experiment 1 in Sect. 6.

First step, divide the 64-bit simhash code $A$ into 8 parts $(A_1, A_2, \ldots, A_8)$ of which every part consists of 8 bits. 8 new simhash codes with 64 bits (represented as $\{(A_i, B_i)|0 \leq i \leq 8\}$) are formed with the method of a transposition function $Trans(A, i)$, moving the $i^{th}$ part to the head of the code. According to the demonstration above, we can just find the Hamming Distance of $B_i$ regarding $A_i$ as an index to find records whose Hamming Distance is no more than 7. Accordingly, the key-value pairs are created in the form of $(A_i, B_i)$ as Fig. 2.

Selecting 7 as the Hamming Distance, dividing the simhash code only once is not able to reduce the searching space sufficiently. Thus in the second step, we do the same thing to the rest 56 bits $B_i(0 \leq i \leq 8)$. As shown in Fig. 2, the key-value pairs are created in the form of $\left(B_{ij}, C_{ij}\right)$.

As a result, the 64-bit simhash code generates $8 * 8 = 64$ new simhash codes after the second dividing. As Fig. 3 shown, it can be represented as $\{(A_i, B_{ij}, C_{ij})|0 \leq i \leq 8, 0 \leq j \leq 8\}$. With $A_i$ and $B_{ij}$ regarded as the matching index, the number of index bits is $8 + 7 = 15$ and each simhash code increases to 64 codes. The Hamming Distance needs to be searched only in 49-bit $C_{ij}$. With 15-bit index, it reduces the searching space to $1/(2^{15}/64) = 1/512$ of the former one on ideal conditions and compressing the complexity. As a consequence, the computing time can decrease from millions to tens of

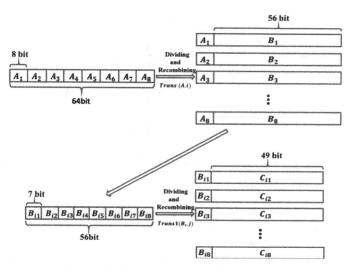

**Fig. 2.** Divide and recombine Simhash record

thousands. In the last step, we find the Hamming Distance of each record pair successively in the Reduce procedure. The MapReduce algorithm is explicated in Algorithm 2. Though we reduced the searching space of citations, the load in the reduce phase is still heavy because it is responsible for the matching task. Adding the number of reducers properly improves efficiency evidently. In additional, another MapReduce Job is needed for duplicates removing. This job is simple so we omit the introduction of it.

**Fig. 3.** The form of new Simhash record

## 6 Experimental Evaluation

Our framework is fully implemented in Java 1.7. Experiment 1 and 2 were performed on a PC with Intel Pentium(R) Dual-Core E6700 3.2 GHz, running Windows 7. Experiment 3 was ran on our local cluster with 5 nodes, and each of them consists of a E5-2620 6(12) @ 2.3GHZ CPU running Centos 6.0 with 64 GB memory and 2X 500 GB SATA disks. Our experiment is based on Hadoop 2.2.0.

### 6.1 Data Sets

Our experiment datasets consist of two parts, one of which is Chinese medicine citations recorded by a Chinese Medicine Digital Library, and the other is Cora corpus (McCallum's citation matching test set).

The size and description of datasets are as follows (Table 1).

**Table 1.** The size and description of data set

| Dataset No | Size of Dataset | The Description of Dataset |
|---|---|---|
| **Dataset1** | 15000 | Citations selected randomly |
|  | 9,914 | Cited paper data records |
| **Dataset2** | 4,097 | Citations with wrong title |
|  | 9,914 | Cited paper data records |
| **Dataset3** | 1879 | **Cora corpus** (McCallum's citation matching test set) |
| **Dataset4** | 7,555,857 | All Citations |
|  | 5,942,858 | All Cited paper data records |

Experiment 1 is for verifying the validity of every part of the framework using dataset1 and 2. Experiment 2 is the comparative experiment, in which we use dataset3, a citation matching benchmark test set. In experiment 3 we use dataset4 which consists of millions of citations and paper records so as to verify the validity, and efficiency of the framework. Besides, dataset1 and 2 are subsets of dataset4.

### 6.2    Experiment 1 Framework Experiment

**Title Matching Experiment.** We use dataset1 to do title exact matching experiment. The accuracy is 98.63 % and the recall is 72.69 %. Because of the high accuracy, we can use title exact matching as first processing.

The reason why only 72.69 % of the citation is matched when the title is the only element in exact matching is probably on account of the spelling mistakes in titles, the inconsistency between the citation title field and the paper title field, etc. Therefore, our framework exactly matches the titles for the given citation data for the first step.

**Hamming Distance Experiment.** In this experiment, we use dataset2 to find the optimal Hamming Distance. Dataset2, it was sampled from dataset1 for 4097 citations with wrong spelling which means we cannot use title field for exact matching. We set the weights of citation fields equally, and then calculate the simhash value of the segmented citations. Finally we match the citations to the paper records by choosing different Hamming Distance. The results are show in Fig. 4.

According to the results, this framework achieves best performance with the recall of 68 % and the accuracy of 96 % when selected Hamming Distance is 7.

In [8], it shows that Charikar's simhash [3] is practically useful for identifying near-duplicates in web documents and experimentally validate that for a repository of 8B webpages, 64-bit simhash fingerprints and k = 3 are reasonable. However, citation records are much shorter than webpages and a few noise words may cause the increment of Hamming Distance between two similar records. That's why the empirical value of 3 is not suitable for short text similarity. As what can be seen from Fig. 5, through authentic experiments, setting the Hamming Distance as a relative larger value still leads to a satisfactory result. That is, with appropriate Hamming Distance, Charikar's simhash [3] is also available for short text similarity.

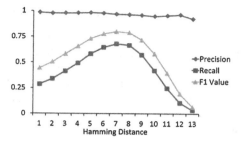

**Fig. 4.** Result of different Hamming Distance

**Citation Block Weight Experiment.** The matching rate and the precision of results can be improved by selecting the optimal field vector and the field weights in the framework. In this experiment, we use dataset1 consisting of 7 fields that are title, authors, publisher, published year, month, volume and page. The Hamming Distance of the simhash is selected as 7. Then we pick one field and set its weight as from 0 to 6 with the rest fields weights fixed as 1. The experiment results are as Fig. 5.

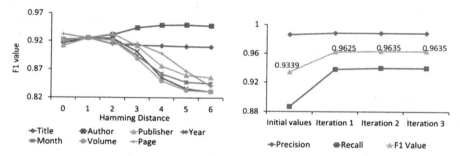

**Fig. 5.** F1 Values with citation fields weighted differently

**Fig. 6.** Iteration results of heuristic algorithm

From the Fig. 5, we can learn that the weight of author field is heavy, implying that the author field is accurate relatively and the names of Chinese authors have a high degree of distinction for different citations. The title field which is used for citation matching in general does not occupy a heavy weight and it is probably because the words of the title are usually more than that of the other fields so that simhash is biased to the title field naturally. Thus, increasing the weight of the title field doesn't affect the performance significantly. For the page field, the weight gets its local optimization when it is 0, which means we may abandon this field.

When applying the heuristic algorithm, we initially set the weights as {1, 1, 1, 1, 1, 1, 0} for {title, authors, publisher, year, month, volume, page}, the results of iterative computation is shown in Fig. 6. With the final acquired weights{1, 5, 2, 3, 1, 1, 0}, we got the precision of 0.9884, the recall of 0.9397 and the F1 value of 0.963467, which is a much better result than any local optimization of fields.

### 6.3    Experiment 2: Comparative Experiment of Public Dataset

The Cora corpus (McCallum's citation matching test set) has been frequently used in citation matching researches. The Cora corpus includes 1879 citation recodes related to artificial intelligence. We use it as dataset3 to do the experiment and compare the results with those of other methods. Through the analysis of the dataset, publisher field is made up of book title field, journal field and publisher field. If the year field is missing, it is likely to be drawn from date field.

With Hamming Distance set as 7, we select author field, title field, publisher field, year field and page field, and determine their weights through the heuristic algorithm. The weight of title field is set as 6 while the weights of other fields are all set as 1 (Table 2).

**Table 2.** Results of comparative experiment

| Precision | Recall | F1 value |
|-----------|--------|----------|
| 0.9662    | 0.8646 | 0.9128   |

In this experiment, we got the F1 value of 0.9128. Compared with the methods in other literatures, such as correlation clustering method [14] which is less than 0.8, [6] which is 0.8926, efficient clustering method [13] which is 0.839, our framework has a better performance, proved to be valid. The experiments using datasets with different languages verify the generality of the framework as well.

### 6.4    Experiment on MapReduce

There is a huge collection of papers in a digital library. Parallel computation is a valid solution for matching the massive citations effectively. For this experiment, we use dataset 4 which has over 7 million citations and almost 6 million cited paper data records. The parameters are the same as those in Experiment 1. With exact matching for title, 6,269,810 citations are matched, in which 5,850,579 citations are correct. For the rest 1,286,047 citations, we use MapReduce to match simhash records.

As the Hamming Distance set as 7, we match 1,068,195 citations and 926,362 are correct. For the whole dataset, 7,338,005 citations are matched and 6,776,941 are correct. The precision is 92.35 %. The recall is 89.69 %. The F1 value is 0.91.

In order to achieve the performance of algorithm, we randomly divide the citation data into 4 parts, whose number of citations ranges from 1 million to 7 million and we set the number of reducer as 1, 3, 5. The experiment results are shown in Fig. 7.

From the performance experiment results, we can see that when the number of reducers is 1, the time consumed is longer than that under any other setting. In our framework, reducers are responsible for the matching between citations and cited paper after the process of indexing. Although the searching space ought to be reduced to 1/512 of the former one under ideal conditions, the searching space is reduced to nearly 1/100 in practice, still having a heavy demand on reducers. However, as can be seen from the results, when the number of reducers increases to 3, time consumed can be

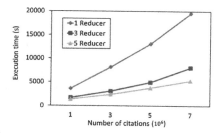

**Fig. 7.** Performance experiment in MapReduce

reduced to a large degree. In addition, as the data volume increases, time increases relatively gently. When the number of reducers is 5, the trend is gentler. As a result, adding the number of reducers properly to improve running efficiency is applicable in this framework. Furthermore, it can be seen that the running time increases linearly with the increase of citations. This is to say, our framework is able to be applied to dispose a larger scale of dataset. In these MapReduce experiments, the datasets are extracted from a real-dataset in a digital library and there are some noisy records, even though, we can still get high recall, precision and F1 values, showing that the framework is efficient and effective.

## 7 Conclusion and Future Work

This paper presents a generalized citation matching framework based on simhash. Through customizing citation fields, citation field weights, segmentation weights and heuristic algorithm, the generality and effectiveness of proposed framework is obviously improved.

In order to obtain high efficiency, we make a lot of improvements. Firstly, so as to reduce the searching space of similarity matching and accomplish the simhash similarity matching of mass data, we divide the 64-bit simhash strings into parts on the basis of Pigeonhole Principle and a certain Hamming Distance. Secondly, we implement our framework in MapReduce to adapt to large-scale data computing.

In the future, we will focus on enhancing the generality of our framework and using it in a wider range of applications such as duplicate record detection, spam messages identification, author names disambiguation and so on. In terms of parallelization, optimizing our framework in MapReduce or implementing it in a more effective parallel computation platform like Spark are considered to improve the efficiency.

**Acknowledgments.** This work is supported in part by the National Key Basic Research and Department (973) Program of China (No. 2013CB329606), and the Co-construction Project of Beijing Municipal Commission of Education.

# References

1. Councill, I.G., Li, H., Zhuang, Z., et al.: Learning metadata from the evidence in an on-line citation matching scheme. In: JCDL, pp. 276–285 (2006)
2. Pasula, H., Marthi, B., Milch, B., et al.: Identity uncertainty and citation matching. In: Advances in Neural Information Processing Systems, pp. 1425–1432 (2003)
3. Charikar, M.S.: Similarity estimation techniques from rounding algorithms. In: STOC, pp. 380–388 (2002)
4. Hitchcock, S., et al.: Citation linking: improving access to online journals. In: Proceedings of the Second ACM International Conference on Digital Libraries, pp. 115–122 (1997)
5. Liao, Z., Zhang, Z.: A generalized joint inference approach for citation matching. In: Wobcke, W., Zhang, M. (eds.) AI 2008. LNCS (LNAI), vol. 5360, pp. 601–607. Springer, Heidelberg (2008)
6. Koo, H.K., Kim, T., Chun, H.W., et al.: Effects of unpopular citation fields in citation matching performance. In: ICISA, pp. 1–7 (2011)
7. Kan, M.Y., Tan, Y.F.: Record matching in digital library metadata. Commun. ACM **51**(2), 91–94 (2008)
8. Manku, G.S., Jain, A., Das Sarma, A.: Detecting near-duplicates for web crawling. In: WWW, pp. 141–150 (2007)
9. Fedoryszak, M., Tkaczyk, D., Bolikowski, Ł.: Large scale citation matching using Apache Hadoop. In: Aalberg, T., Papatheodorou, C., Dobreva, M., Tsakonas, G., Farrugia, C. J. (eds.) TPDL 2013. LNCS, vol. 8092, pp. 362–365. Springer, Heidelberg (2013)
10. Liu, Y., Wu, Q., Han, Y., et al.: The fingerprint analysis technique-oriented research on microblog for public opinion analysis. In: ICIMCS, pp. 372–375 (2013)
11. Pham, T.A.N, Nguyen, V.K.: A simhash-based scheme for locating product information from the web. In: SoICT, pp. 199–206 (2011)
12. Bilenko, M., Mooney, R.J.: Adaptive duplicate detection using learnable string similarity measures. In: KDD, pp. 39–48 (2003)
13. McCallun, A., Nigam, K., Ungar, L.: Efficient clustering of high-dimensional data sets with application to reference clustering. In: KDD, pp. 169–179 (2000)
14. Chierichetti, F., Dalvi, N., Kumar, R.: Correlation clustering in MapReduce. In: KDD, pp. 641–650 (2014)

# A Cloud Based Type-2 Diabetes Mellitus Lifestyle Self-Management System

Shih-Hao Chang[✉] and Chih-Ning Li

Department of Computer Science and Information Engineering, Tamkang University,
New Taipei, Taiwan
shhchang@mail.tku.edu.tw, 401410591@s01.tku.edu.tw

**Abstract.** In this paper, we designed a patient-centric cloud based diabetes lifestyle management system. It is composed of three layers namely sensing, communication and user interface. The goal of this cloud based diabetes lifestyle management system is to provide Type-2 diabetes mellitus patients useful information to remind user's blood sugar level. The function of the sensor networks in this framework is to collect the data from human body and human activity as well as environmental information that may have effects on the healthy statement of the diabetes patients. The communication and central server part will handle the data exchange and data analysis that help to generate a final decision data and sent to user interface to remind the user of valuable information. Different from traditional e-health system, due to the diabetes patients are prone to effect by weather and environment varying. Therefore, the presented approach provide a rule algorithm which enables the rescue decision in the cloud server and transmit through the communication level, and finally provide a integrated user interface for diabetes users. An early warning user interface for diabetes patents has been designed and presented in this paper.

**Keywords:** Type-2 diabetes mellitus · u-Health · Cloud computing · Wireless sensor networks (WSNs) · Machine-to-Machine (M2M)

## 1 Introduction

Type 2 diabetes mellitus (T2DM) is a metabolic disorder that results in hyperglycemia (high blood glucose levels) due to the body being ineffective at using the insulin or unable to produce enough insulin. T2DM was formerly known as non-insulin-dependent or adult-onset diabetes due to its occurrence mainly in people over 40. However, in recent years, T2DM is now becoming more common in young adults, teens and children and accounts for approximately 90 % of all affected patients worldwide. According to the International Diabetes Federation (IDF) figure [1], more than 387 million people across the globe have diabetes and this figure is predicted to rise to over 550 million by 2030. T2DM is a serious medical condition that often requires the use of anti-diabetic medication, or insulin to keep blood sugar levels under control.

A diagnosis of T2DM is made if a fasting plasma glucose concentration is >7.0 mmol/L (>126 mg/dl) or plasma glucose 2 h after a standard glucose challenge is

© Springer International Publishing Switzerland 2015
X.-L. Li et al. (Eds.): PAKDD 2015, LNCS 9441, pp. 91–103, 2015.
DOI: 10.1007/978-3-319-25660-3_8

>11.1 mmol/L (>200 mg/dl). The development of T2DM and its side effects, such as heart, kidney eye diseases, can be prevented if detected and treated at an early stage. Many factors affect how well T2DM is controlled and most of these factors are controlled by the person with diabetes, including how much and what is eaten, how frequently the blood sugar is monitored, physical activity levels, and accuracy and consistency of medication dosing [2–4].

Nevertheless, to effectively prevent or manage T2DM, it is important to understand how to balance dietary, physical activity, and medication. The lifestyle improvement is one of the most important issues in the prevention and management of T2DM. An efficient T2DM lifestyle management system can sustain positive effects on weight and cardiovascular risk factors [5]. To achieve well protect and control T2DM, the continuous recognition of dietary activities from patients, balance dietary, physical activity, and medication every day have immediate and long-term effects to the patient to prevent with type-2 diabetes. However, lifestyle management for patients to prevent and control T2DM is difficult in routine primary care and traditional face-to-face specialty care solutions are not feasible for immediate and long-term implementation.

Recently research found that T2DM and climate change are directly and indirectly interconnected [6]. For example, climatic extremes such as drought, disasters and long periods of extreme heat increase people's exposure to diabetes risk factors. Therefore, supporting a better quality diabetes lifestyle self-management system (DLSMS) may need to conduct using a range of Machine-to-Machine (M2M) communication technologies. Due to self-management strategies to be sustainable in the long term, patients require a sense of having a stake in their management that is appropriate for their beliefs and perceptions, timely information and support, and an overall sense of empowerment in managing their diabetes in relation to other aspects of their life. Thanks to the Micro-Electro-Mechanical-Systems (MEMS) technology, its combined low power integrated circuits and wireless communication and made this new generation of body sensor networks (BSNs) possible. The wearable body sensor device could allow inexpensive and continuous healthcare monitoring health condition of the diabetes patient, and

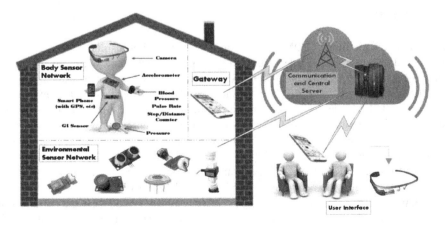

**Fig. 1.** Diabetes lifestyle management system diagram

human activities with real-time updates of body signs via Internet. Moreover, the environment sensor will be deployed to collect surrounding environment conditions, for instance, climate sensors, humidity sensors and air-condition sensors.

As shown in Fig. 1, with integrate these body and environment sensors nodes with Machine-to-Machine (M2M) [7] technology, our DLSMS system can provide patient-centric e-health system and delivering actionable information with minimal human intervention. The e-health is the use of information and communication technologies (ICT) to enable health improvement and healthcare service. Remainder of this paper is organized as follows: a brief review of background and related works is presented in Sect. 2. Rule based diabetes lifestyle management system architecture is described in Sect. 3. Our design outline will be present in Sect. 4 and finally conclusions and future work are explored in Sect. 5.

## 2   Related Work

In this section, we provide an overview of a selection of related mechanism and algorithm that have been developed to e-health system related to diabetes management. To the best of our knowledge so far, only limited papers have tried to address T2DM issue in e-health application. Van Puffelen et al. [8] have developed the 'Living with diabetes' course: a group-based self-management support program specifically tailored to T2DM patients and their partners in the first years of living with diabetes. They aim to support both patients and partners in successfully integrating diabetes (care) into their daily lives and, hereby, enhancing self-management and diabetes-specific health-related quality of life in T2DM patients. Given the importance to intervene at an early stage in T2DM and the promising results of previous studies based on the Common-Sense Model, psychological and social aspects, including perceptions and attitudes, empowerment and social support, are integrated in the course because of their known important role in behavior change.

Sumi [9] proposed a new concept "SODA", representing service oriented device architecture. It provides us an attractive and detailed scenario of the application of the architecture to display the fancy outcome of the proposed idea. It expounds the device integration in "SODA" with DDL (device description language) and propagates a clear and comprehensive framework of personal tele-health management system. While it ignores the inspection of the environmental factor which may has decisive effects on the data collected by the M2M communication system and the detailed solution for certain kind of healthy topic, for instance diabetes, has not been mentioned.

Lupu [10] proposed a framework for automatic management of body-area sensor networks. It utilizes the concept of self-managed cell, which consists of event bus, discovery service, role service, and policy service. The event-bus design, however, risks at detecting unnecessary events lead to more power consumption and they do not clarify who should be responsible for producing the policies. Sebestyen [11] proposed a web service-based data transfer solution for remote patient monitoring. It adopts a gateway (e.g. a PDA or smart phone) to bridge the body area network and the central server. Communications are web service based, ensuring modularity and interoperability.

This work, however, is designed for passive monitoring of health conditions, rather than actively providing context aware advices to patients.

Forjuoh [12] carried out an experiment with PDA (personal digital assistant) to assist diabetes patients on self-care. Their study observed a significant glycosylated hemoglobin (HbA1c) decrease among patients who reported using their PDA more often, suggesting a positive role that PDA like information technology tools play in glycemic control. Jensen [13], they proposed a DiasNet Mobile, which is a personalized advisory service targeting at type-1 diabetics. It is implemented using a Bluetooth enabled blood glucose meter and a mobile phone. This service could estimate patients' blood glucose level based on three factors: insulin, carbohydrate intake and BMI (Body Mass Index) measurements. Based on the estimated blood pressure, glucose, BMI and waist circumference advices are shown in Table 1. Table 1 display of each evaluative result which is in accordance to the range of measurement values for blood pressure, blood glucose, BMI, and waise circumference.

**Table 1.** Classifications of blood pressure, diabetes and obesity

| Risk factors | | Normal | Pre stage | Stage 1 | Stage 2 | Stage 3 |
|---|---|---|---|---|---|---|
| Blood pressure | SBP | <120 | 120–139 | 140–159 | ≥160 | |
| | DBP | <80 | 80–89 | 90–99 | ≥100 | |
| Glucose | FPG | <100 | 100–125 | ≥126 | | |
| | 2h-PG | <140 | 140–199 | ≥200 | | |
| BMI | | 18.5–24.9 | 25.0–29.9 | 30.0–34.9 | 35.0–39.9 | ≥40 |
| Wait circumference | | ≤40, ≤35 | >40, >35 | | | |

**FPG** Fasting Plasma Glucose, **2h-PG** 2 h Plasma Glucose, **BMI** Body Mass Index

Unlike existing systems, we propose a cloud-based e-healthcare service model that can enable environment sensor nodes and wearable m-health devices to recognize the relationship between mutual diseases and risk factors and apply the autonomous assistant model to helping T2DM patients take care of themselves in their living environment. Our framework tries to achieve the following two goals:

- Make the system autonomous by reducing user input as much as possible.
- Be context aware by bring in additional information of human activity and surrounding environment.

In addition, our framework not only offers a monitoring platform but also actively provides feedbacks to patients on the context base.

# 3 Diabetes Lifestyle Self-Management System Model

In this section, we introduce the design architecture of the proposed DLSMS. The DLSMS would be merged into patients' daily lives, collecting, analyzing, body sensors information. At the same time, we also collect surrounding environment information such as climate sensors, air condition sensors to care a patient health from various aspects in his/her daily life then deliver this sensing information with M2M communication to the back end for further data analyze. Hence, there are three information entrances in our DLSMS: user input, body sensor input and environment sensor input. Body sensor input includes body sugar test result, the GSP information, video sensors input, etc., while environment sensor input includes temperature, humidity and so on. Users can communicate with the smart phone to record the intake food and physical exercise through voice controlling, photograph or even word typing.

## 3.1 Rule Structure

There are three information entrances in the DLSMS: body sensor input, environment sensor input and user input. For example, body sensor input includes body sugar test result, such as the Glycosylated Serum Protein (GSP) information, while environment sensor input includes temperature, humidity and so on. Users can record the eating food and physical exercise through voice controlling as his/her personal input data. Most of all, our system adopts the event-driven paradigm. Major activities are triggered by certain events. In the context of diabetes management, these events include, but not limited to, high blood glucose, low blood glucose, severe exercise, and purchasing high sugar food. When one of the aforementioned events occurs, certain corresponding conditions are checked. If the conditions are satisfied, one or more actions may be taken. Otherwise, no actions will be taken. We bind the three elements: triggering event, conditions and actions together to form a set of rules. Functions of our system are based on the rule evaluations. Figure 2 illustrates the rule composition of our system.

| Device Identity | Event Message | Case List | Validation Period |
|---|---|---|---|

**Fig. 2.** Rule composition format

Figure 2 shows the rule composition. To ensure flexible and platform-independent evaluation of rules, all rule elements are described using XML language. An interpreter should be used for rule evaluation.

- Device Identity: Each device identity is represented as a sensing function which enables connection to the machine-to-machine (M2M) network. In terms of the blood pressure glucose (M2MBG), only the measured blood glucose is not displayed. Instead, the data on obesity measured by the weight scale (M2MOB) are requested to acquire the result.
- Event Message: Each rule has one and only one predefined event. For instance, the sample rule will be evaluated when the blood glucose is >7.0 mmol/L. The event

element would be feed into an event detect, which will trigger the rule evaluation when the specified event occurs.

- Case list: The case list consists of at least one case. Cases are indeed conditions and actions pairs. Each case consists of a nonnegative number of conditions. All conditions are jointed by the "AND" operator, implying that all conditions have to be satisfied in order for the corresponding actions to be performed. There has to be at least one actions associated with each case. Furthermore, we can specify whether the actions are executed sequentially or concurrently with the <sequential> or <concurrent> tag. Note that all cases have to be evaluated. Furthermore, it is the responsibility of the entity, which generates the rule, to ensure that different cases do not contradict with each other.
- Validation period: This element specifies a time period, during which the rule is considered valid. For instance, the sample rule will be valid forever since its creation. The <repeat> element defines which the rule should be evaluated repeatedly or not. If its value is equal to false, the rule will only be evaluated once. Figure 3 sketches a sample rule, which will be used to illustrate the detailed rule definition. Each rule is composed of the following three elements:

### 3.2  Event Driven Model

Event-driven model is appropriate for many intelligent applications, especially in M2M network since it has to take measurement by different sensor devices while collecting data by the use of network. Therefore, as it is displayed in Fig. 4, the application is constructed as 5 major events and their event handlers for processing. The first event is a boot event; this boot event will occur when the power is turned on and it initializes the M2M device and broadcasts the "join message". In the measurement event which occurs when measurement button is pressed to measure the medical data, Data.Req message is sent and measurement function is activated.

Data Acquisition event occurs when the measurement becomes terminated and the measurement data is acquired from the sensor. Furthermore, Receive event also occurs when Data_Ack or Data_Nak sent from other device becomes received. Accordingly, Receive event must make progressing according to the types of received message. Join and Leave messages cause for M2M Member list available from the network to become added or deleted. Additionally, if the type of the received message is Data_Req, it is the request to send risk factors (measurement value or assessment result) of the patient designated in the Payload. Therefore, risk factor table is searched and Data.Ack (or Data.Nak) message is composed and sent. Moreover, this algorithm was structured so that it does not suggest measurement value immediately upon the occurrence of Data-Acquisition event and pass through assessment process after fixed timeout. In order to receive all the messages from other IOT devices in the network, time delay is needed.

### 3.3  System Architecture

As the diagram shows in Fig. 5, the entire system consists of two parts: the server and the mobile application. Communications between the mobile app and the server is facilitated by web service. In the rest of this section, we are going to introduce each

```
<rule name="highBloodGlucose" version="1.0">
   <event>
      <bloodGlucose comparator="gt">
         7.0 mmol/L
      </bloodGlucose>
   </event>
   <cases>
      <case>
         <conditions>
           <sinceLastMeal comparator="gt">
              2 hours
           </sinceLastMeal>
           <whether>
              sunny
           </whether>
         </conditions>
         <actions>
           <sequential>
              <voiceReminder>
                 blood glucose is too high,
                 consider doing some exercise
                 to lower the blood glucose.
              </voiceReminder>
              <timerTask>
                 <alarm>2 hours</alarm>
                 <work>
                 <voiceReminder>
                    Test the blood glucose again
                 </voiceReminder>
                 </work>
              </timerTask>
           </sequential>
         </actions>
      </case>
   <cases>
   <validation>
      <repeat>true</repeat>
      <from>creationTime</from>
      <to>infinite</to>
   </validation>
</rule>
```

**Fig. 3.** Sample rule diagram

system components and their corresponding functionality. The server provides four services for the mobile app:

- History update service: the mobile app could use this service to commit historical sensor readings to the history database (DB), which locates on the server. Instead, on the mobile phone, we only cache short-term sensor readings. The historical sensor readings can be utilized to generate, say weekly health report. Furthermore, we can apply machine learning or data mining techniques on the historical data for rule generation. Rule generation based on historical data could provide personalization features [13].
- Report generates service: this service is used to generate personal health report, this healthy report can be weekly or monthly basis.
- Condition check service: during rule evaluation, the mobile application may call this service to validate some condition clauses. The reason why we need this service is

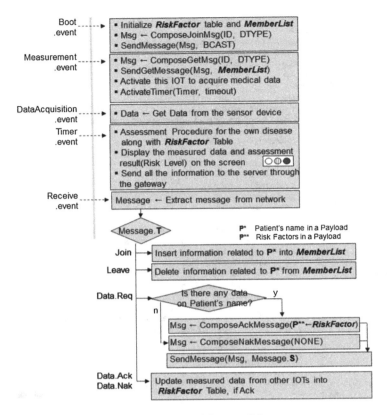

**Fig. 4.** Event driven model

because some conditions clauses may need to be validated based on data which is not available on the mobile phone, e.g., some historical sensor data and whether information. If the conditions can be checked with local data, which is available at the mobile phone, this service would not be used.

- Rule update service: the mobile application uses this service to retrieve new rules or update old rules.

Apart from the four services provided by the server, it is worth mentioning the rule generator, which automatically generates a set of rules based on historical sensor data, and information stored at the hospital customer relationship management (CRM) system. For instance, the rule generator discover a treatment in the CRM system, it should generate rules to reminder the patient to take the treatment on time. Automatic rule generation, however, is not the only way of rule update. We also allow manual rule update. Doctors or researchers may manually code their experience or research results into rules and dispatch the rules to patient. On the mobile phone side, it consists of the following components to carry out rule evaluations:

- Local rule DB: it stores a set of rules to be evaluated.

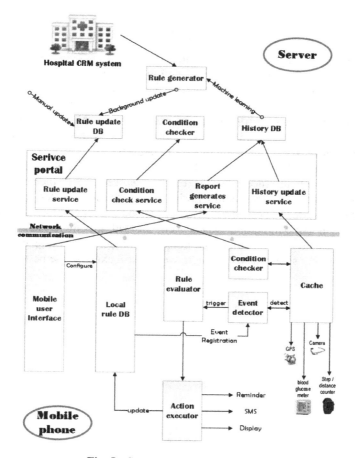

**Fig. 5.** System architecture diagram

- Mobile user interface: users could use this interface to configure the rule DB, e.g., disable some rules or change the notification methods. Furthermore, users can also retrieve and view the health report through the interface.
- Event detector: when a rule is added into the local rule DB, it should register its event to the event detector, signaling which event it is interested in. Accordingly, when the rule is disabled or removed, appropriate deregistration should be carried out. The event detector is responsible to monitor the sensor readings and detect those registered events. Note that only registered events will be detected, but not others
- Rule evaluator: when the event detector detects an event, the rules that register the event will be triggered for evaluation, which is coordinated by the rule evaluator.
- Condition checker: this component is used to check each condition clause. In case, the local data is not enough to validate the condition, it should contact the condition check service at the server to evaluation the condition.
- Action executor: it the conditions clause is valid, the corresponding actions should be executed, which is carried out by the action executor. Apart from noticing users

through either multimedia message, or phone display, the action executor may also adaptively update the local rule DB by adding new rules or modify rule parameters.

With the aforementioned system architecture, actions are trigger by contextual events, reducing the amount of human intervention. More importantly, it shifts the advisory system from the pull-based paradigm to the push-based paradigm. The right advices can be delivered to users based on the current context without user awareness. The extensive adoptions of sensors free users from manual input, which is quite inconvenient for handhold devices such as smart phones. Furthermore, with sensor, we can acquire data at a much faster speed, allowing more accurate advices.

The system capability is limited by the sensor capability. For instance, the system can only get intermittent glucose sensor readings, as the most of the current glucose meters cannot achieve continuous monitoring. With the modular design, our system, however, allows gradually upgrading of sensor and incorporation of new sensors. Note that our system is not a mission critical system. Instead, it is more likely an assistant system, which provides users with suggestions or reminders. Therefore, even if in case some sensors are not sophisticated enough, we can still exercise the best effort to help users.

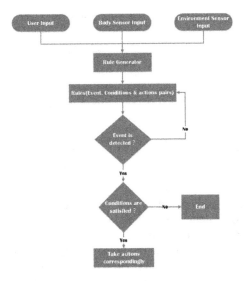

**Fig. 6.** Logical diagram of system architecture

We use a real life scenario to illustrate how our system architecture works. Suppose we have a rule as shown in Fig. 6, which is generated based on good medical practices and updated manually to the rule update DB located on the server. The mobile client periodically poll new rules from the server using the rule update service. When this new rule is synchronized to the local rule DB located on the mobile client. The local rule DB will register the event specified by this rule to the event detector. In this particular case, the event that this rule is interested in is high blood glucose (>7.0 mmol/L).

Next the event detector will detect the registered event. It periodically poll sensor readings, based on which events are detected. The sensor that triggers this particular event is the blood glucose meter. Unlike normal sensor, which can monitor patient's condition continuously, most existing blood glucose meters require patients to prick the skin manually. We could overcome this shortcoming by continuously simulate the blood glucose level based on the discrete glucose meter reading input. When the blood glucose exceeds 7.0 mmol/L, the rule evaluation is triggered.

The rule evaluator component is responsible for coordinating the rule evaluation. It enumerates each case element of the rule, and uses the condition checker to check the corresponding conditions. For instance, in the first case of the example rule, we have three conditions to check. If all three conditions are satisfied, say the last blood glucose value is less than or equal to 7.0 mmol/L (otherwise, the actions will be constantly fired whenever the glucose level is larger than 7.0 mmol/L), it is 2 h after the last meal, and today is sunny, the corresponding actions specified by the case element will be executed by the actions executor.

The action executor executes the actions in the designated order. In this case, it would reminder the patient that his/her blood glucose level is too high, and suggest him/her doing some exercise to lower down the glucose level. Meanwhile, the action executor will schedule a timer task, which reminder the patient to re-test his/her blood glucose in 2 h.

With the above scenario, we could see clearly how different system component interact with each other. The whole process is largely automated and event triggered. In the above example, the only two steps that involves user input is the rule generation based on good medical practice and the blood glucose measurement by pricking the skin. The rule generation, however, is once and for all. The manual blood glucose measurement can be improved with non-intrusive glucose measurement equipment when they get into the market. Furthermore, new features in our system are added into the name or rules, which do not require system upgrade and reboot, making it very easy to use for non-technical users.

# 4 Evaluation

This system can be divided into two parts namely sensing and communication. In sensing part, body sensors will attached around the human body to collect the information on the healthy statement of the user and environmental sensors aiming at those surrounding factors which will affect the patient's healthily condition. In the communication part, these body sensors will communicate to each other by utilizing ZigBee or Wi-Fi standards to transmit or relay the sensing result to the gateway. A gateway can be mobile devices such as smart phone to coordinate the operation of the body sensor network and collect environment information as well as communicate with the central server via 3G communication system. Once the central server received the information from DLSMS, the central server is in charge of data analysis and decision making support. Ultimately, these analyzed data will be sending back to user interface to remind the user of useful information.

## 5   Conclusion and Future Works

In this paper, the proposed concept of diabetes lifestyle management system is a patient-centric e-health care system. Its aim at provides a friendly user interface to provide useful information and alert user while they need. This system can be divided into two parts namely sensing and communication. In sensing part, body sensors will attach around the human body to collect the information on the healthy statement of the user. Weather and environmental sensors aim at those surrounding factors which will affect the patient's healthily condition. In our future work, we consider to implement our system and integrate hospital customer relationship management (CRM) system to provide a better complete solution for diabetes patients. And through user interface, the diabetes patients can also adjust the reminding mechanism according to their preference. The communication and central server part will handle the data exchange and data analysis, which help to generate a final decision data and sent to user interface to remind the user of valuable information.

## References

1. The 6th Revision Edition of the IDF Diabetes Atlas. http://www.idf.org/diabetesatlas
2. International Diabetes Federation (IDF), What is diabetes? http://www.idf.org/diabetesatlas/7e/what-is-diabetes
3. Tama, B.A., Rodiyatul, F.S., Hermansyah, D.: An early detection method of type-2 diabetes-mellitus, public hospital. TELKOMNIKA 9(2), 287–294 (2011)
4. Delahanty, L.M., McCulloch, D.K.: Patient information: type 2 diabetes mellitus and diet (Beyond the Basics). http://www.uptodate.com/contents/type-2-diabetes-mellitus-and-diet-beyond-the-basics
5. Danaei, G., Finucane, M.M., et al.: National, regional, and global trends in fasting plasma glucose and diabetes prevalence since 1980: systematic analysis of health examination surveys and epidemiological studies with 370 country-years and 2·7 million participants. Lancet 378, 31–40 (2011)
6. Dain, K., Hadley, L.: Diabetes and climate change-two interconnected global challenges. Diabetes Res. Clin. Pract. 97(2), 337–339 (2012)
7. Niyato, D., et al.: Machine-to-machine communications for home energy management system in smart grid. IEEE Commun. Mag. 49(4), 53–59 (2011)
8. Van Puffelen, A.L., Rijken, M., Heijmans, M.J., Nijpels, G., Rutten, G.E.H.M., Schellevis, F.G.: Living with diabetes: a group-based self-management support programme for T2DM patients in the early phases of illness and their partners, study protocol of a randomised controlled trial. BMC Health Serv Res. 14, 144 (2014)
9. Helal, S., Bose, R., Chen, C.: STEPSTONE: an intelligent integration architecture for personal tele-health. J. Comput. Sci. Eng. 5(3), 269–281 (2011)
10. Lupu, E., Dulay, N., Sloman, M., Sventek, J., et al.: AMUSE: autonomic management of ubiquitous e-Health systems. Concurrency Comput. Pract. Exper. 20, 277–295 (2008)
11. Sebestyen, G., Krucz, L.: Remote monitoring of patients with mobile healthcare devices. In: 2010 IEEE International Conference on Automation Quality and Testing Robotics (AQTR), pp. 1–6 (2010)
12. Forjuoh, S.N., Reis, M.D., Couchman, G.R., Ory, M.G.: Improving diabetes self-care with a PDA in ambulatory care. Telemed. J. E Health. 14(3), 273–279 (2008)

13. Jensen, K.L., Pedersen, C.F., Larsen, L.B.: Diasnet mobile - a personalized mobile diabetes management and advisory service. In: Proceedings of the Second International Workshop on Personalisation for e-Health in conjunction with User Modelling, Corfu, Greece (2007)
14. Ratnasamy, S., Karp, B., Shenker, S., Estrin, D., et al.: Data-centric storage in sensornets with GHT, a geographic hash table. ACM Mob. Netw. Appl. (MONET) 8(4), 427–442 (2003)

# Construction of a Prediction Model for Nephropathy Among Obese Patients Using Genetic and Clinical Features

Guan-Mau Huang[1], Yi-Cheng Chen[3], and Julia Tzu-Ya Weng[1,2(✉)]

[1] Department of Computer Science and Engineering,
Yuan Ze University, Taoyuan, Taiwan
koko5696@gmail.com, julweng@saturn.yzu.edu.tw
[2] Innovation Center for Big Data and Digital Convergence,
Yuan Ze University, Taoyuan, Taiwan
[3] Department of Computer Science and Information Engineering,
Tamkang University, Tamsui, Taiwan
ycchen@mail.tku.edu.tw

**Abstract.** Obesity is a complex disease arising from an excessive accumulation of body fat which leads to various complications such as diabetes, hypertension, and renal diseases. The growing prevalence of obesity is also becoming a major risk factor for nephropathy. When patients are diagnosed with nephropathy, their progression towards renal failure is usually inevitable. Therefore, a prediction tool will help medical doctors identify patients with a higher risk of developing nephropathy and implement early treatment or prevention. In this study, we attempted to construct a diagnostic support system for nephropathy using clinical and genetic traits. Our results show that prediction models involving the use of both genetic and clinical features yielded the best classification performance. Our finding is in accordance with the complex nature of obesity-related nephropathy and support the notion of using genetic traits to design a personalized diagnostic model.

**Keywords:** Obesity · Nephropathy · Prediction · Personalized diagnostic support system

## 1 Introduction

Obesity is the result of an excessive accumulation of body fat. Despite the advancement in diet and lifestyle awareness, the prevalence of obesity is still on the rise. In fact, the number of obese adults is expected to reach from the current 300 million to 700 million by 2015 in the world [1]. Increasing evidence suggests that obesity is a major risk factor for diabetes, cardiovascular and kidney diseases [2–4]. Thus, the surveillance and control of obesity, as well as its complications, are becoming increasingly important.

Obesity results in serious metabolic problems, leading to persistent elevated levels of albumin in the urine, progressive decline in the glomerular filtration rate, increased arterial blood pressure, and ultimately nephropathy [4]. Generally, the symptoms of

© Springer International Publishing Switzerland 2015
X.-L. Li et al. (Eds.): PAKDD 2015, LNCS 9441, pp. 104–112, 2015.
DOI: 10.1007/978-3-319-25660-3_9

nephropathy are not obvious, but as the major cause of end stage renal disease (ESRD), this disease can inflict serious and adverse effects on morbidity, mortality and the patients' quality of life [5]. However, when patients are diagnosed with abnormal urinary protein level, it is often difficult to reverse the significant damages or prevent their progression towards ESRD [5]. Hence, a user-friendly prediction model that considers various kidney-related factors (e.g. gender, comorbid diseases, body mass index, etc.) would be beneficial for early diagnosis.

To date, decision support systems are emerging as useful tools in medicine, not only for assisting clinicians in diagnosing cardiovascular disease, chronic diseases, and cancers, but also for making decisions in intensive care units [6]. However, very few diagnostic support models make use of genetic features to achieve personalized risk predictions. Yet, recent evidence suggests that genes play important roles in nephropathy [7]. In fact, our group has previously combined genetic and clinical features to successfully construct a personalized diabetic nephropathy prediction tool for Taiwanese diabetic patients [8].

In the present study, we utilized the data generated by Wu et al. [9, 10] from genetic association analyses performed on 527 obese patients with and without nephropathy. We integrated the genetic and clinical information collected from this previous study to build a classification model for nephropathy risk prediction among obese patients. Our results indicate that the inclusion of genetic features yielded better performance in distinguishing those with a higher risk of developing nephropathy.

## 2    Methods and Materials

### 2.1    Participants

527 Taiwanese patients with obesity were recruited from the Tri-Service General Hospital in Taipei, Taiwan, in 2002 under the approval of the hospital's institutional review board. These data were previously published by Wu et al. [9, 10]. The case group and the control group consisted of 232 obese patients with nephropathy and 295 obese patients without nephropathy. The clinical and genetic attributes, as well as the demographic data of the patients, used in this study are shown in Tables 1 and 2, respectively.

### 2.2    System Flow

The system flow of our work is illustrated in Fig. 1. The training dataset consisted of 140 positive and 211 negative data, and the testing dataset, 92 positive and 84 negative data. Features were selected based on their information gain scores for decision tree and naïve Bayes, or F-scores for SVM. The classification performance was evaluated by a five-fold cross-validation approach for decision tree, random forest, SVM and naïve Bayes methods in models with only clinical features or genetic features, and those with both clinical and genetic features.

**Table 1.** Clinical and genetic attributes used in this study

| Attribute | Description | Attribute type | Attribute value |
|---|---|---|---|
| BMI | Body Mass Index | Numeric | |
| Gender | The gender of patients | Text | Male/Female |
| Diabetic | The history of diabetic | Text | Y/N |
| Hypertension | High blood pressure | Text | Y/N |
| Hyperlipidemia | Lips in the blood43 | Text | Y/N |
| Age | The age of patients | Numeric | |
| Fpg | Fasting plasma glucose | Numeric | |
| Stc | Serum total cholesterol | Numeric | |
| St | Serum triglyceride | Numeric | |
| BUN | Blood urea nitrogen | Numeric | |
| BC | Blood creatinine | Numeric | |
| SGOT | The level of liver function tests | Numeric | |
| SGPT | The level of liver function tests | Numeric | |
| PPAR | Gene name (SNP: rs1801282) | Text | CC/CG/GG |
| GNB3 | Gene name (SNP: rs5443) | Text | CC/CT/TT |
| FTO | Gene name (SNP: rs9939609) | Text | TT/AT/AA |
| ADRB2 | Gene name (SNP: rs1042714) | Text | CC/CG/GG |
| ADRB3 | Gene name (SNP: rs4994) | Text | TT/TC/CC |
| UCP1 | Gene name (SNP: −3826 A > G) | Text | AA/AG/GG |
| UCP2 | Gene name (SNP: rs659366) | Text | CC/CT/TT |
| UCP3 | Gene name (SNP: rs1800849) | Text | AA/AG/GG |
| IL6R | Gene name (SNP: rs8192284) | Text | AA/CA/CC |
| PCSK1 | Gene name (SNP: rs6235) | Text | CC/CG/GG |
| AGT | Gene name (SNP: rs699) | Text | AA/AG/GG |
| PLIN | Gene name (SNP: rs894160) | Text | AA/AG/GG |
| ENPP1 | Gene name (SNP: rs1044498) | Text | AA/AC/CC |
| ADIPOQ | Gene name (SNP: rs266729) | Text | CC/CG/GG |
| TCF7L2 | Gene name (SNP: rs7903146) | Text | CC/CT/TT |
| IGF2BP2 | Gene name (SNP: rs4402960) | Text | CC/CG/GG |
| SREBP | Gene name (SNP: rs11868035) | Text | AA/AG/GG |
| GHSR | Gene name (SNP: rs9819506) | Text | CC/CT/TT |
| GHSR | Gene name (SNP: rs490683) | Text | CC/CG/GG |
| LPIN2 | Gene name (SNP: rs3745012) | Text | AA/AG/GG |

## 2.3    Feature Selection

Experiments were conducted in LibSVM (version 3.12) [11] and WEKA, or Waikato Environment for Knowledge Analysis (version 3.6.5) [12]. Features were selected based on their F-scores for support vector machine (SVM), and information gain scores for decision tree and naïve Bayes.

**Table 2.** Demographic and clinical characteristics of the patients.

| Parameter | Nephropathy | No nephropathy |
|---|---|---|
| Number of people | 232 | 295 |
| BMI | 25.2 ± 3.8 | 24.3 ± 3.6 |
| Gender (M/F) | 129/103 | 117/178 |
| Age | 57.6 ± 10.3 | 55.6 ± 9.6 |
| Diabetic (Y/N) | 185/47 | 160/135 |
| Hypertension (Y/N) | 211/21 | 125/170 |
| Hyperlipidemia (Y/N) | 180/52 | 220/75 |
| Fpg | 162 ± 67.2 | 132 ± 48.7 |
| Blood urea nitrogen | 40.3 ± 24.1 | 14.3 ± 3.6 |
| Blood creatinine | 3.6 ± 3.5 | 0.9 ± 0.2 |
| Stc | 202.7 ± 50.8 | 201.6 ± 35.3 |
| Serum triglyceride | 212.8 ± 168.8 | 131.9 ± 85.7 |
| SGOT | 22.7 ± 15.8 | 22.3 ± 11.1 |
| SGPT | 21.3 ± 19.5 | 23 ± 13.8 |

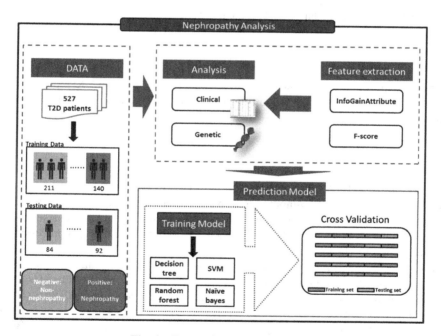

**Fig. 1.** System flow of our analysis

$F$-score [13] is a feature selection technique that measures the ability of a certain attribute to discriminate a dataset into different groups. For training vectors $x_k$, if k = 1,2,3 …, m, and if $n_-$ and $n_+$ denote the number of positive and negative instances, respectively, then the $F$-score of the $i^{th}$ feature can be computed by:

$$F(i) = \frac{(\bar{x}_i^{(+)} - \bar{x}_i)^2 + (\bar{x}_i^{(-)} - \bar{x}_i)^2}{\frac{1}{n_+ - 1} \sum_{k=1}^{n_+} (x_{k,i}^{(+)} - \bar{x}_i^{(+)})^2 + \frac{1}{n_- - 1} \sum_{k=1}^{n_-} (x_{k,i}^{(-)} - \bar{x}_i^{(-)})^2} \tag{1}$$

The average of the $i^{th}$ feature of the whole, positive, and negative datasets are represented by $\bar{x}_i, \bar{x}_i^{(+)}, \bar{x}_i^{(-)}$, respectively; $x_{k,i}^{(+)}$ indicates the $i^{th}$ feature of the $k^{th}$ positive instance, while $x_{k,i}^{(-)}$ is the $i^{th}$ feature of the $k^{th}$ negative instance.

The InfoGainAttribute tool [14] in WEKA evaluates the extent by which an attribute can accurately and specifically classify a dataset by measuring its information gain according to the following:

$$IG(A, S) = H(S) - \sum_{t \in T} p(t)H(t) \tag{2}$$

where information gain IG(A) is the measure of the difference in entropy from before to after the dataset S is split by an attribute A, while t is the subsets created from the splitting, such that $S = \underset{t \in T}{\cup} t$, and p(t) is the proportion of the number of elements in t to the number of elements in dataset S. H is the information entropy, which is calculated by:

$$H(S) = - \sum_{x \in X} p(x) \log_2 p(x) \tag{3}$$

where S is the dataset for which entropy is being calculated, and X represents the classes in S, while p(x) is the proportion of the number of elements in class x to the number of elements in set S.

## 2.4   Classification

Next, we used the C4.5 decision tree algorithm [15] to perform classification among obese patients with and without nephropathy. Tree induction in C4.5 involves: (1) construction of a large tree from the training data according to attribute selection by information gain scores; (2) removal of branches to avoid overfitting; (3) processing of the pruned tree to enhance its interpretability [15].

SVM was also used for classification. The SVM algorithm attempts to find a hyperplane that best differentiate the data into one category or the other [16]. We selected features for SVM classification by ranking them according to their F-scores.

Next, Naïve Bayes [17, 18] was evaluated for its performance in classifying patients with and without nephropathy in the dataset. The formula of Naïve Bayes follows Bayes' theorem of probability,

$$P(C_k|x) = P(C_k) \times \frac{P(x|C_k)}{P(x)} \tag{4}$$

where $P(C = C_k | X = x)$ is the probability that an item set belongs to class $C_k$, given that $C_k$ has a feature vector x. $C_k$ and x are values taken on by random variables; therefore, C and X simplify notation by omitting those random variables.

Random forest was also included as one of the classifiers for building the risk prediction model. The random forest algorithm [19] outputs a collection of decision trees based on the random selection of features.

## 3  Results and Discussions

Multiple environmental and genetic factors affect the disease progression of kidney complications related to obesity [9]. The aim of the present study was to develop an effective personalized risk assessment model combining genetic and clinical parameters, so as to assist clinicians in the identification of obese patients with nephropathy. The ultimate goal was to facilitate efficient monitoring of patients and cost-effective use of medical resources.

Through a 5-fold cross-validation approach, we compared the performance of prediction models using only clinical features, or only genetic features, with those employing both genetic and clinical features in different classifiers. The performance for classification among obese patients with and without nephropathy using variable number of the top ranking clinical measures via different classification approaches is shown in Table 3. Model built with the Naïve Bayes algorithm appeared to generate the poorest performance, while those constructed with decision tree, SVM, and random forest were comparable in their prediction performance. We obtained similarly disappointing results with classification models constructed using only genetic features (Table 4).

**Table 3.** Performance of using variable numbers of clinical features to predict nephropathy among obese patients.

| Parameter | DT | RF | SVM | NB |
|---|---|---|---|---|
| #Features | 5 | 5 | 7 | 5 |
| Training dataset (P:140,N:211) | | | | |
| Accuracy | 71.79 % | 71.79 % | 70.37 % | 68.09 % |
| Sensitivity | 75.71 % | 63.38 % | 91.43 % | 42.14 % |
| Specificity | 69.19 % | 77.51 % | 56.40 % | 85.31 % |
| Precision | 61.99 % | 65.69 % | 58.18 % | 65.56 % |
| Independent testing dataset (P:92,N:84) | | | | |
| Accuracy | 72.77 % | 73.30 % | 76.14 % | 63.64 % |
| Sensitivity | 64.13 % | 64.13 % | 90.22 % | 36.96 % |
| Specificity | 82.14 % | 83.33 % | 60.71 % | 92.86 % |
| Precision | 79.73 % | 80.82 % | 71.55 % | 85 % |

DT = Decision Tree; RF = Random Forest; NB = Naive Bayes; SVM = support vector machine; P = positive data; N = negative data Sensitivity: TP/(TP + FN); Specificity: TN/(TN + FP); Precision: TP/(TP + FP)

**Table 4.** Performance of using variable numbers of genetic features to predict nephropathy.

| Parameter | DT | RF | SVM | NB |
|---|---|---|---|---|
| #Features | 7 | 7 | 10 | 9 |
| Training dataset (P:140,N:211) | | | | |
| Accuracy | 63.25 % | 64.10 % | 66.95 % | 65.53 % |
| Sensitivity | 26.43 % | 30.71 % | 40.71 % | 38.57 % |
| Specificity | 87.68 % | 86.26 % | 84.36 % | 83.41 % |
| Precision | 58.73 % | 59.72 % | 63.33 % | 60.67 % |
| Testing dataset (P:92,N:84) | | | | |
| Accuracy | 63.07 % | 63.64 % | 65.34 % | 60.80 % |
| Sensitivity | 39.13 % | 41.30 % | 47.83 % | 46.74 % |
| Specificity | 89.29 % | 88.10 % | 84.52 % | 76.19 % |
| Precision | 80 % | 79.17 % | 77.19 % | 68.25 % |

DT = Decision Tree; RF = Random Forest; NB = Naive Bayes; SVM = support vector machine; P = positive data; N = negative data Sensitivity: TP/(TP + FN); Specificity: TN/(TN + FP); Precision: TP/(TP + FP)

Because the development of nephropathy is associated with both genetic and environmental factors, perhaps by separating clinical and genetic features, we have overlooked the possible interactions between genes and clinical traits. Thus, we tried integrating both clinical and genetic attributes for classification and evaluated the accuracy, sensitivity, and specificity of including genetic features in the prediction for nephropathy among obese patients. Table 5 shows the performance comparison of implementing variable numbers of the top ranking features in different classifiers. The best performance was achieved by the seven-, six-, and eleven-attribute model in decision tree, random forest, Naïve Bayes and SVM, respectively. Overall, this approach outperformed previous attempts utilizing only clinical or genetic attributes for classification. The Naïve Bayes model, again, was the lowest in performance.

Though the SVM model seemed to exhibit the highest accuracy, it required 11 attributes for classification. In contrast, the decision tree and random forest models were able to utilize fewer attributes to output comparable results. To facilitate a cost-effective diagnostic pipeline involving biochemical testing and genetic screening, decision tree and random forest may be more efficient than SVM. Also, from a clinician's point of view, a model that offers the visualization of a tree as a prediction output may be more user-friendly and easier to convince patients to take necessary measures to prevent or slow down the progression towards ESRD.

Since a slight increase in performance was achieved after the clinical and genetic features were combined for classification, for complex diseases like obesity and nephropathy, accurate early identification may require the consideration of various risk factors. Equally possible is that each genetic and environmental determinant may contribute minor effects to nephropathy, but together, these factors may significantly influence the risk of developing nephropathy in obese patients.

**Table 5.** Performance of using variable numbers of clinical and genetic features to predict nephropathy among obese patients.

| Parameter | DT | RF | SVM | NB |
|---|---|---|---|---|
| #Features | 7 | 6 | 11 | 6 |
| Training dataset (P:140,N:211) | | | | |
| Accuracy | 76.35 % | 76.35 % | 74.93 % | 72.08 % |
| Sensitivity | 69.29 % | 70 % | 75.71 % | 57.14 % |
| Specificity | 81.04 % | 80.57 % | 74.41 % | 81.99 % |
| Precision | 70.80 % | 70.50 % | 66.25 % | 67.80 % |
| Independent testing dataset (P:92,N:84) | | | | |
| Accuracy | 75.57 % | 76.70 % | 78.98 % | 70.45 % |
| Sensitivity | 65.22 % | 70.65 % | 83.70 % | 57.61 % |
| Specificity | 86.90 % | 83.33 % | 73.81 % | 84.52 % |
| Precision | 84.50 % | 82.28 % | 77.78 % | 80.30 % |

DT = Decision Tree; RF = Random Forest; NB = Naive Bayes; SVM = support vector machine; P = positive data; N = negative data Sensitivity: TP/(TP + FN); Specificity: TN/(TN + FP); Precision: TP/(TP + FP)

## 4 Conclusion

To our knowledge, this study was the first to combine genetic and clinical features in the construction of a personalized nephropathy risk prediction model for obese patients. Our results show that the decision tree or random forest classifiers may outperform other classification methods in terms of cost, efficiency, and user-friendliness. Further refinements and improvements of the models in a larger sample size are required to increase the prediction performance and validate the usefulness of the proposed approach. Overall, our study suggests that combining interdisciplinary research efforts to build diagnostic support systems involving the use of genetic features may have the potential to enhance the performance of disease risk prediction.

**Acknowledgements.** Julia Tzu-Ya Weng are supported by the Ministry of Science and Technology of the Republic of China, Taiwan, under the Contract Number of MOST 103-2221-E-155-038, while Yi-Cheng Chen is supported with funding from MOST 104-2221-E-032-037-MY2.

## References

1. Ji, C.Y., Cheng, T.O.: Epidemic increase in overweight and obesity in Chinese children from 1985 to 2005. Int. J. Cardiol. **132**, 1–10 (2009)
2. Iseki, K., Tokashiki, K., Iseki, C., Kohagura, K., Kinjo, K., Takishita, S.: Proteinuria and decreased body mass index as a significant risk factor in developing end-stage renal disease. Clin. Exp. Nephrol. **12**, 363–369 (2008)

3. Kramer, H., Luke, A., Bidani, A., Cao, G., Cooper, R., McGee, D.: Obesity and prevalent and incident CKD: the hypertension detection and follow-up program. Am. J. Kidney Dis. Official J. Nat. Kidney Found. **46**, 587–594 (2005)
4. Maric, C., Hall, J.E.: Obesity, metabolic syndrome and diabetic nephropathy. Contrib. Nephrol. **170**, 28–35 (2011)
5. Sharifiaghdas, F., Kashi, A.H., Eshratkhah, R.: Evaluating percutaneous nephrolithotomy-induced kidney damage by measuring urinary concentrations of β2-microglobulin. Urol. J. **8**, 277–282 (2011)
6. Belle, A., Kon, M.A., Najarian, K.: Biomedical informatics for computer-aided decision support systems: a survey. Sci. World J. **2013**, 769639 (2013)
7. Thorsby, P.M., Midthjell, K., Gjerlaugsen, N., Holmen, J., Hanssen, K.F., Birkeland, K.I., Berg, J.P.: Comparison of genetic risk in three candidate genes (TCF7L2, PPARG, KCNJ11) with traditional risk factors for type 2 diabetes in a population-based study–the HUNT study. Scand. J. Clin. Lab. Invest. **69**, 282–287 (2009)
8. Huang, G.M., Huang, K.Y., Lee, T.Y., Weng, J.: An interpretable rule-based diagnostic classification of diabetic nephropathy among type 2 diabetes patients. BMC Bioinform. **16**, S5 (2015)
9. Lin, E., Pei, D., Huang, Y.J., Hsieh, C.H., Wu, L.S.: Gene-gene interactions among genetic variants from obesity candidate genes for nonobese and obese populations in type 2 diabetes. Genet. Test Mol. Biomarkers **13**, 485–493 (2009)
10. Wu, L.S., Hsieh, C.H., Pei, D., Hung, Y.J., Kuo, S.W., Lin, E.: Association and interaction analyses of genetic variants in ADIPOQ, ENPP1, GHSR, PPARgamma and TCF7L2 genes for diabetic nephropathy in a Taiwanese population with type 2 diabetes. Nephrol. Dial. Transplant. **24**, 3360–3366 (2009)
11. Chang, C.-C., Lin, C.-J.: LIBSVM: A Library for Support Vector Machines (2001)
12. Hall, M., Frank, E., Holmes, G., Pfahringer, B., Reutemann, P., Witten, I.H.: The WEKA data mining software: an update. SIGKDD Explor. **11**(1), 10–18 (2009)
13. Akay, M.F.: Support vector machines combined with feature selection for breast cancer diagnosis. Expert Syst. Appl. **36**, 3240–3247 (2009)
14. Firouzi, F., Rashidi, M., Hashemi, S., Kangavari, M., Bahari, A., Daryani, N.E., Emam, M. M., Naderi, N., Shalmani, H.M., Farnood, A., Zali, M.: A decision tree-based approach for determining low bone mineral density in inflammatory bowel disease using WEKA software. Eur. J. Gastroenterol. Hepatol. **19**, 1075–1081 (2007)
15. Quinlan, J.R.: Improved use of continuous attributes in C4.5. J. Artif. Intell. Res. **4**, 77–90 (1996)
16. Cortes, C., Vapnik, V.: Support-vector networks. Mach. Learn. **20**, 273–297 (1995)
17. Chen, J., Huang, H.: Feature selection for text classification with Naïve Bayes. Expert Syst. Appl. **36**, 5432–5435 (2009)
18. Guh, R.-S., Wu, T.-C.J., Weng, S.-P.: Integrating genetic algorithm and decision tree learning for assistance in predicting in vitro fertilization outcomes. Expert Syst. Appl. **38**, 4437–4449 (2011)
19. Breiman, L.: Random Forests (2001)

# A Research of Applying Association Rules and Decision Tree to Endometriosis

Lin Hui[1]([✉]), Huan-Chao Keh[2], Nan-Ching Huang[3],
Chiung-Tzu Chang[2], and Yi-Fan Yang[1]

[1] Department of Innovative Information and Technology,
Tamkang University, Tamsui, Taiwan
{amar0627,ssyyfss}@gmail.com
[2] Department of Computer Science, Tamkang University, Tamsui, Taiwan
Keh@mail.tku.edu.tw
[3] Institute of Clinical Medicine NYMMC,
National Yang-Ming University, Taipei, Taiwan
kingsleynch@gmail.com

**Abstract.** With the medical technology getting developed day by day, medical quality has been playing a significant role in treatment achievement evaluation, recurrence evaluation and complication disease differentiation. However, the variety and complexity of medical data type makes it possible to cause some deviations of results by subjective judgments and affect the medical decision. So, it is necessary to choose the appropriate data analyzing methods. When it comes to strategy selection, we can find that categorized data type is superior to helping to make a decision. Through medical records, taking the method of data mining to analyze the association relations among certain diseases and then we can generalize the characteristics and dig out the hidden information. This research is to take use of association rules and decision tree to analyze the association relationship among endometriosis, barrenness and alcohol treatment. By analyzing the recorded medical associated data, we will find out the potential information as well as useful knowledge. That can provide references for physician when carry out the medical treatment.

**Keywords:** Association rules · Data mining · Endometriosis · Barrenness · Alcohol treatment

## 1 Introduction

Due to the widely using of medical information system, the scale of data which saved in database has been increasing a lot. Although doctors can access the history data of patients rapidly and seize control on the treatment, that just means the diagnosis of doctor and the medical history of patient were recorded. However, it will do a great contribution to improve medical knowledge if we add some analysis and processing to such huge amount of those data and find out the association rules among diseases. There's no doubt that data mining and knowledge diggings are getting more and more popular. Lots of expects, enterprises as well as scholars have been making use of data

X.-L. Li et al. (Eds.): PAKDD 2015, LNCS 9441, pp. 113–124, 2015.
DOI: 10.1007/978-3-319-25660-3_10

mining technology to analyze data and achieve the potentially useful data in all kinds of field. In clinical treatment, data mining is also a good assistant to check the results of operation methods, medical experiments and exploring the association rules between clinical data and pathological data [1, 8, 9].

With the technology of laparoscope popularizing, it is found that some women showed no clinical signs on endometriosis but some of them suffered a lot with huge discomfort and pains resulting in barrenness. Although these symptoms can be cured by medicine or operations, the research shows that the treatments always come with hurts and adhesion. According to reports delivered by scholars, without considering other special conditions of patients, it is better to cure these with alcohol treatments than other traditional methods. And in such treatment, it would be the best to cure the patients with alcohol for 10–15 min. However, it indicates that when we add into certain conditions of patients such as barrenness, some situations goes against the results from researchers by analyzing the screened samples.

Due to the finding showed above, this paper will carry out a deeper research on the curative effect of alcohol treatment and some other symptoms using the methods of association rules and decision tree in data mining to find out the association among endometriosis, other diseases (like barrenness), operations (like laparotomy, Laparoscopic operation) and alcohol treatment. The specialty of medical data will be analyzed and recorded, and the potential data will be found out. Based on these, we will come up with important decision factors related to detection data and clinic symptoms, assisting doctors to do treatment as references, aiming to ensure the best curing method and reduce hurts, improving treating efficiency.

This paper will discuss the background related work, outline the definition and causes of endometriosis, and introduce what are data mining, association rules and decision tree in second section. In third section, research method will be explained. It will introduce the research framework and steps, and process of operating analysis which is developed basing on the process of data mining. The whole forth section is going to find out the medical rules which are clinically meaningful by making use of the results coming from the analyzing implementation of seizing association rules on relative data collecting from patients of endometriosis. The fifth section will base on the result from implementations and analyzing process to explain and investigate the conclusions and future directions of research.

## 2  Related Work

### 2.1  Endometriosis

Endometriosis is a gynecological disease that cells from the lining of uterus (endometrium) appear and flourish outside the uterine cavity, coming with Primary tissue cell biological function. There are two main kinds of endometriosis:

1. Adenomyosis: similar to original histiocyte growing in uterine muscle layers
2. Endometriosis of pelvis: occupy the most part, happening in ovary or abdominal film. Like endometrium, it will shed and bleed when stimulated by estrus hormone. For these endometrium tissue are in cavum pelvis, they cannot be eliminated from

body and would inflame, then puff up forming reticular scar tissue. This is called adhesions. Contents of some of these endometria are liquid which is similar to tar cyst or chocolate; if this liquid flow into cavum pelvis, it will cause peritonitis.

About 10 % of normal women who once been pregnant would form lesions and the probability would even reach to 80 % for women who have barrenness or feel painful during menses. It is still unclear how the endometriosis forms, but there are many hypotheses and the most popular are "Endometrial tissue planted theory" and "peritoneal epithelium metaplasia deformation theory" which are most widely accepted by gynecological doctors [2, 3].

Normally, endometriosis can be caused by the followings [3–5]:

1. Regurgitation: uterine contraction happens during menses, besides eliminating scaled endometrium out of body through cervix, it also pulls endometrium into peritoneal cavity.
2. Import through lymphatic system: many endometrium cells may be transported to other parts in body like bellows, umbilicus and lymph gland through openings of fallopian and uterine vessels.
3. Autoimmune defects: it is so common that during menses, endometrium travels all around and these fragments will be engulfed by leucocytes; only a small number of women whose body cannot deal with too much these cells, as a result, the left cells will attach to other organs like: ovary, fallopian tubes, bladder, large intestine and Douglas pouch.

According to the classifications of American Society for Reproductive Medicine, there are 4 levels of endometriosis: 1. Mild (1–5 points); 2. Low-grade (6–15 points); 3. Moderate (16–40 points); 4. Severe (above 40 points). For 1 and 2 level, the best solution is to get pregnant immediately or take Dannazol for 3–6 months making problem cells shrivel then get pregnant as soon as possible; for 3–4 levels, doctors would advise to accept operation assisted with medicine or injection for 3–6 months. Also they need to get pregnant within one year after drug withdrawal in avoid of recrudescence.

The treatment of endometriosis need to take in many considerations, such as level of disease, whether ever accepted operations or pharmacotherapy and what is the expectation of keeping fertility. The most thorough solution is total hysterectomy ovariectomy for that endometriosis would relapse any time, but some couples expect to keep fertility so they must accept operations or pharmacotherapy or alcohol treatment.

Drugs which are often used in pharmacotherapy include: Danazol (Ladogal), Gestrnone (Dimetriose), GnRHa (GnRH analogs), Progesterone and oral contraception [2, 4, 5]. Pharmacotherapy has a good effect on easing the pain bringing from endometriosis and can reduce the activity making problem cells narrowing. When the size of cells reduces to 5–6 mm, they will be controlled and regulated by peritoneal fluid.

Through operation, niduses can be cut off completely. Although it really costs time, but 80 % patients can reduce their pain for longer than 5 years, and probability of getting pregnant will reach or exceed 67 % [2, 4, 5]. There are two main operations: 1. Laparoscope surgery 2. Laparotomy.

Alcohol treatment is to cut a small incisional and inject absolute alcohol in guided by ultrasonic wave or CT [11–13]; for that absolute alcohol has a strong deaquation, once injected capsular space, the inner cells will lose their secretion function and the cyst will shrivel then disappear. Compared to other treatment, there's less side effects and lower probability of complication as well as safety. In this treatment, the taboo is relative not absolute for there are few taboos for alcohol injection and less hurt for body, effective and cheap. This is also a considerable treatment for patients. This paper will mainly talk about alcohol treatment and divide the treatment as: less than 1 min, 1–9 min, 10–15 min and keep alcohol in with deeper research.

### 2.2    Data Mining

Facing large scale and dispersive data but hard to find out the wanted is "Data-rich but information-poor situation" introduced by Han and Kanber. In order to solve this problem, people applied a lot of computer technologies on it to help to deal with those data and developed data mining.

Data mining means finding relevant patterns and extract information automatically from large database [5]. The most important part in data mining is the word "automatically". So Berry and Linoff define data mining as realizing to analyze and extract valuable data from database automatically or semi automatically through algorithm [6]. However, Witten and some others consider it as a process of finding patterns automatically or semi automatically with meaning and proceeds.

The functionality of data mining can be classified as classification, estimation, prediction, affinity, clustering and description. According to data characteristics, the mining methods are mainly divided as association rules, classification, clustering analysis and sequential pattern analysis. Because this paper mainly use association rule and decision tree these two methods, we just introduce these two following.

**Apriori Algorithm.** Association rule is one of the main methods in data mining and usually defined as market-basket analysis (MBA). The main purpose of association rule is to discover the related associations and potential knowledge among dataset.

An association rule is usually represented as $A \Rightarrow B$, A and B are two unions of trading items, $A \cap B = \phi$, and association rule is to find out the associations which have high support and confidence from trading data. The definitions of support and confidence are showed below:

$$\text{support}(A \Rightarrow B) = P(A \cup B) \tag{1}$$

$$\text{confidence}(A \Rightarrow B) = P(B|A) \tag{2}$$

Before analyzing association rules, we need to define the minimum of support and confidence in order to select proper items and rules. However, the threshold value of minimum is defined by users subjectively; if too high, there may miss some meaningful rules; oppositely, there may be some weak rules. So they are two important indexes.

**Decision Tree.** Decision tree is a kind of tool which is suitable for users to do data mining. The main functionality is to develop models through classified dataset and forecast and classify the untreated data using established models. We can analyze the characteristics of data by decision tree. For decision tree, each node represents a predicate storing class, and leaf node represents the decision goal we reached.

The most popular decision tree algorithm was developed by Breman et al. 1984 known as CART algorithm also called Classification and Regression Trees [14]. The main advantages of this algorithm is that it can be applied on dispersive and continuous data. The establishing progress is to prepare a classified training dataset and classify data at each node constructing a whole decision tree.

Compared to others, decision tree contains the advantages with easy to understand and realize, the preparation of data is easy or even unnecessary, easy to come up with relative logical expression and easy to evaluate the model by static testing.

## 3  Process of Analyzing Implementation

### 3.1  Process of Analyzing Implementation

According to U.M. Fayyad [10], data mining is kind of repeated communicating operation which led by users: from screening data from database, selecting target data which is preprocessed and do analysis, transforming data to reduce the scale, displaying the results after mining to evaluating the out coming and some other operations; then build up a mining model and trace whether the result reach the requiring level. In order to show the process more clear, this research designs the operating process basing on the process developed by U.M. Fayyad with little changes see in Fig. 1.

As is showed in Fig. 1, firstly we define and analyze the problems from the starting point of medical science, we will learn the resource and the species of data which is required during the data mining through this step and then define the goal of data mining basing on these related data.

After defining the goal of data mining, we will do data preprocessing and data transforming in order to build up the data for data mining. Since there may contain many unordered or wrong values in original data, such data would affect the efficiency and the accuracy. So it is necessary to do the operations like preprocessing. Besides, with the changes of data mining goals, the original columns may have the limitation in data expressing; in that case, another significant point is to set up the derived columns, and all these procedures should be done in the period of data preprocessing.

When preprocessing is done, directing towards different analyzing goal, we select the proper columns as the goal of mining algorithm or additional columns. After this, data mart in small scale and tailor made is formed. The selection in this part will affect the interpretability and accuracy of whole mining result. Next step is to deal with or eliminate the missing data and noisy data in data mart, and transform the different data formats according to the certain analytic goal and requirements of some data mining technology.

Completing the steps above, then comes the most important part selecting data mining algorithm. In this research, the emphasis point is to analyze if the CA exponent

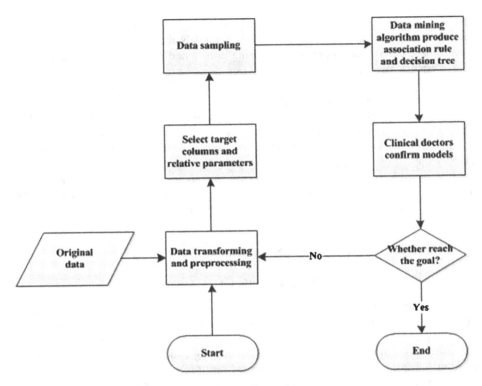

**Fig. 1.** Flow chart of operating process

is in the normal range after diagnosis and treatment. Association rules in data mining will be applied here. However, the association rules involved here is too many to define, so the ultimate rules will be defined after factitious screening.

Once the mining model is produced, it will be tested with the assistance of clinic doctors and the result will be presented with words and diagram because of the small scale of samples considering the accuracy and the applicability in clinic practice instead of testing immediately after model formed.

### 3.2   Preparations of Analytic Data

During the analyzing process, this research will take the data from a medical center as the sample data finding out the association rules basing on the association among diseases. We will preprocess the data before analyzing including: unifications of missing value and noisy value, transformation of data formats, discretion of data, calculating the derived attributes, selecting data sample space; so that we can keep up the accuracy.

- A. Unifications of missing value or noisy value: Missing value and noisy value will affect the accuracy of analytic results. Because of this, such values need to be unified as a certain value. For records of huge mistake, if they share little percentage, they can be deleted directly.

- B. Transformation of data formats: During the period of loading original data into database, the data format of table columns is displayed as character. But in the period of data analyzing, it is necessary to transform the columns into proper data format to keep algorithm function well.
- C. Discretion of data: The original data is continuous value needing to be changed into discrete one. Discrete means cut the continuous value into discrete value for a convenient calculating; it is necessary to concentrate on how to divide the value, because even a wispy change of continuous value will lead to a great effect on probability distribution. In this research, the divide line will be defined by doctors, so the probability is accurate in certain level.
- D. Calculating the derived attributes: In order to analyze data, sometimes the original attributes of data cannot be used directly. Thus, we have to calculate the original attributes and produce new attributes. It would be clearer to describe the characteristic of data and better to produce results by data mining algorithm through derived data.
- E. Selecting data sample space: For the data mining planning with forecasting goal, usually we divide original data into several dataset pro rata mainly sampling the original data, dividing into two parts:

Training dataset: a dataset to build forecasting model

Testing dataset: a dataset to test the accuracy of built model; in this research, we change that into clinic doctor assisted verifying forecasting model.

## 3.3 Description of Analytic Data

This research takes the goal of find in what situation will patients' CA exponents stay in normal range which means lower than 35 U/ml. Under the condition of hospital rules, medical ethics and protecting patients' privacy, 104 data of endometriosis is collected as researching targets eliminating others which has problems with columns.

**Table 1.** Explanations of columns and data formats

| Column name | Column explanations | Data formats |
|---|---|---|
| Yr | Have barrenness or not | Y: yes N: no |
| Para | Ever been pregnant or not | Y: yes N: no |
| Laparotomies | Ever took laparotomies or not | Y: yes N: no |
| Laparoscope | Ever took laparoscope and how many times | Y: yes N: no |
| | | 2: twice or more than twice |
| CA normal | CA exponents before operation | Y: normal range |
| | | N: abnormal range |
| ASP time | Alcohol treatment | 1: less than 1 min then out |
| | | 2: 1–9 min then out |
| | | 3: 10–15 then out |
| | | 4: remain in body |

Going through the preparation of data analyzing and processing, we screen out the missing value, null value and value which may cause noise; then communicate with clinic doctors and select the original data according to patients' basic data, clinically examining data and treating related data. At last, the data will be screened by human beings; those which are not proper to deal with association rules would be deleted. The only reference index to evaluate the curative effect will be the CA exponents after operation. Explanations of columns and data formats showed in Table 1.

## 4  Result and Discussion

Although endometriosis is defined as a benign tumor in clinic, if CA exponents keeps going up or exceeding the normal range, patients still have a certain probability to get other complications. The so called CA exponents means the value of CA-125 in blood which refers to a kind of ovarian epithelial tumor antigen whose value can be used to judge the severity of endometriosis or evaluate the result of treatment. Normally, the CA exponents of women should be lower than 35 U/ml. But when tissues got damaged or paraplasm, CA-125 will increase. Even though the value of CA-125 is lack of accuracy and sensitiveness that is not suitable for a clear judgment, and there will be inaccuracy during menses, it is still an index of treatment when it is discovered. During the operational treatment, if CA-125 decreases, that means a positive impact occurs; oppositely, the current treatment should be shut down, and a new treating plan need to be drew up. Thus, through the communication with clinic doctors, we decided to analyze the association between CA exponents after operation and alcohol treatment.

Firstly, we analyzed part of columns in Table 1 and we found that:

- ASP time: When taking normal CA exponents as index, there would reach a certain percentage in getting better after alcohol treatment. Although ASP:2 (inject alcohol in for 1–9 min then take out)seemed to get a better result than ASP:3 (inject in for 10–15 min then take out); however, this result doesn't go same with some other researches [4, 6, 7]: alcohol treatment lasting for more than 10 min would reach the best impact. When we have a detail observation, we'll find that ASP:4 (inject in without taking out)shares the best impact with percentage of 60.71 %,; but only basing on the number of patients, ASP:3 with 18 patients has the best impact. The reason of reaching such a result might be the small number of samples and unbalanced distribution of each class. We have faith to achieve a clearer display of results if we increase the number of samples. In fact, the following discussion will stay in the same state once the alcohol treatment is involved. Meaning while, we will only have a partly discussion on the probability which have improvement after alcohol treatment, because alcohol treatment has 4 types with the condition of less samples and unbalanced distribution.
- CA normal: Probability of patients who had a normal range of CA exponents before operation taking a turn for better is 1.69 times compared to those who had an abnormal range. The proportion is 72.97–43.28.
- Barrenness: Probability of patients without barrenness taking a turn for better is 1.69 times compared to those who had barrenness. The proportion is 64.62–35.9.

Till now, we find that the curative effect is mainly affected by CA exponents before operation and barrenness these two parameters.

- Laparotomies: It seems to have little influence in whether patients ever taken a laparotomy.

## 4.1    Analysis Directed Towards Barrenness, CA Normal Range and Alcohol Treatment

After basic analysis, we did analyses exploiting association rules integrating barrenness, CA normal range value, alcohol treatment and some other columns together. As is shown following Table 2.

**Table 2.** Association rules one

| Yr | CA normal | ASP time | |
|----|-----------|----------|---|
| Y | Y | 1 → Y (100 %) (N: 0, Y: 1) | 2 → Y (66.67 %) (N: 1, Y: 2) |
| | | 3 → Y (0 %) (N: 3, Y: 0) | 4 → Y (0 %) (N: 1, Y: 0) |
| Y | N | 1 → Y (20 %) (N: 4, Y: 1) | 2 → Y (33.33 %) (N: 4, Y: 2) |
| | | 3 → Y (33.33 %) (N: 8, Y: 4) | 4 → Y (42.86 %) (N: 4, Y: 3) |
| N | Y | 1 → Y (71.43 %) (N: 2, Y: 5) | 2 → Y (85.71 %) (N: 1, Y: 6) |
| | | 3 → Y (80 %) (N: 1, Y: 4) | 4 → Y (80 %) (N: 2, Y: 8) |
| N | N | 1 → Y (30 %) (N: 7, Y: 3) | 2 → Y (33.33 %) (N: 2, Y: 1) |
| | | 3 → Y (69.23 %) (N: 4, Y: 9) | 4 → Y (60 %) (N: 4, Y: 6) |

In analytical rules, the left side of "→"is parameters, while the other side means whether the CA exponents are in normal range. For we are interested in the normal CA exponents after operation, the value of normal CA after operation in all rules is represented as Y; the first "()"means the probability of CA exponents remaining in normal range after operation, the second one represents the results calculating from support value in association rules; N is number of patients who are not in the normal range and Y means number of those are in.

Taking an example of Yr: Y, CA_normal: Y, ASP_time: 1 → Y (100 %) (N: 0, Y:1). Patients in the condition of barrenness with normal CA value, the result is that each of those patients had a normal CA value after alcohol treatment; for this rule, patients with CA exponents which are in normal range occupied 100 %, so does the other rules by the parity of reasoning.

According to the result found above, we form the Table 3. Base on Table 3, we find that the only patients group who are not suitable for alcohol treatment is those who have barrenness with normal CA value, going through the opposite way from other published researches. This is worthwhile to carry out a continuous research.

**Table 3.** Analytical result explanation one

| Condition | Explanation |
|---|---|
| Patients who have barrenness with normal CA value | Although the number of samples is limited, from 100 % recovery without alcohol treatment to 0 % recovery with alcohol treatment for more than 10 min, we know that these patients are not suitable for alcohol treatment, not conforming to other researches |
| Patients who have barrenness with abnormal CA value | Although the percentage of recovery is low; we still discover that the longer the treatment lasts, the higher the probability of recovery would be agreeing with other researches. So these patients are suitable for alcohol treatment lasting longer than 10 min |
| Patients who have no barrenness with normal CA value | There are little differences among patients. However, patients who took the alcohol treatment longer than 10 min share a higher recovery than those who didn't. So this group is suitable for treatment longer than 10 min |
| Patients who have no barrenness with abnormal CA value | Having big differences in recovery. When treating time less than 10 min, the percentage of recovery shares only 30.77 % comparing to 65.22 % those treated longer than 10 min with clear curative effect. Thus, these patients need to accept treatment for longer than 10 min |

## 4.2 Doing Analysis Among Barrenness, Gravidity and Alcohol Treatment

We carried out a deeper research in barrenness, the rules are shown below Table 4.

After analyzing rules, we draw the following Table 5. From Table 5 we know that only patients who have barrenness and once have been pregnant are not suitable for alcohol treatment, going through the opposite way from other published researches. This is worthwhile to carry out a continuous research.

**Table 4.** Associationl rules two

| Yr | Para | ASP time | |
|---|---|---|---|
| Y | Y | 1 → Y (40 %) (N: 3, Y: 2) | 2 → Y (100 %) (N: 0, Y: 1) |
| | | 3 → Y (12.5 %) (N: 7, Y: 1) | 4 → Y (33.33 %) (N: 2, Y: 1) |
| Y | N | 1 → Y (0 %) (N: 1, Y: 0) | 2 → Y (37.5 %) (N: 5, Y: 3) |
| | | 3 → Y (50 %) (N: 4, Y: 4) | 4 → Y (40 %) (N: 3, Y: 2) |
| N | Y | 1 → Y (44.44 %) (N: 5, Y: 4) | 2 → Y (100 %) (N: 0, Y: 3) |
| | | 3 → Y (77.78 %) (N: 2, Y: 7) | 4 → Y (80 %) (N: 2, Y: 8) |
| N | N | 1 → Y(44.44 %) (N: 5, Y: 4) | 2 → Y (57.14 %) (N: 3, Y: 4) |
| | | 3 → Y(66.67 %) (N: 3, Y: 6) | 4 → Y (60 %) (N: 4, Y: 6) |

**Table 5.** Analytical result explanation two

| Condition | Explanation |
|---|---|
| Patients who have barrenness without being pregnant before | Although the number of samples is limited and it is hard to evaluate the result, comparing the recovery probability of 23.08 % who take the alcohol treatment with 40 % who don't take we will find these patients are not suitable for the treatment. However, when it comes to 50 % who take the treatment for less than 10 min and 18.18 % who take the treatment for long than 10 min, we know that these patients are not suitable for taking alcohol treatment longer than 10 min, not conforming to other researches |
| Patients who have barrenness with being pregnant before | Although the percentage of recovery is low; we still discover that when the treatment lasts for longer than 10 min, the probability of recovery would reach to 46.15 % higher than those limited in 10 min with 33.33 % agreeing with other researches. So these patients are suitable for alcohol treatment lasting longer than 10 min |
| Patients who have no barrenness with being pregnant before | Although the recovery of being treated for less than 10 min reaches 100 %, there still need to collect more data to ensure this result. The more is that patients who take more than 10 min get a better recovery. So this group is suitable for treatment longer than 10 min |
| Patients who have no barrenness without being pregnant before | Having big differences in recovery. When treating time less than 10 min, the percentage of recovery shares only 50 % comparing to 63.15 % those treated longer than 10 min with clear curative effect. Thus, these patients need to accept treatment for longer than 10 min |

## 5   Conclusion

According to the integrating result from last section, patients who have barrenness with normal CA value and patients who have barrenness but used to be pregnant are not suitable for alcohol treatment. For other patients, it seems to be effective to cure the disease while taking alcohol treatment for longer than 10 min. However, is it the best to take the treatment for longer than 10 min? or is there a time line for treatment when exceeds the line, the curative effect comes to be best? Whether there exist side-effects in this treatment or exceeds how many minutes would form a side-effect? All these questions may be answered if we can access more samples and carry out a deeper research with analyses on more research columns.

We plan to continue the cooperation with hospitals, program to construct a data mining oriented database, develop software which helps to collect data increasing the number of samples to find out the characteristics of clinical diseases and make use of the following indexes to do analyses, including: improving CA exponent within normal range, second-time extraction rate, second-time operation rate, tumor size within normal size, improving tumor size within normal range, ache within normal range, improving ache within normal range and so on. By transforming all the above indexes and some other data into useful results, we have faith to make it a good reference for clinical doctors to achieve a higher percentage of curative effect and a better medical quality.

# References

1. Prather, J.C., Lobach, D.F., Goodwin, L.K., Hales, J.W., Hage, M.L., Hammond, W.E.: Medical data mining: knowledge discovery in a clinical data warehouse (1997)
2. Yu, K.-Y.: Taipei Veterans General Hospital gynecology area. http://www.vghtpe.gov.tw
3. Kuo, C.: Health library. http://health.wedar.com
4. Huang, S.-P.: To Analysis the Relapse of Endometriosis's Patient Treated with Ultrasound Guided Aspiration of Ovarian Endometrioma and Ethanol Sclerotherapy by Using Decision Tree, June 2007
5. Huang, T.L.: The application of data mining in the study of customer relationship management in life insurance — using t assurance broker company as an example (2001)
6. Berry, M.J., Linoff, G.: Data Mining Techniques: for Marketing, Sales, and Customer Support. Wiley, New York (1997)
7. Ho, T.: Discovering and using knowledge from unsupervised data. Decis. Support Syst. **21**, 29–42 (1997)
8. Chen, C.-Y.: An Efficient Algorithm for Association Rule with Disjunctive Consequent- The Case of the Insurance Industry, June 2006
9. Yang, Y.-K.: Use Closed Itemset Lattices for Mining and Analyzing the Users' Browsing Behavior, pp. 6–7 (2001)
10. J. Pract. Med. **20**(11) (2004)
11. Guangdong Med. J. **22**(1) (2001)
12. Guangxi Med. J. **24**(9) (2001)
13. Wu, K.-C.: The Application of Data Mining fo Medical Database (2000)
14. Lai, S.-P.: Analyzing Behaviors of WIFLY customers using Data Mining techniques, June 2007

# A Dynamic Feature Selection Based LDA Approach to Baseball Pitch Prediction

Phuong Hoang[1]([✉]), Michael Hamilton[2], Joseph Murray[3], Corey Stafford[2], and Hien Tran[1]

[1] North Carolina State University, Raleigh, NC 27695, USA
{phoang,tran}@ncsu.edu
[2] Columbia University, New York, NY 10027, USA
jmurray@zerofox.com, {mh346,css2165}@columbia.edu
[3] ZeroFOX, Baltimore, MD 21230, USA

**Abstract.** Baseball, which is one of the most popular sports in the world, has a uniquely discrete gameplay structure. This stop-and-go style of play creates a natural ability for fans and observers to record information about the game in progress, resulting in a wealth of data that is available for analysis. Major League Baseball (MLB), the professional baseball league in the US and Canada, uses a system known as PITCHf/x to record information about every individual pitch that is thrown in league play. We extend the classification to pitch prediction (fastball or nonfastball) by restricting our analysis to pre-pitch features. By performing significant feature analysis and introducing a novel approach for feature selection, moderate improvement over published results is achieved.

**Keywords:** Machine learning · Hypothesis testing · Feature selection · Pitch prediction · PITCHf/x · MLB · LDA · ROC

## 1 Introduction

One area of statistical analysis of baseball that has gained attention in the last decade is pitch analysis. Studying pitch performance allows baseball teams to develop more successful pitching routines and batting strategies. To aid this study, baseball pitch data produced by the PITCHf/x system is now widely available for both public and private use. PITCHf/x is a pitch tracking system that allows measurements to be recorded and associated with every pitch thrown in Major League Beaseball (MLB) games. The system, which was installed in every MLB stadium circa 2006, records useful information for every pitch thrown in a game such as the initial velocity, plate velocity, release point, spin angle, spin rate, and pitch type (e.g., fastball, curveball, changeup, knuckleball, etc.). The pitch type is a value reported by PITCHf/x using a proprietary classification algorithm. Because of the large number of MLB games (2430) in a season and the high number of pitches thrown in a game (an average of 146 pitches), PITCHf/x

© Springer International Publishing Switzerland 2015
X.-L. Li et al. (Eds.): PAKDD 2015, LNCS 9441, pp. 125–137, 2015.
DOI: 10.1007/978-3-319-25660-3_11

system provides a rich data set on which to train and evaluate methodologies for pitch classification and prediction. The pitch analysis can either be performed using the measurements provided by PITCHf/x in their raw forms or using features derived from the raw data. Because each of the recorded pitches has a pre-assigned pitch classification provided with measurement data, a comparison between the proprietary PITCHf/x classification algorithm, which is assumed to generally represent truth, and other classification methods is possible. For example, in [2,3], several classification algorithms including support vector machine (SVM) and Bayesian classifiers were used to classify pitch types based on features derived from PITCHf/x data. The authors evaluated classification algorithms both on accuracy, as compared to the truth classes provided by PITCHf/x, and speed. In addition, linear discrimination analysis and principal component analysis were used to evaluate feature dimension reduction useful for classification. The pitch classification was evaluated using a set of pitchers' data from the 2011 MLB regular season. Another important area of ongoing research is pitch prediction, which could have significant real-world applications and potentially provides MLB managers with the statistical competitive edge to make crucial decisions during the game. One example of research on this topic is the work by [7], who use a linear support vector machine (SVM) to perform binary (*fastball* vs. *nonfastball*) classification on pitches of unknown type. The SVM is trained on PITCHf/x data from pitches thrown in 2008 and tested on data from 2009. Across all pitchers, an average prediction accuracy of roughly 70 percent is obtained, though pitcher-specific accuracies vary.

In this paper, we provide a machine learning approach to pitch predictions, using linear discriminant analysis (LDA) to predict binary pitch types (*fastball* vs. *nonfastball*). A novel and distinct feature of our approach is the introduction of an adaptive strategy to features selection to mimic portions of pitchers' cognition. This allows the machine learning algorithm to select different sets of features (depending on different situations) to train the classifiers. Features that are used contain not only original features but also hybrid features (that are created to better resemble the way of *data processing* by pitchers). Finally, cross validation is implemented to detect and avoid overfitting in our predictions. Overall, the prediction accuracy has been significantly improved by approximately 8 % from results published in [7]. A report of our initial effort in this study can be found in [8].

It is noted that the proposed methodology can be applied for pitch prediction of various pitch types (other than fastball or nonfastball). However, for other pitch types (curveball, slider, knuckleball, etc.) the data set is not sufficiently large to carry out the analysis. Hence, in this paper, we only study pitch prediction for fastball versus nonfastball.

This paper is organized as follows. Section 2 describes pitch data that are used in this study. In Sect. 3, we present our adaptive approach to feature selection and dimension reduction. Pitch prediction results are presented in Sect. 5 and conclusion is presented in Sect. 6.

## 2   Pitch Data

In this study, we used pitch data created by Sportvision's PITCHf/x pitch tracking system. We conduct our analysis over the period of 5 seasons from 2008 to 2012 with over 3.5 millions observations (pitches); each contains about 50 features (quantitative and qualitative). We only use 18 features from the raw data (see Table 1), and create additional features that we believed to be more relevant to pitch prediction. The reason is simply that classification uses post-pitch information about a pitch to determine which type it is, whereas prediction uses pre-pitch information to classify its type. We may use features like pitch speed and curve angle of that pitch to determine whether or not it was a fastball. These features are not available pre-pitch; in that case we use information about prior results from the same scenario to judge which pitch can be expected. Some created features are: the percentage of fastballs thrown in the previous inning,

**Table 1.** Description of original attributes selected for pitch prediction

| No | Variable | Description |
|----|----------|-------------|
| 1 | *atbat_num* | number of pitchers recorded against a specific batter |
| 2 | *outs* | number of outs during an at-bat |
| 3 | *batter* | batter's unique identification number |
| 4 | *pitcher* | pitcher's unique identification number |
| 5 | *stand* | dominant hand of batter; left/right |
| 6 | *p_throws* | pitching hand of pitcher; left/right |
| 7 | *des* | out come of one pitch from pitcher's perspective; ball/strike/foul/in-play, etc. |
| 8 | *event* | outcome of at-bat from batter's perspective; ground-out/double/single/walk, etc. |
| 9 | *pitch_type* | classification of pitch type; FF= Four-seam Fastball, SL = Slider, etc., |
| 10 | *sv_id* | date/time stamp of the pitch; YYMMDD_ hhmmss |
| 11 | *start_speed* | pitch speed, miles per hour |
| 12 | *px* | horizontal distance of the pitch from the home plate |
| 13 | *pz* | vertical distance, of the pitch from the home plate |
| 14 | *on_first* | binary column; display 1 if runner on first, 0 otherwise |
| 15 | *on_second* | binary column; display 1 if runner on second, 0 otherwise |
| 16 | *on_third* | binary column; display 1 if runner on third, 0 otherwise. |
| 17 | *type_confidence* | likelihood of the pitch type being correctly classified |
| 18 | *ball_strike* | display either ball or strike |

the velocity of the previous pitch, strike result percentage of previous pitch, and current game count (score). For a full list of features that were used in our study, see Appendix.

## 3  Adaptive Feature Selection

A key difference between our approach and former research of [7] is the feature selection methodology. Rather than using one static set of optimal features (for example, [7]), an adaptive set of features is used for each pitcher/count pair. This allows the algorithm to adapt to achieve the best prediction performance result as possible on each pitcher/count pair of data.

In baseball there are a number of factors that influence the pitcher's decision (consciously or unconsciously). For example, one pitcher may not like to throw curveballs during the daytime because the increased visibility makes them easier to spot; however, another pitcher may not make his pitching decisions based on the time of the game. In order to maximize accuracy of a prediction model, one must try to accommodate each of these factors. For example, a pitcher may have particularly good control of a certain pitch and thus favors that pitch, but how can one create a feature to represent its favorability? One could, for example, create a feature that measures the pitcher's success with a pitch since the beginning of the season, or the previous game, or even the previous batter faced. Which features would best capture the true effect of his preference for that pitch? The answer is that each of these approaches may be best in different situations, so they all must be considered for best accuracy. Pitchers have different dominant pitches, strategies and experiences; in order to maximize accuracy our model must be adaptable to various pitching situations.

Of course, simply adding many features to our model is not necessarily the best choice because one might run into issues with curse of dimensionality. In addition, some features might not be relevant to the pitch prediction. Our approach is to change the problem of predicting a pitch into predicting a pitch for each given pitcher in a given count. Count, which gives the number of balls and strikes in a at bat situation, has a significant effect on the pitcher/batter relationship. For example, study by [10] showed that average slugging percentage (a weighted measure of the on-base frequency of a batter) is significantly lower in counts that favor the pitcher; however, for neutral counts or counts that favor the batter, there is no significant difference in average slugging percentage. In addition, [7] concluded that pitcher are much more predictable when there are more balls than strikes. These studies showed that count is an important factor in making pitch prediction. In order to maximize accuracy in pitch prediction, in our study we took an additional step by choosing (for each pitcher/count pair) a most relevant pool of features from the entire available set. This allows us to maintain our adaptive strategy while controlling dimensionality.

## 3.1 Implementation

As discussed above, our feature selection algorithm is adaptive; that is, finding a good set of features for each pitcher/count situation. The implementation of this adaptive strategy mainly consists of the following 3 steps.

1. First, we select a subset of features (18) from the raw data and create additional features (59) from the data that are deemed more relevant to pitch prediction. This set of 76 features is further divided into 6 groups of similar features. The number of features from each group varies from as small as 6 to 22 features (see the full list in the Appendix).
2. Second, we then compute the receiver operating characteristic (ROC) curve for each group of features, then select the most useful features for pitch prediction. In practice, selecting only the best feature provides worse prediction than selecting the best two or three features. Hence, at this stage, the size of each group is reduced from 6–22 features to 1–10 features.
3. Third, we remove all redundant features from our final feature set. From our grouping, features are taken based on their relative strength. There is the possibility that a group of features might not have good predictive power. In those instances, we want to prune them from our feature set before we begin to predict. The resulting set of features is pruned by conducting hypothesis testing to measure significance of each feature at the $\alpha = .01$ level.

The above 3 steps in our adaptive feature selection approach is summarized and depicted in Fig. 1.

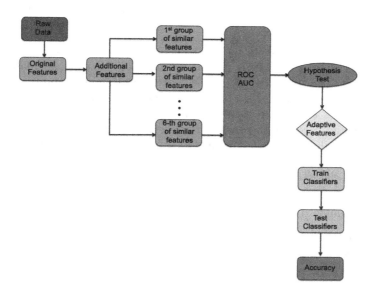

**Fig. 1.** Schematic diagram of the proposed adaptive features selection.

## 3.2   ROC Curves

Receiver operating characteristic (ROC) curves are two-dimensional graphs that are commonly used to visualize and select classifiers based on their performance [6]. They have been used in many applications including signal detection theory [5] and diagnostic tools in clinical medicine [11,12]. It is noted that a common method to determine the performance of classifiers is to calculate the area under the ROC curve, often denoted by AUC [4]. An example of a ROC curve using data from PITCHf/x pitch tracking system is depicted in Fig. 2.

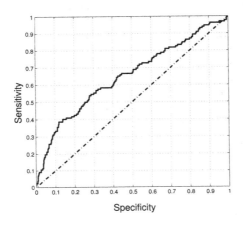

**Fig. 2.** ROC curve for a specific feature selected for pitch prediction

In this study, ROC curves are used for each individual feature in order to measure how useful a feature is for the pitch prediction. We calculate this by measuring the area between the single feature ROC curve and the diagonal line represents the strategy of random guessing. This value of area quantifies how much better the feature is at distinguishing the two classes, compared to random guessing. Because the area under the diagonal line from (0,0) to (1,1) is 0.5, these area values are in the range of $[0, 0.5)$, where a value of 0 represents no improvement over random guessing and 0.5 would represent perfect distinction between both classes.

## 3.3   Hypothesis Testing

The ability of a feature to distinguish between two classes can be verified by using a hypothesis test. Given any feature $f$, we compare $\mu_1$ and $\mu_2$, the mean values of $f$ in Class 1 (*fastballs*) and Class 2 (*nonfastballs*), respectively. Then we consider

$$H_0 : \mu_1 = \mu_2, \tag{1}$$

$$H_A : \mu_1 \neq \mu_2, \tag{2}$$

and conduct a hypothesis test using the student's $t$ distribution. We compare the $p$-value of the test against a significance level of $\alpha = .01$. When the $p$-value is less than $\alpha$, we reject the null hypothesis and conclude that the studied feature means are different for each class, meaning that the feature is significant in separating the classes. In that sense, this test allows us to remove features which have insignificant separation power.

## 4 Linear Discriminant Analysis

Classification is the process of taking an unlabeled data observation and using some rule or decision-making process to assign a label to it. In this study, we use classification for pitch prediction (fastball or nonfastball) using pre-pitch features. There are several classifications one can use to accomplish this task, we selected Linear Discriminant Analysis (LDA) [9] for this binary classification study.

The Linear Discriminant Analysis (LDA) classifier assumes that the observations within each class $k$ are generated from a Gaussian (or normal) distribution with a class-specific mean vector $\mu_k$'s and a common variance $\sigma_k^2$'s. Estimates for these parameters are substituted into the Bayes classifier results in LDA.

Assume that we only have one predictor (or feature) in a $K$-class classification problem. Then Bayes' theorem states that

$$\Pr(Y = k | X = x) = \frac{\pi_k f_k(x)}{\sum_{l=1}^{K} \pi_l f_l(x)} \tag{3}$$

where

1. $\pi_k$ represent the prior probability that a randomly chosen observation is associated with the $k$-th class,
2. $f_k(X) \equiv \Pr(X = x | Y = k)$ denotes the density function of $X$ for an observation that comes from $k$-th class
3. We will use the abbreviation $p_k(X) = \Pr(Y = k | X)$ is referred as the posterior probability that an observation $X = x$ belongs to the $k$-th class.
4. If we can compute all the terms for (3), we would then easily classify an observation to the class for which $p_k(X)$ is largest.

Since $f_k(x)$ is Gaussian, the normal density takes the form

$$f_k(x) = \frac{1}{\sqrt{2\pi}\sigma_k} \exp\left( -\frac{1}{2\sigma_k^2} (x - \mu_k)^2 \right). \tag{4}$$

Substitute (4) into (3) under assumption that $\sigma_k^2 \equiv \sigma^2$, taking the log and rearranging the terms, we find that this is equivalent to

$$\delta_k(x) = x \cdot \frac{\mu_k}{\sigma^2} - \frac{\mu_k^2}{2\sigma_k^2} + \log(\pi_k). \tag{5}$$

The LDA method approximates the Bayes classifier by substitute the following estimates for $\pi_k$, $\mu_k$ and $\sigma^2$ into (5)

$$\hat{\pi}_k = \frac{n_k}{n}$$

$$\hat{\mu}_k = \frac{1}{n_k} \sum_{i:y_i=k} x_i$$

$$\hat{\sigma}^2 = \frac{1}{n-K} \sum_{k=1}^{K} \sum_{i:y_i=k} (x_i - \hat{\mu}_k)^2,$$

where $n$ is the total number of training observations and $n_k$ is the number of training observations in $k$-th class. After the LDA procedure, (5) becomes

$$\hat{\delta}_k(x) = x \cdot \frac{\hat{\mu}_k}{\hat{\sigma}^2} - \frac{\hat{\mu}_k^2}{2\hat{\sigma}_k^2} + \log(\hat{\pi}_k). \tag{6}$$

The LDA classifier can be extended to multiple predictors. To do this, we assume that $X = (X_1, X_2, ..., X_p)$ is drawn from a multivariate Gaussian distribution with a class-specific mean vector and common covariance matrix.

The formulas for estimating the unknown parameters $\pi_k$, $\mu_k$, and $\Sigma$ are similar to the one dimensional case. To assign an observation $X = x$, LDA assigns the class label for which discrimination function $\hat{\delta}_k(x)$ is largest. The word *linear* in the classifier's name comes from the fact that these discrimination functions are linear functions of $x$.

## 5    Results

To form a baseline for our prediction results, we compare our prediction model against the naive guess model. The naive guess simply return the most frequent pitch type thrown by each pitcher, calculated from the training set, see [7]. The improvement factor $I$ is calculated as follow

$$I = \frac{A_1 - A_0}{A_0} \times 100, \tag{7}$$

where $A_0$ and $A_1$ denotes the accuracies of naive guess and our model, respectively.

In order to avoid possible overfitting issue, we applied cross validation, a common strategy for model validation and selection [1]. In specific, the repeated subsampling cross validation was used in our baseball pitch prediction as follows: in each pitcher-count training set with more than 15 pitches in the training set we split the training set randomly in half (e.g., if there are 20 pitches, we randomly pick ten of them. The remaining ten becomes the test set.) We then predict with this training set and compare to the actual class membership. We do this ten times for each pitcher-count training set and take the average accuracy of the ten tests.

We conduct prediction for all pitchers who had at least 750 pitches in both 2008 and 2009. After performing feature selection (see Sect. 3) on each data subset, each classifier is trained on each subset of data from 2008 and tested on each subset of data from 2009. The average classification accuracy for each classifier is computed for test points with a type confidence of at least 80 %.

**Table 2.** Baseball pitch prediction results comparison. Note that percentage improvement is calculated on a per-pitcher basis rather than overall average

| Author | Training | Testing | Classifier | Accuracy | Cross Validation | Improvement |
|--------|----------|---------|------------|----------|------------------|-------------|
| J.Guttag | 2008 | 2009 | SVM | 70.00 | . | 18.00 |
| This study | 2008 | 2009 | LDA | 77.97 | 77.21 | 21.00 |
| This study | 2011 | 2012 | LDA | 76.08 | 75.20 | 24.82 |
| This study | 2010 and 2011 | 2012 | LDA | 76.27 | 75.54 | 24.07 |

Table 2 depicts the average accuracy among all pitches in 2008–2009 season, our model attained 78 %. Compared to the naive model's natural prediction accuracy, our model on average performs 21 % improvement. In previous work, the average prediction accuracy of 2008–2009 season is 70 % with 18 % improvement over naive guessing [7]. It should be noted that previous work only use SVM classifier and considers 359 pitchers who threw at least 300 pitches in both 2008 and 2009 seasons.

With cross validation implemented, the prediction accuracy slightly decreased by less than 1 %. In addition, applying this model on new data set from 2010, 2011 and 2012 season, the performance remain stable within ±2 % of the original results. This serves as an important confirmation that our results are reliable and our methods would perform well when applied to a newly introduced data set.

**Table 3.** Prediction results by Type Confidence (TC) levels (for a description of TC see Table 1).

| TC (%) | 50 | 60 | 70 | 80 | 90 | 95 | 99 |
|--------|-----|-----|-----|-----|-----|-----|-----|
| Test size | 355,755 | 344,300 | 332,238 | 312,574 | 196,853 | 24,412 | 7,150 |
| Accuracy | 77.19 | 77.17 | 77.13 | 77.13 | 77.97 | 83.19 | 81.76 |

As shown in Table 3, higher (better) type confidence cut-off thresholds reduces the sizes of testing sets. In fact, majority of test points have 80 % or higher type confidence. There is not a significant reduction in test sizes from 50 % level (355,755) to 80 % level (312,574), hence prediction performances from all methods remain stable throughout these intervals. Only when the cut-off threshold of type confidence are raised to 90 % level, we can notice the reduction in test sizes and the increase in average prediction accuracies among all methods. We obtain even higher average prediction accuracy, 83 % accurated at 95 % level.

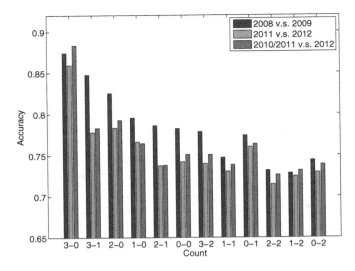

**Fig. 3.** Prediction accuracy by count.

However, there is only 24, 412 pitches at this level, less than 7 % of all pitches from original test set of about 360, 000 pitches, at 0 % level. Hence, we choose 80 % level to be the most reasonable choice to cut-off, which contains more than 50 % of the original test points. Notice that even a low type confidence level of 50 %, this model still outperform formal study [7], results in 77 % accurate.

Figure 3 depicts average prediction accuracy per each count situation. Accuracy is significant higher in batter-favored counts and approximately equal in neutral and pitcher-favored counts. Prediction is best at 3-0 count (89 %) and worst at 1–2 and 2-2 counts (73 %).

**Table 4.** Pitch prediction results for selected pitchers in 2008–2009 season

| Pitcher | Training Size | Testing Size | Prediction Accuracy | Naive Guess | Improvement |
|---------|---------------|--------------|---------------------|-------------|-------------|
| Park | 1309 | 1178 | 72.40 | 52.60 | 37.62 |
| Rivera | 797 | 850 | 93.51 | 89.63 | 0.04 |
| Wakefield | 2110 | 1573 | 100.00 | 100.00 | 0.00 |
| Weathers | 943 | 813 | 77.76 | 35.55 | 118.72 |
| Vaquez | 2412 | 2721 | 73.05 | 51.20 | 42.68 |
| Fuentes | 919 | 798 | 80.15 | 71.05 | 12.81 |
| Meche | 2821 | 1822 | 74.83 | 50.77 | 47.39 |
| Madson | 975 | 958 | 81.85 | 25.56 | 220.23 |

We randomly selected 8 pitchers from 2008 and 2009 seasons to examine in details. Table 4 illustrates average prediction accuracy per pitcher in comparison with Naive guess. For pitchers with only one dominant pitch type such as Wakefield with knucle-ball (nonfast) or Rivera with cutter-ball (fastball), Naive Guess is sufficient to reach almost perfect prediction. However, for pitchers having various pitch types at their disposals such as Weathers or Madson, our model adapt much better with accuracy improvements of 100 % to 200 %. Overall, our model outperforms naive guessing significantly.

## 6   Conclusion

Originally our scheme developed from consideration of the factors that affect pitching decisions. For example, the pitcher/batter handedness matchup is often mentioned by sports experts as an effect ([7,10]), and it was originally included in our model. However, it was discovered that implementing segmentation of data based on handedness has essentially no effect on the prediction results. Thus, handedness is no longer implemented as a further splitting criterion of the model, but this component remains a considered feature. In general, unnecessary data segmentations have negative impact solely because it reduce the size of training and testing data for classifiers to work with.

Most notable is our method of feature selection which widely varies the set of features used in each situation. Features that yield strong prediction in some situations fail to provide any benefit in others. In fact, it is interesting to note that in the 2008 v.s. 2009 prediction scheme, every feature is used in at least one situation and no feature is used in every situation.

It is also interesting to note that the LDA classification algorithm of this model is supported by our feature selection technique. In fact, as a Bayesian classifier, LDA relies on a feature independence assumption, which is realistically not satisfied. However, our model survives this assumption because although the features within each of the 6 groups are highly dependent across groups, the features which are ultimately chosen are highly independent. The model represents a significant improvement over simple guessing. It is a useful tool for batting coaches, batters, and others who wish to understand the potential pitching implications of a given game scenario. For example, batters could theoretically use this model to increase their batting average, assuming that knowledge about a pitch's type makes it easier to hit. The model, for example, is especially useful in certain intense game scenarios and achieves accuracy as high as 90 percent. It is in these game environments that batters can most effectively use this model to translate knowledge into hits.

**Acknowledgements.** Part of this research was supported by NSA grant H98230-12-1-0299 and NSF grants DMS-1063010 and DMS-0943855. The authors would like to thank Lori Layne, David Padget , Brian Lewis and Jessica Gronsbell, all from MIT LL, for their helpful advices and constructive inputs and Mr. Tom Tippett, Director of Baseball Information Services for the Boston Red Sox, for meeting with us to discuss this research and providing us with useful feedback, and Minh Nhat Phan for helping us scrape the PITCH f/x data.

# A    Appendix

From the original 18 features given in Table 1, we generated a total of 76 features and arranged them into 6 groups as follows:

**Group 1**
1. Inning
2. Time (day/afternoon/night)
3. Number of outs
4. Last at bat events
5-7. Pitcher v.s. batter specific: fastball or nonfastball on previous pitch/ lifetime percentage of fastballs/ previous pitch's events
8. Numeric score of previous at bat event
9-11. Player on first base/ second base/ third base (true/false)
12. Number of base runners
13. Weighted base score

**Group 2**
1-3. Percentage of fastball thrown in previous inning/game/at-bat
4. Lifetime percentage of fastballs thrown to a specific batter over all at bats
5-8. Percentage of fastballs over previous 5/10 /15/ 20 pitches
9-10. Previous pitch in specific count: pitch type/ fastball or nonfastball
11-12. Previous 2 or 3 pitches in specific count: fastball/nonfastball combo
13-14. Previous pitch: pitch type/ fastball or nonfastball
15. Previous 2 pitches: fastball/nonfastball combo
16. Player on first base (true/false)
17-18. Percentage of fastballs over previous 10/15 pitches thrown to a specific batter
19-21. Previous 5 /10 /15 pitches in specific count: percentage of fastballs

**Group 3**
1. Previous pitch: velocity
2-3. Previous 2 pitches/ 3 pitches: velocity average
4. Previous pitch in specific count: velocity
5-6. Previous 2 pitches/ 3 pitches in specific count: velocity average

**Group 4**
1-2. Previous pitch: horizontal/ vertical position
3-4. Previous 2 pitches: horizontal/ vertical position average
5-6. Previous 3 pitches: horizontal/vertical position average
7. Previous pitch: zone (Cartesian quadrant)
8-9. Previous 2 pitches/3 pitches: zone (Cartesian quadrant) average
10-11. Previous pitch in specific count: horizontal/vertical position
12-13. Previous 2 pitches in specific count: horizontal/vertical position average
14-15. Previous 3 pitches in specific count: horizontal/vertical position average
16. Previous pitch in specific count: zone (Cartesian quadrant)
17-18. Previous 2 or 3 pitches in specific count: zone (Cartesian quadrant) average

**Group 5**

    1. SRP[1] of fastball thrown in the previous inning

    2. SRP of fastball thrown in the previous game

 3-5. SRP of fastball thrown in the previous 5 pitches/ 10 pitches/ 15 pitches.

    6. SRP of fastball thrown in previous 5 pitches thrown to a specific batter

 7-8. SRP of nonfastball thrown in the previous inning/ previous game

9-11. SRP of nonfastball thrown in the previous 5 pitches/ 10 pitches/ 15 pitches

  12. SRP of nonfastball thrown in previous 5 pitches thrown to a specific batter

**Group 6**

    1. Previous pitch: ball or strike (boolean)

 2-3. Previous 2 pitches/ 3 pitches: ball/strike combo

    4. Previous pitch in specific count: ball or strike

 5-6. Previous 2 pitches/ 3 pitches in specific count: ball/strike combo

# References

1. Arlot, S.: A survey of cross-validation procedures for model selection. Stat. Surv. **4**, 40–79 (2010)
2. Attarian, A., Danis, G., Gronsbell, J., Iervolina, G., Layne, L., Padgett, D., Tran, H.: Baseball pitch classification: a Bayesian method and dimension reduction investigation. IAENG Transactions on Engineering Sciences, pp. 392–399 (2014)
3. Attarian, A., Danis, G., Gronsbell, J., Iervolino, G., Tran, H.: A comparison of feature selection and classification algorithms in identifying baseball pitches. In: International MultiConference of Engineers and Computer Scientists 2013. Lecture Notes in Engineering and Computer Science, pp. 263–268. Newswood Limited (2013)
4. Bradley, A.: The use of the area under the ROC curve in the evaluation of machine learning algorithms. Pattern Recogn. **30**(7), 1145–1159 (1997)
5. Egan, J.: Signal detection theory and ROC analysis. Cognition and Perception. Academic Press, New York (1975)
6. Fawcett, T.: An introduction to ROC analysis. Pattern Recogn. Lett. **27**(8), 861–874 (2006)
7. Ganeshapillai, G., Guttag, J.: Predicting the next pitch. In: MIT Sloan Sports Analytics Conference (2012)
8. Hamilton, M., Hoang, P., Layne, L., Murray, J., Padget, D., Stafford, C., Tran, H.: Applying machine learning techniques to baseball pitch prediction. In: 3rd International Conference on Pattern Recognition Applications and Methods, pp. 520–527. SciTePress (2014)
9. Hastie, T., Tibshirani, R.: The Elements of Statistical Learning. Springer, New York (2009)
10. Hopkins, T., Magel, R.: Slugging percentage in differing baseball counts. J. Quant. Anal. Sports **4**(2), 1136 (2008)
11. Swets, J., Dawes, R., Monahan, J.: Better decisions through science. Sci. Am. **283**, 82–87 (2000)
12. Zweig, M.H., Campbell, G.: Receiver-operating characteristic ROC plots: a fundamental evaluation tool in clinical medicine. Clin. Chem. **39**(4), 561–577 (1993)

---

[1] Strike-result percentage (SRP): a metric we created that measures the percentage of strikes from all pitches in the given situation.

# Quality Issues, Measures
# of Interestingness and Evaluation
# of Data Mining Models

# A Study of Interestingness Measures for Associative Classification on Imbalanced Data

Guangfei Yang[✉] and Xuejiao Cui

School of Management Science and Engineering,
Dalian University of Technology, Dalian, China
gfyang@dlut.edu.cn, xjcui@mail.dlut.edu.cn

**Abstract.** Associative Classification (AC) is a well known tool in knowledge discovery and it has been proved to extract competitive classifiers. However, imbalanced data has posed a challenge for most classifier learning algorithms including AC methods. Because in the AC process, Interestingness Measure (IM) plays an important role to generate interesting rules and build good classifiers, it is very important to select IMs for improving AC's performance in the context of imbalanced data. In this paper, we aim at improving AC's performance on imbalanced data through studying IMs. To achieve this, there are two main tasks to be settled. The first one is to find which measures have similar behaviors on imbalanced data. The second is to select appropriate measures. We evaluate each measure's performance by AUC which is usually used for evaluation of imbalanced data classification. Firstly, based on the performances, we propose a frequent correlated patterns mining method to extract stable clusters in which the IMs have similar behaviors. Secondly, we find 26 proper measures for imbalanced data after the IM ranking computation method and divide them into two groups with one especially for extremely imbalanced data and the other suitable for slightly imbalanced data.

**Keywords:** Associative classification · Imbalanced data · Interestingness measure · Stable clusters · Ranking computation

## 1 Introduction

Associative Classification (AC) is a branch of a larger area of scientific study known as data mining. In the last few years, association rule discovery methods have been successfully used to build accurate classifiers, which have resulted in a branch of AC mining [1, 2]. One of the main advantages of AC approaches is that the output is represented in simple if-then rules, which makes it easy for the end-user to understand and interpret it. Moreover, unlike decision tree algorithms, one can update or tune a rule in AC without affecting the complete rule sets. However, imbalanced data has posed a serious difficulty to AC algorithms [2–4], which assume a relatively balanced class distribution. Data can be divided into imbalanced data and balanced data according to their class distributions. For binary class data, class distribution can be defined as the ratio of the number of rare class samples to that of the prevalent class.

© Springer International Publishing Switzerland 2015
X.-L. Li et al. (Eds.): PAKDD 2015, LNCS 9441, pp. 141–151, 2015.
DOI: 10.1007/978-3-319-25660-3_12

Although existing knowledge discovery and data engineering techniques have shown great success in many real-world applications, the problem of learning from imbalanced data is a relatively new challenge that has attracted growing attention from both academic and industry [5, 6].

During the AC process, Interestingness Measure (IM) plays an important role to discover interesting rules. It can be applied to rule generation, filtering and ranking phases to generate good classifiers. So it is very important to select proper IMs for improving AC method in dealing with imbalanced data. In this paper, we select Classification Based on Associations (CBA) [2] as the basic algorithm to complete the associative classification process. It is a classical associative classification method. To improve its performance on imbalanced data, two main tasks should be settled. The first one is to find those measures with similar behaviors in imbalanced data classification. The second is to select appropriate measures for imbalanced data. What's more, different from relevant researches, we adopt AUC as the classifier evaluation measure instead of the traditional measure Accuracy, which assumes a balanced framework and has a bias to the majority classes. AUC is usually used for imbalanced data classification and it can be directly regarded as the performance of a classifier generated by a certain IM. So we can select IMs according to their AUC values rather than the domain knowledge. In our paper, we propose a frequent correlated patterns mining process and a IM ranking computation method to extract stable clusters in which the IMs have similar behaviors in the condition of imbalanced data, and proper IMs for imbalanced data.

The rest of the paper is organized as follows. In Sect. 2, related work will be described. In Sect. 3, we will introduce our method in detail. In Sect. 4, the experiment is conducted and subsequent analysis will be given. In Sect. 5, a conclusion about our work will be summarized and a further study will be introduced.

## 2   Related Work

A number of studies, theoretical, empirical, or both, have been conducted to provide insight into the properties and behaviors of IMs. Tan et al. [7] analyzed the correlations among IMs, introduced new measures and presented some properties to select measures in 2004. In 2007, Huynh et al. [8] proposed the clustering of IMs based on ranking behavior. In the same year, Lallich et al. [9] analyzed IMs' relationships from a theoretical standpoint. Lenca et al. [10] designed a multi-criteria decision system to select IMs based on both theoretical properties and empirical results in 2008. Abe and Tsumoto [11] studied IMs' behaviors in the context of classification, proposed a different approach where they average interestingness values over sets of rules first and computed correlations in 2008. Sahar [12] made a distinction between objective and subjective IMs in 2010. In the same year, Wu et al. [13] argued against the sensitivity of IMs to null transactions. In 2010, the analysis of Jalali-Heravi and Zaïane [14] was in the context of association classifiers. They focus on the impact of the choice of IMs in each phase: rule generation/pruning and rule selection. Tew et al. [15] analyzed the rule-ranking behavior of IMs. They highlighted and proved unreported equivalences among IMs in 2014. In 2006, Arunasalam and Chawla [16] proposed a new measure, the "Complement Class Support (CCS)" which can guarantee the generated rules positively correlated. It is the first IM for imbalanced data. For imbalanced data classification, most researches focus on data preprocessing, algorithm improvement and cost-sensitive learning [6, 7]. There are no relevant conclusions about IMs for imbalanced data. Because of the significant role of IMs at improving AC's performance, it is more necessary to study IMs in the context of imbalanced data.

# 3   Method

## 3.1   Stable Clusters Mining

This part discusses mining stable clusters in different imbalanced data sets. First, the Graph-based Clustering [17] is adopted here to deliver clustering for IMs on different imbalanced data sets. As graphs are a good means to offer relevant visual insights on data structure, the correlation matrix of IMs is used as the relation of an undirect and valued graph, called "Correlation Graph" (*CG*). In a correlation graph, a vertex represents an IM and an edge value is the correlation between two vertices. When the absolute correlation value between two IMs is greater than or equal to a minimal threshold $\tau$ (0.9 is widely accepted in the literature), they are regarded to be $\tau - correlated$. These $\tau - correlated$ edges are retained and the formed subgraphs are denoted by *CG+*. Then each cluster of IMs is defined as a connected subgraph. This IMs deliver a close point of view on data. After using the graph-based clustering method, we can get *CG+* graphs of different data sets. In order to filter those stable clusters which occur frequently in different data sets, we propose a frequent correlated patterns mining method which borrows the thought of frequent item mining from Apriori algorithm and is illustrated in Fig. 1.

However, the frequent items mining process is computationally demanding, because the database is scanned in each iteration. To enhance efficiency, we divide this frequent correlated patterns mining process into two stages: (1) each distinct cluster is counted first according to its frequency in different *CG+* graphs. (2) in frequent $k$-item patterns mining process, the support of each candidate pattern can be calculated by using the results of step (1) rather than scanning the whole database. For instance, there are two clusters {I1, I2, I5} and {I1, I2, I3}. Their frequencies are separately 2 and 3. Then the support of candidate {I1, I2} is 5, which is the sum of the frequencies of its supersets. So in this process, we need to scan the database only once, which saves a lot of calculation.

In Fig. 1, each distinct subgraph (cluster) is counted according to its frequency in $G$ from line 1–2. In line 3, the candidate one item patterns are selected from $G$. From line 4 to 6, each candidate is counted according to the support values of the clusters which it belongs to, and only those with support values greater than or equal to *minsup* can be retained in $L_1$. When $k \geq 2$, the candidate $k$-item patterns set $C_k$ is generated from $L_{k-1}$ through *apriori_gen*() method in line 14–22. In *apriori_gen*(), $C_k$ is created through $L_{k-1}$'s self-join. During the candidate generation process, the Apriori property indicated in *has_* inf *requent_subset*() from line 23 to 26 is applied to prune those candidates with infrequent subsets. From line 9 to 11, we can get each candidate's

**Input:** $G$: the set of $CG+$ graphs from different data sets; *minsup*: the minimum frequency that a pattern of IMs occur in $G$.

```
1. for each distinct subgraph g ∈ G
2.    g.count++;
3.  C₁ = find _ candidate _ 1 _patterns(G);
4. for each candidate c ∈ C₁
```
5.    $c.count = \sum g.count$, where $c = subset\ (g)$;

6.  $L_1 = \{c \mid c \in C_1 \wedge c.count \geq \min sup\}$;

7. for $(k=2; L_{k-1} \neq \emptyset; k++)\{$

8.    $C_k = apriori\_gen\ (L_{k-1})$;

9.    for each candidate $c \in C_k$

10.      $c.count = \sum g.count$, where $c = subset\ (g)$;

11.    $L_k = \{c \mid c.count \geq \min sup\}$;

```
12. }
```
13. return $L = \cup_k L_k$;

procedure $apriori\_gen\ (L_{k-1} : frequent\ (k-1)\ pattern)$

14. for each pattern $l_1 \in L_{k-1}$

15.    for each pattern $l_2 \in L_{k-1}$

16.      if $(l_1[1] = l_2[1]) \wedge \cdots \wedge (l_1[k-2] = l_2[k-2]) \wedge (l_1[k-1] \prec l_2[k-1])$ then

17.        { $c = l_1 \bowtie l_2$;

18.          if $has\_inf requent\_subset\ (c, L_{k-1})$ then

```
19.             delete c;
```
20.          else add $c$ to $C_k$;

```
21.      }
```
22. return $C_k$;

```
Procedure
has_infrequent_subset(
```
$c : candidate\ \ k\ pattern;\ L_{k-1} : frequent\ (k-1)\ pattern)$

23. for each $(k-1)$ subset $s$ of $c$

24.    if $s \notin L_{k-1}$ then

```
25.       return TRUE;
26.    return FALSE;
```
**Output:** $L$: frequent correlated patterns.

**Fig. 1.** Pseudocode of the frequent correlated patterns mining algorithm

support according to $G$ and only those with frequency above or equal to *minsup* can be kept in $L_k$. In line 13, all the frequent correlated patterns are generated. Then stable clusters can be gotten after integrating the frequent patterns in $L$.

### 3.2    Interestingness Measures Selection

In this section, we give a method for selecting suitable IMs for imbalanced data and analyzing the relationship among these measures. Our method comes from the common sense that an IM with the best performance can be selected for a certain application. We give the IM ranking computation process in Fig. 2. From line 1 to 6, ten subsets with different class distributions are sampled from each data set $d \in D$. To get more reliable experiment results, such sampling process will be repeated for ten times for $d$. Then we can get 100 sampled subsets from $d$ just like $d_{s_k}$, which means the subset with the class distribution $0.1 \times s$ and sampled at the $k_{th}$ time. In line 7–12, the performances of classifiers with certain measures are evaluated by AUC on each sampled data set. From line 13 to 17, $p_{i,s}$, which is the average AUC value of measure $i$ under class distribution $0.1 \times s$ is calculated. From this process, we can get all the IMs' average performances over $D$ under each class distribution. For each class distribution, we rank such IMs according to their performances in line 18. Since we will study how an IM performs compared with others when class distribution ranges from 0.1 to 1.0, we opt to change the absolute performance values into relative performance ranks. In a ranking list $P_s$, the IMs with the same performance value are assigned with an average value of what

---

**Input:** $D$: a set of data sets; $I$: a set of Interestingness Measures.
```
1.  for d∈ D
2.    for (k=1;k<=10;k++)
3.      for (s=1;s<=10;s++) d_{s_k} =sample(d);
4.      end
5.    end
6.  end
7.  for d∈ D
8.    for i ∈ I
9.       Classifier(i, d_{s_k}) ← CBA(i, d_{s_k});
10.      AUC(i, d_{s_k}) ← utilize Classifier(i, d_{s_k});
11.  end
12. end
13. for (s=1;s<=10;s++) do
14. for i ∈ I
15.    p_{i,s} ←Average over D of AUC(i, d_{s_k});
16.  end
17. end
18. Order P_s = (p_{1,s}, p_{2,s}, p_{3,s}, ..., p_{n,s})^T;
19. Create rank list R_s of I by replacing the above
values by the corresponding ranks.
```
**Output:** Ranking lists of IMs under ten different class distributions.

**Variables:** $0.1 \times s$ is a certain class distribution; $n$ is the number of IMs in $I$.

**Fig. 2.**  Interestingness measure ranking computation

their ranks would be. For example, if the AUC values are 0.9, 0.7, 0.7, 0.6, 0.6, and 0.5, then the resulting ranks would be 1, 2.5, 2.5, 4.5, 4.5, and 6. In line 19, the rank lists $R_s$ can be obtained by replacing the average AUC values by rank values. After this process, the top ten IMs under each class distribution will be chosen for imbalanced data classification.

## 4  Experimental Results

### 4.1  Experimental Set-Up

In this work, nine typical imbalanced data sets are selected from UCI repository [18]. The features of these data sets will be described from the number of items (#item) (which represents attribute threshold), the number of instances (#instance) and Class Distribution (the ratio of minor class to major class) in Table 1. To make our results more reliable, we conduct a sampling process from the nine data sets and get 100 sampled subsets with different class distributions for each data set and finally have 900 subsets.

**Table 1.** Data sets description

| Dataset | #item | #instance | Class distribution |
|---|---|---|---|
| breast | 20 | 699 | 0.53 |
| cylBands | 124 | 540 | 0.73 |
| hepatitis | 56 | 155 | 0.26 |
| pima | 38 | 768 | 0.54 |
| ticTacToe | 29 | 958 | 0.53 |
| adult | 97 | 48842 | 0.31 |
| mushroom | 90 | 8124 | 0.93 |
| ionosphere | 157 | 351 | 0.56 |
| horseColic | 85 | 368 | 0.59 |

In this paper, we select 55 well known IMs just as summarized in Appendix. In our work, we have been careful to go back to and read the relevant papers about the measures and select 55 classical IMs with different formulas. Because of the limitation of the paper length, the detailed information and references are not listed.

### 4.2  Analysis of Results

(A)  Stable Clusters and Analysis. After using the graph-based clustering method, we get *CG+* graphs of different data sets in Fig. 3. In a *CG+* graph, a vertex represents an IM and an edge value is the correlation between two vertices. Each subgraph represents a cluster in which the IMs are $\tau - correlated$ ($\tau = 0.9$). From this figure, we can see that the number of clusters and the inner-connection structures of IMs for different data sets are different. Considering that there may be some such measures which are strongly correlated under most of the cases, we conduct the frequent correlated patterns mining method in Fig. 1 to get those generally strongly correlated IMs, called as stable clusters. In this process, we borrow the thought of frequent items mining from Apriori to find those measures frequently occurring in one cluster in the nine $CG+$ graphs in Fig. 3. We set the frequency threshold *minsup* as 8 and mine those patterns of IMs which have occurred in the same cluster for at least eight times. Finally, we can obtain seven stable clusters illustrated in Table 2. They represent seven patterns of IMs which occur at least eight times in nine CG+ graphs and the IMs of a stable cluster are $\tau - correlated$ ($\tau = 0.9$).

In cluster $C_1$, $C_2$, $C_3$ and $C_4$, we can find the equivalent IMs which have been proved by Tew et al. [15], indicating the correction of our clustering result. They are separately {CON, ECR, GAN}, {JAC, KU1}, {YQ, YY, OR}, {IG, LIF}. Apart from that, we can supply something new among the IMs' correlations in the

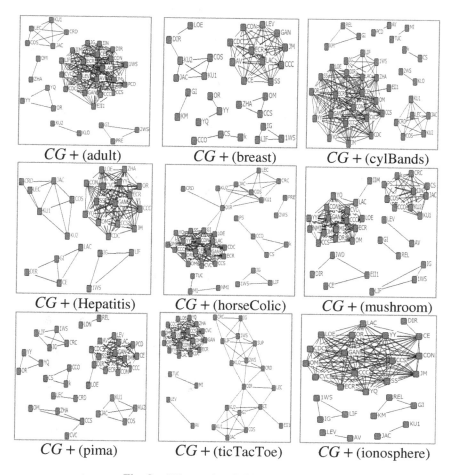

**Fig. 3.** $CG+$ graphs of different data sets

**Table 2.** Stable clusters of IMs on imbalanced data

| Stable clusters | Equivalent IMs |
|---|---|
| $C_1$:{CON, ECR, JM, CCC, GAN, LAC} | {CON, ECR, GAN} |
| $C_2$:{JAC, KU1, COS} | {JAC, KU1} |
| $C_3$:{YQ, YY, OR} | {YQ, YY, OR} |
| $C_4$:{IG, LIF, 1WS} | {IG, LIF} |
| $C_5$:{CE, DIR} | |
| $C_6$:{OM, CCS} | |
| $C_7$:{CVC, CCS} | |

context of imbalanced data. For instance, the measure OM and CCS in $C_6$ are strongly correlated, which means that they have similar behaviors in dealing with imbalanced data.

(B)  Interestingness Measures Selection Result and Analysis. After IM ranking computation process, we can select 26 proper IMs for imbalanced data. The abbreviations of the measures are CCO, CS, k, PS, PCD, ZHA, IIM, CRC, GK, EII1, IIN, LEV, AV, OM, CCS, CVC, YQ, SS, YY, OR, CDC, CCC, ECR, GAN, JM and CON. Here we use Hierarchical Agglomerative Clustering (HAC) [19] to make clustering analysis to see the relationships among them. The advantage of HAC is that it can produce a complete sequence of nested clusters, by starting with each interestingness measure in its own cluster and successively merging the two closest clusters into a new cluster until a single cluster containing all of the IMs is obtained. The clustering result is shown in Fig. 4(a). The 26 IMs are divided into two groups when the cut point is equal to 25. To analyze the relationship among the IMs of each group, we draw the star map of each IM under ten class distributions in Fig. 4(b). In a star, there are ten sectors and the radius of each

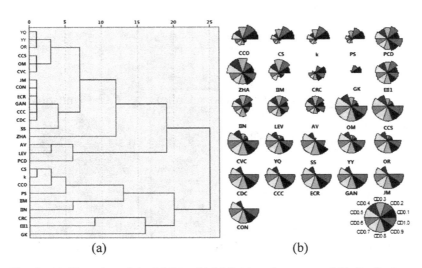

(a)                                                      (b)

**Fig. 4.** (a) Clustering of the 26 IMs; (b) 26 IMs' performances of 10 distributions.

sector means the measure's performance of the current class distribution. The longer is the arc length, the higher is the performance. In the bottom right of the map, a standard star is used to show different class distributions by different sectors. We find that CCO, CS, k, PS, PCD, ZHA, IIM, CRC, GK, EII1, IIN, LEV and AV perform better when class distribution is less than 0.4, while OM, CCS, CVC, YQ, SS, YY, OR, CDC, CCC, ECR, GAN, JM and CON are more suitable for those data with class distribution more than 0.4.From Fig. 4(b), we can also find that CCO, CS, k, PS, IIM, CRC, GK, IIN, LEV and AV perform worse with data more balanced, meanwhile the left do better with data more balanced. So combining Fig. 4(a) and (b), we can classify the 26 IMs into two groups with different characteristics.

- **group** *A* {CCO, CS, k, PS, PCD, ZHA, IIM, CRC, GK, EII1, IIN, LEV, AV} The measures can deal well with extremely imbalanced data and most of them perform better with data more imbalanced.
- **group** *B* {OM, CCS, CVC, YQ, SS, YY, OR, CDC, CCC, ECR, GAN, JM, CON} The measures perform well in slightly imbalanced data and do better with data more balanced.

## 5  Conclusion

In this paper, we aim at improving associative classification's performance on imbalanced data through studying interestingness measures. As to task 1, we propose a frequent correlated patterns mining method to find those stable clusters of IMs in general imbalanced data. In terms of task 2, 26 IMs are selected as the proper IMs for imbalanced data relatively. After a further analysis, we get two groups of IMs with different characteristics.

From the above results, we know that to select IMs, class distribution of data should be considered. What's more, our study finds appropriate IMs which can offer candidates for decision makers and help them to find the most suitable measure more efficiently for a certain application. In the future, we will further study the relations among IMs based on the above experiment results and explain why certain IMs behave similarly, especially as it related to degree of class imbalance.

**Acknowledgements.** This work is supported by the National Natural Science Foundation of China (71001016).

## Appendix

See Table 3.

**Table 3.** Interestingness measures for association patterns

| # | Interestingness measure | # | Interestingness measure |
|---|---|---|---|
| 1 | Complement Class Support (CCS) | 29 | J-measure (JM) |
| 2 | 1-way Support (1WS) | 30 | Kappa (k) |
| 3 | 2-way Support (2WS) | 31 | Klosgen (KLO) |
| 4 | Added Value (AV) | 32 | K-measure (KM) |
| 5 | Confirmed Confidence Causal (CCC) | 33 | Kulczynski 1 (KU1) |
| 6 | Confidence Causal (CDC) | 34 | Kulczynski 2 (KU2) |
| 7 | Chi-square ($\chi^2$) | 35 | Laplace Correction (LAC) |
| 8 | Collective Strength (CS) | 36 | Least Contradiction (LEC) |
| 9 | Conditional Entropy (CE) | 37 | Leverage (LEV) |
| 10 | Conviction (CVC) | 38 | Lift (LIF) |
| 11 | Correlation Coefficient (CCO) | 39 | Loevinger (LOE) |
| 12 | Cosine (COS) | 40 | Logical Necessity (LON) |
| 13 | Coverage (COV) | 41 | Mutual Information (MI) |
| 14 | Confirm Causal (CRC) | 42 | Normalized Mutual Information (NMI) |
| 15 | Confirm Descriptive (CRD) | 43 | Odd Multiplier (OM) |
| 16 | Dilated Chi-square ($D\chi^2$) | 44 | Odds Ratio (OR) |
| 17 | Directed Information Ratio (DIR) | 45 | Putative Causal Dependency (PCD) |
| 18 | Example and Counterexample Rate (ECR) | 46 | Prevalence (PRE) |
| 19 | Entropic Implication Intensity 1 (EII1) | 47 | Piatetsky-Shapiro (PS) |
| 20 | Entropic Implication Intensity 2 (EII2) | 48 | Relative Risk (REL) |
| 21 | Ganascia (GAN) | 49 | Sebag-Schoenauer (SS) |
| 22 | Gini Index (GI) | 50 | Support (SUP) |
| 23 | Goodman-Kruskal (GK) | 51 | Theil Uncertainty Coefficient (TUC) |
| 24 | Information Gain (IG) | 52 | Confidence (CON) |
| 25 | Intensity of Implication (IIM) | 53 | Yule's Q (YQ) |
| 26 | Implication Index (IIN) | 54 | Yule's Y (YY) |
| 27 | Interestingness Weighting Dependency (IWD) | 55 | Zhang (ZHA) |
| 28 | Jaccard (JAC) | 56 | – |

# References

1. Ali, K., Manganaris, S., Srikant, R.: Partial classification using association rules. In: KDD-97, pp. 115–118 (1997)
2. Liu, B., Hsu, W., Ma, Y.: Integrating classification and association rule mining. In: KDD, pp. 80–86 (1998)

3. Antonie, M.L., Zaïane, O.R.: Text document categorization by term association. In: Proceedings of the IEEE 2002 International Conference on Data Mining, pp. 19–26, Maebashi City, Japan (2002)

4. Li, W., Han, J., Pei, J.: CMAR: accurate and efficient classification based on multiple class-association rules. In: IEEE International Conference on Data Mining (ICDM 2001), San Jose, California, 29 November–2 December 2001

5. He, H., Garcia, E.A.: Learning from imbalanced data. IEEE Trans. Knowl. Data Eng. **21**(9), 1263–1284 (2009)

6. Chawla, N.V.: Data mining for imbalanced datasets: an overview. In: Maimon, O., Rokach, L. (eds.) Data Mining and Knowledge Discovery Handbook, pp. 875–886. Springer, New York (2010)

7. Tan, P., Kumar, V., Srivastava, J.: Selecting the right objective measure for association analysis. Inf. Syst. **29**(4), 293–313 (2004)

8. Huynh, X.H., Guillet, F., Blanchard, J., Kuntz, P., Briand, H., Gras, R.: A graph-based clustering approach to evaluate interestingness measures: a tool and a comparative study. In: Guillet, F., Hamilton, H. (eds.) Quality Measures in Data Mining. SCI, vol. 43, pp. 25–50. Springer, Heidelberg (2007)

9. Lallich, S., Teytaud, O., Prudhomme, E.: Association rule interestingness: measure and statistical validation. In: Guillet, F., Hamilton, H. (eds.) Quality Measures in Data Mining. SCI, vol. 43, pp. 251–275. Springer, Heidelberg (2007)

10. Lenca, P., Meyer, P., Vaillant, B., Lallich, S.: On selecting interestingness measures for association rules: user oriented description and multiple criteria decision aid. Eur. J. Oper. Res. **184**(2), 610–626 (2008)

11. Abe, H., Tsumoto, S.: Analyzing behavior of objective rule evaluation indices based on a correlation coefficient. In: Lovrek, I., Howlett, R.J., Jain, L.C. (eds.) KES 2008, Part II. LNCS (LNAI), vol. 5178, pp. 758–765. Springer, Heidelberg (2008)

12. Sahar, S.: Interestingness measures-on determining what is interesting. In: Maimon, O., Rokach, L. (eds.) Data Mining and Knowledge Discovery Handbook, 2nd edn., pp. 603–612. Springer, New York (2010)

13. Wu, T., Chen, Y., Han, J.: Re-examination of interestingness measures in pattern mining: a unified framework. Data Min. Knowl. Discov. **21**(3), 371–397 (2010)

14. Jalali-Heravi, M., Zaïane, O.: A study on interestingness measures for associative classifiers. In: Proceedings of the 25th ACM Symposium on Applied Computing, pp. 1039–1046 (2010)

15. Tew, C., Giraud-Carrier, C., Tanner, K., Burton, S.: Behavior-based clustering and analysis of interestingness measures for association rule mining. Data Min. Knowl. Discov. **28**(4), 1004–1045 (2014)

16. Arunasalam, B., Chawla, S.: CCCS: a top-down associative classifier for imbalanced class distribution. In: Proceedings of the 12th ACM SIGKDD International Conference on Knowledge Discovery and Data Mining, pp. 517–522, New York, NY, USA (2006)

17. Huynh, X.-H., Guillet, F., Briand, H.: ARQAT: an exploratory analysis tool for interestingness measures. In: ASMDA 2005, Proceedings of the 11th International Symposium on Applied Stochastic Models and Data Analysis, pp. 334–344, Brest, France (2005)

18. Asuncion, A., Newman, D.: UCI machine learning repository. School of Information and Computer Sciences, University of California, Irvine. http://www.ics.uci.edu/mlearn/mlrepository.html (2007)

19. Johnson, S.: Hierarchical clustering schemes. Psychometrika **2**, 241–254 (1967)

# Evaluation of Community Mining Algorithms in the Presence of Attributes

Reihaneh Rabbany[✉] and Osmar R. Zaïane

Department of Computing Science, University of Alberta, Edmonton, Canada
{rabbanyk,zaiane}@ualberta.ca

**Abstract.** Grouping data points is one of the fundamental tasks in data mining, commonly known as clustering. In the case of interrelated data, when data is represented in the form of nodes and their relationships, the grouping is referred to as *community*. A community is often defined based on the connectivity of nodes rather than their attributes or features. The variety of definitions and methods and its subjective nature, makes the evaluation of community mining methods non-trivial. In this paper we point out the critical issues in the common evaluation practices, and discuss the alternatives. In particular, we focus on the common practice of using attributes as the ground-truth communities in large real networks. We suggest to treat these attributes as another source of information, and to use them to refine the communities and tune parameters.

**Keywords:** Network clusters · Community mining · Networks with attributes · Community evaluation · Community validation

## 1  Introduction and Related Works

One fundamental property of real networks is that they tend to organize according to an underlying modular structure [9]. Clustering networks (a.k.a community mining) has direct application such as module identification in biological networks; for example clusters in protein-protein interaction networks outline protein complexes and parts of pathways [47]. Clustering networks is also an intermediate step for further analyses of networks such as link and attribute prediction which are the basis of targeted advertising and recommendation systems; for example clusters of hyperlinks between web pages in the WWW outline pages with closely related topics, and are used to refine the search results [2].

A cluster in a network a.k.a community is loosely defined as groups of nodes that have relatively more links between themselves than to the rest of the network. This definition is interpreted in the literature in many different ways, e.g. a group of nodes that: have structural similarity [48], are connected with cliques [33], within them a random walk is likely to trap [34], follow the same leader node [36], coding based on them gives efficient compression of the graph [43], are separated from the rest by minimum cut, or conductance [22], the number of links between them is more than chance [1,29].

© Springer International Publishing Switzerland 2015
X.-L. Li et al. (Eds.): PAKDD 2015, LNCS 9441, pp. 152–163, 2015.
DOI: 10.1007/978-3-319-25660-3_13

Fortunato [8] shows that the different community mining algorithms discover communities from different perspective and may outperform others in specific classes of networks. Therefore, an important research direction is to evaluate and compare the results of different community mining algorithms. An intuitive practice is to validate the results partly by a human expert [24]. However, the community mining problem is NP-complete; the human expert validation is limited, and is based on narrow intuition rather than on an exhaustive examination of the relations in the given network, specially for large real networks.

There is a congruence relation between defining communities and evaluating community mining results. In fact, the well-known Q-modularity by Newman and Girvan [28] which is commonly used as an objective function for community detection, was originally proposed for quantifying the goodness of the community structure, and is still used for evaluating the algorithms [4,41]. More generally, the *internal evaluation* practice verifies whether a clustering structure produced by an algorithm matches the underlying structure of the data, using only information inherent in the data [13]. The main problem with this type of evaluation is the assumption it makes about what are good communities, and hence is not appropriate to validate results of algorithms built upon different assumptions. In our earlier works in Rabbany et al. [35,38], we presented an extensive set of general objectives for evaluation of network clustering algorithms, mostly adapted from clustering background such as Variance Ratio Criterion, Silhouette Width Criterion, Dunn index, etc. Our experiments revealed that the ranking of these measures depends on the experiment settings, and there is not one to rule them all. This is not surprising as an evaluation criterion encompasses the same non-triviality as of the community mining task itself.

Another common evaluation practice is the *external evaluation*, which involves measuring the agreement between the discovered communities and the ground-truth structure in benchmark datasets [3,7,12,17,32]. There are few and typically small real world benchmarks with known communities available. Therefore the external evaluation is usually performed on synthetic benchmarks or on large networks with explicit or predefined communities. In the following, we discuss the issues and considerations with these types of evaluation.

The external evaluation is not applicable in real-world networks, as the ground-truth is not available. However we assume that the performance of an algorithm on the synthetic benchmarks, is a predictor of its performance on real networks. For this assumption to hold, we need realistic synthetic benchmarks, with tunable parameters for different domains; since it has been shown that the characteristics of clusters in networks are remarkably similar between networks from the same domain [19,30]. However, the current common generators used for synthesizing benchmarks, such as the LFR benchmarks [18], are domain-independent and also overlook some characteristics of the real networks [27,31]. Consequently, there are recent studies which try to improve the synthetic benchmark generators, including our recent works in [20].

Alternative to generating benchmarks for the community detection task, large real world benchmarks are often used where the ground-truth communities are defined based on some explicit properties of the nodes such as user

memberships in social network. Notably Yang and Leskovec [49] adapt this approach to compare different community detection algorithms based on their performance on large real world benchmarks; where characteristics such as social
groups are considered "reliable and robust notion of ground-truth communities".
For example, in a collaboration network of authors obtained from DBLP, venues
are considered as the ground-truth communities, or in the Amazon product
co-purchasing network, product categories are considered as the ground-truth.
A similar analysis is performed in Yang et al. [51], including a comparison
between the result on large real social networks and the LFR benchmarks, argu-
ing that the former is better indicator of the performance of the algorithms.
However as Lee and Cunningham [21] elaborate, this ground-truth data is imperfect and incomplete and should be rather considered as metadata or labeled
attributes correlated with the underlying communities.

In this paper we first investigate the correlations between attributes and
community structure using our network specific agreement/external indexes proposed recently in [40]. Then we present the concept of *community guidance by
attributes*, where we adapt our previously proposed TopLeaders [37] community
detection method, to find the right number of communities in the given network,
based on the available attributes information.

## 2    Correlation of Communities and Attributes

Traud et al. [45] show that a set of node attributes can act as the primary
organizing principle of the communities; e.g. House affiliation in their study of
Facebook friendship network of five US universities. In computing the correlation between attributes and relations, Traud et al. [45] use the basic clustering
agreement indices for communities comparison. They observe that the correlation significantly depends on this agreement index and differs significantly even
between those indices that have been known to be linear transformation of each
other. Here we perform similar experiments, but in the context of evaluating
community mining algorithms. In more details, we compare the agreements of
the results from four different community mining algorithms, with each attribute
in the dataset; see Fig. 1 for a visualized example. First, the community mining algorithms are applied on the dataset, which are InfoMap [42], WalkTrap
[34], Louvain [1], and FastModularity [29]. Then the correlations between the
resulted communities from these algorithms and the attributes are measured
using clustering agreement indices[1]. More specifically, we measure the agreement assuming the unique attribute values are grouped together and formed a
clustering. For example for the attribute 'year', all nodes that have value '2008'
are in the same group or cluster. Figure 2 shows the agreements of the community mining algorithms with each attribute averaged over all the networks in the
Facebook 100 dataset. The agreements, between two groupings/clusterings of the
dataset, are measured with eight different agreement indices: Jaccard Index, F-
measure, Variation of Information(VI), Normalized Mutual Information(NMI),

---

[1] Code available at: https://github.com/rabbanyk/CommunityEvaluation.

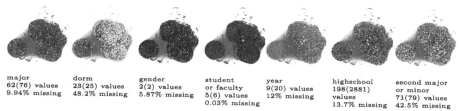

| major | dorm | gender | student | year | highschool | second major |
|---|---|---|---|---|---|---|
| 62(76) values | 23(25) values | 2(2) values | or faculty | 9(20) values | 198(2881) | or minor |
| 9.94% missing | 48.2% missing | 5.87% missing | 5(6) values | 12% missing | values | 71(79) values |
| | | | 0.03% missing | | 13.7% missing | 42.5% missing |

(a) Attributes: nodes are colored the same if they have the same value for the corresponding attribute; nodes with a missing value for the attribute are white. The number of unique attribute values, i.e. different colours, and the percentage of missing values are also reported. The number outside the parentheses is the number of main values which have at least five nodes, whereas the total number of unique values is reported inside the parentheses.

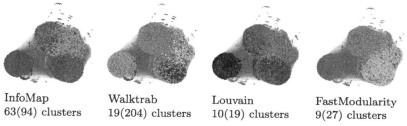

| InfoMap | Walktrab | Louvain | FastModularity |
|---|---|---|---|
| 63(94) clusters | 19(204) clusters | 10(19) clusters | 9(27) clusters |

(b) Communities: nodes are colored the same if they belong to the same community in the results of corresponding community mining algorithms. The number of clusters, i.e. colours, with at least five members is reported, whereas the total number of clusters in the result is given inside the parentheses.

**Fig. 1.** Visualization of correlations between attributes and communities for the American75 dataset from *Facebook 100 dataset*[46]. This network has 6386 nodes and 217662 edges (friendships which are unweighted, undirected). Visualization is done with Gephi, and an automatic layout is used which positions nodes only based on their connections.

Rand Index(RI), Adjusted Rand Index(ARI), and two structure based extensions of ARI tailored for comparing network clusters: with overlap function as the sum of weighted degrees($\mathcal{ARI}_{x^2}^{\Sigma d}$), and the number of common edges($\mathcal{ARI}_{x^2}^{\xi}$) [38].

Unlike the previous study, we observe very similar rankings with different agreement indexes. The most agreements are observed with the attribute 'year', followed not so closely by 'dormitory'. We can however see that the ranking across different attributes is not the same, whereas Walktrap is the winner according to the 'year', and Infomap performs the best if we consider the agreement with the 'dormitory'. Therefore, although we observe a correlation between the attributes and the communities, it is not wise to compare the general performance of community mining algorithms based on their agreements with a selected attribute as the ground-truth. Instead one should treat attributes as another source of information. In the next section, for example, we use this information to fine tune the parameters of a community mining algorithm, so that it results in a community

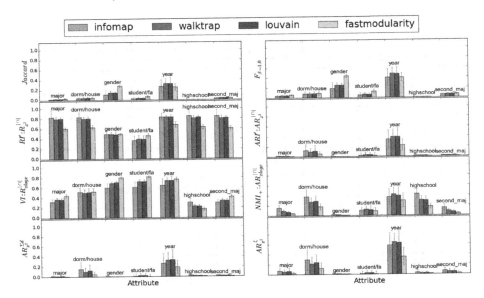

**Fig. 2.** The agreement of different community detection algorithms with each attribute, averaged over datasets from *Facebook 100 dataset.*

structure which compiles most with our selected attribute. Before that we present a discussion on the effect of missing values on the agreement indices.

### 2.1   Missing Values and Agreement Indices

The definitions of original agreement indices assume the two clusterings are covering the same set of datapoints. Therefore to use these indices, nodes with missing values should be either removed, or grouped all as a single cluster. The implementations we use here are based on our generalized formula proposed recently in [40]. Unlike the original definitions, these formulae do not require the assumption that the clusterings cover the whole dataset. Hence they can be directly applied to the cases where we have un-clustered datapoints, which will be ignored. For the sake of comparison, in Fig. 3 three bars are plotted per <attribute, community mining> pair, corresponding to how the missing values can be handled: (i) when nodes with missing values are removed from both groupings before computing the agreement, (ii) when all the nodes with missing attribute value are grouped into a single cluster, and (iii) when computing the agreements with lifting the covering assumption, using the formulations of [40]. This comparison is in particular important here, since we have many nodes with *missing values* for some of the attributes, such as 'dormitory' or 'second major'; which can significantly increase the agreements if missing values are removed altogether, as seen in the Fig. 3.

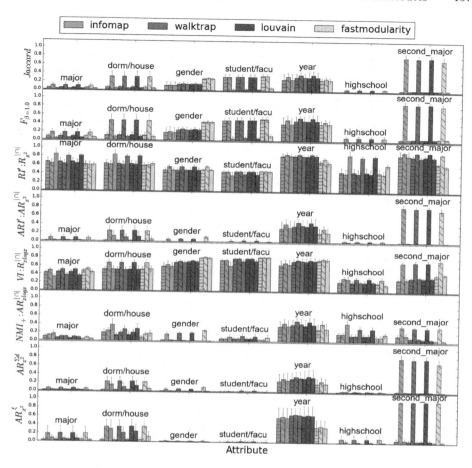

**Fig. 3.** The effect of missing values: bars with horizontal, diagonal, and solid fill correspond respectively to removing missing values, adding missing values as a single cluster, or lifting the covering assumption.

## 3    Community Guidance by Attributes

Many real world applications include information on both attributes of individual nodes as well as relations between the nodes, while there exists an interplay between these attributes and relations [5,16,23]. More precisely, the relations between nodes motivates them to develop similar attributes (influence), whereas the similarities between them motivates them to form relations (selection), a property referred to as homophily. This can also account for the correlation observed between community structure and attributes, i.e. self-identified user characteristics [45]; which has motivated defining ground-truth communities for real networks based on these explicit properties of nodes.

In the presence of attributes, a more plausible viewpoint is finding groups of nodes that are both internally well connected and having their members with homogeneous attributes. This grouping is referred to as structural attribute clustering by Zhou et al. [52] or cohesive patterns mining by Moser et al. [26]. Similar to community mining, several alternative approaches are proposed for this task [6,11,14,15,25,26,50]. Zhou et al. [52] propose clustering an attribute augmented network. The augmented network includes attribute nodes for each <attribute, value> and edges are added between original graph nodes to their corresponding <attribute, value> nodes[2]. The authors show that a straightforward distance function based on a linear combination of the structural and attribute similarities, fails to outperform a similar method that only considers structural or attribute similarities. In Mislove et al. [25], communities are found using a link based approach but are initialized using a clustering based on their attribute similarities. As another example in Cruz Gomez et al. [6], communities found by links are further divided into smaller sub-groups according to the attributes. In more details, the overlap of each community is computed with each cluster in the clustering of the same data according to the attributes. Then larger than average overlaps are cut from the main community to form smaller, more cohesive communities. All these works we have discussed so far further motivate combining attribute and link data, rather than validating one based on the other.

Here, we propose the concept of *community guidance by attributes*, where selected attribute is used to direct a community mining algorithm. More specifically, we guide our TopLeaders [37,39] algorithm to find the right number of communities, based on the agreements[3] of its result with the given attribute[3].

The number of communities, $k$ for short, is the main parameter for the TopLeaders algorithm, similar to the k-means algorithm for data clustering. Figure 4 illustrates an example on the Amherst41 dataset, where the agreements of each attribute with the results of Topleaders are plotted as a function of $k$. For some of the attributes, such as 'student/faculty', we observe a clear peak around the true number of classes. We also plotted where other algorithms land. However, there has not been any parameter tuning for those algorithm, and hence they are indicated with a single point. The vertical lines show the true number of classes for the corresponding attribute, i.e. the distinct values[4].

Consequently, between the communities detected by the TopLeaders for different values of $k$, which only uses the links to discover communities, we select the one that has the most agreement with the given attribute. We used an exhaustive search to find the optimal $k$ for each attribute, in the range of $[2, \sqrt{n}]$, where $n$ is the total number of datapoints. A better optimization method is a future work. Figure 5 shows the agreements obtained through this approach, compared to

---

[2] This graph representation has also been used in link recommendation, e.g. see [10].

[3] The concept is however general and can be applied to fine tune parameters of any community mining algorithm. Which is true for algorithms which are capable of providing different community structure perspectives, based on different values for the algorithm parameters.

[4] For attribute 'highschool', true $k$ is 1075 and out of the plot's scale.

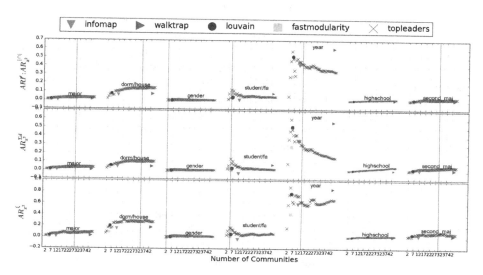

**Fig. 4.** Agreement of attributes with the results of algorithms plotted as a function of number of communities.

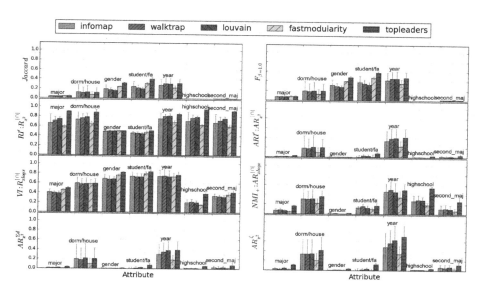

**Fig. 5.** TopLeaders performance when the number of communities are chosen according to the agreement of its results with the given attribute. This result is averaged over a subset of 5 datasets from the 100 Facebook networks, which are: Amherst41, Bowdoin47, Caltech36, Hamilton46, and Haverford76.

the four commonly used community detection algorithms. We can see in Fig. 5 that the communities found by this approach have comparable and in some cases better agreements with the attributes, compared to the methods which do not consider that extra information. This is more significant according to the structure based agreement measures, especially $\mathcal{ARI}_{x^2}^{\xi}$, which considers common edges as the cluster overlaps; and also for less trivial attributes which have a low agreement with the trivial communities, e.g. 'student/faculty', 'second_major', or 'highschool'. One should however note that this is not a comparison for the performance of these algorithms, since TopLeaders used the agreements with the attribute to find the $k$, which is not available to the other methods.

## 4 Conclusions

In this paper we discussed different evaluation approaches for community detection algorithms. In particular, we investigated the evaluation of communities on real-world networks with attributes, where there exist a correlation between the characteristics of individual nodes and their connections. We then proposed the concept of community guidance by attributes, where a community mining algorithm is guided to find a community structure which corresponds most to a given attribute. This is in particular useful in real world applications, since we often have access to both link and attribute information, and an idea of how communities will be used. For example, communities in protein-protein interaction networks are shown to be correlated with the functional categories of their members, which are used to predict the previously uncharacterized protein complexes [44]; in such case, one might be interested to select the community structure that corresponds most with the available functional categories.

## References

1. Blondel, V.D., Guillaume, J.L., Lambiotte, R., Lefebvre, E.: Fast unfolding of communities in large networks. J. Statis. Mech.: Theory Exp. **2008**(10), P10008 (2008)
2. Chen, J., Zaiane, O., Goebel, R.: An unsupervised approach to cluster web search results based on word sense communities. In: IEEE/WIC/ACM International Conference on Web Intelligence and Intelligent Agent Technology, WI-IAT 2008, vol. 1, pp. 725–729, December 2008
3. Chen, J., Zaïane, O.R., Goebel, R.: Detecting communities in social networks using max-min modularity. In: SIAM International Conference on Data Mining, pp. 978–989 (2009)
4. Clauset, A.: Finding local community structure in networks. Phys. Rev. E (Statis., Nonlinear, Soft Matter Phys.) **72**(2), 026132 (2005)
5. Crandall, D., Cosley, D., Huttenlocher, D., Kleinberg, J., Suri, S.: Feedback effects between similarity and social influence in online communities. In: Proceedings of the 14th ACM SIGKDD International Conference on Knowledge Discovery and Data Mining, pp. 160–168. ACM (2008)

6. Cruz Gomez, J.D., Bothorel, C.: Information integration for detecting communities in attributed graphs. In: 2013 Fifth International Conference on Computational Aspects of Social Networks (CASoN), pp. 62–67 (2013)
7. Danon, L., Guilera, A.D., Duch, J., Arenas, A.: Comparing community structure identification. J. Statis. Mech.: Theory Exp. (09), 09008 (2005)
8. Fortunato, S.: Community detection in graphs. Phys. Rep. **486**(35), 75–174 (2010)
9. Fortunato, S., Castellano, C.: Community structure in graphs. In: Computational Complexity, pp. 490–512. Springer (2012)
10. Gong, N.Z., Talwalkar, A., Mackey, L., Huang, L., Shin, E.C.R., Stefanov, E., Song, D., et al.: Jointly predicting links and inferring attributes using a social-attribute network (san). arXiv preprint arXiv:1112.3265 (2011)
11. Günnemann, S., Boden, B., Färber, I., Seidl, T.: Efficient mining of combined subspace and subgraph clusters in graphs with feature vectors. In: Pei, J., Tseng, V.S., Cao, L., Motoda, H., Xu, G. (eds.) PAKDD 2013, Part I. LNCS, vol. 7818, pp. 261–275. Springer, Heidelberg (2013)
12. Gustafsson, M., Hörnquist, M., Lombardi, A.: Comparison and validation of community structures in complex networks. Phys. A Statis. Mech. Its Appl. **367**, 559–576 (2006)
13. Halkidi, M., Batistakis, Y., Vazirgiannis, M.: On clustering validation techniques. J. Intel. Inf. Syst. **17**, 107–145 (2001)
14. Hanisch, D., Zien, A., Zimmer, R., Lengauer, T.: Co-clustering of biological networks and gene expression data. Bioinformatics **18**(suppl. 1), S145–S154 (2002)
15. Hu, B., Song, Z., Ester, M.: User features and social networks for topic modeling in online social media. In: 2012 IEEE/ACM International Conference on Advances in Social Networks Analysis and Mining (ASONAM), pp. 202–209. IEEE (2012)
16. La Fond, T., Neville, J.: Randomization tests for distinguishing social influence and homophily effects. In: Proceedings of the 19th International Conference on World Wide Web, WWW 2010, pp. 601–610. ACM, New York (2010)
17. Lancichinetti, A., Fortunato, S.: Community detection algorithms: A comparative analysis. Phys. Rev. E **80**(5), 056117 (2009)
18. Lancichinetti, A., Fortunato, S., Radicchi, F.: Benchmark graphs for testing community detection algorithms. Phys. Rev. E **78**(4), 046110 (2008)
19. Lancichinetti, A., Kivelä, M., Saramäki, J., Fortunato, S.: Characterizing the community structure of complex networks. PloS One **5**(8), e11976 (2010)
20. Largeron, C., Mougel, P., Rabbany, R., Zaïane, O.R.: Generating attributed networks with communities. PloS One (to appear, 2015)
21. Lee, C., Cunningham, P.: Benchmarking community detection methods on social media data. arXiv preprint arXiv:1302.0739 (2013)
22. Leskovec, J., Lang, K.J., Mahoney, M.: Empirical comparison of algorithms for network community detection. In: Proceedings of the 19th International Conference on World Wide Web, pp. 631–640. ACM (2010)
23. Lewis, K., Gonzalez, M., Kaufman, J.: Social selection and peer influence in an online social network. Proc. Nat. Acad. Sci. **109**(1), 68–72 (2012)
24. Luo, F., Wang, J.Z., Promislow, E.: Exploring local community structures in large networks. Web Intel. Agent Syst. **6**, 387–400 (2008)
25. Mislove, A., Viswanath, B., Gummadi, K.P., Druschel, P.: You are who you know: inferring user profiles in online social networks. In: Proceedings of the Third ACM International Conference on Web Search and Data Mining, WSDM 2010, pp. 251–260. ACM, New York (2010)
26. Moser, F., Colak, R., Rafiey, A., Ester, M.: Mining cohesive patterns from graphs with feature vectors. SDM **9**, 593–604 (2009)

27. Moussiades, L., Vakali, A.: Benchmark graphs for the evaluation of clustering algorithms. In: Proceedings of the Third IEEE International Conference on Research Challenges in Information Science, RCIS 2009, pp. 197–206 (2009)
28. Newman, M.E.J., Girvan, M.: Finding and evaluating community structure in networks. Phys. Rev. E **69**(2), 026113 (2004)
29. Newman, M.E.: Fast algorithm for detecting community structure in networks. Phys. Rev. E **69**(6), 066133 (2004)
30. Onnela, J.P., Arbesman, S., González, M.C., Barabási, A.L., Christakis, N.A.: Geographic constraints on social network groups. PLoS One **6**(4), e16939 (2011)
31. Orman, G.K., Labatut, V.: The effect of network realism on community detection algorithms. In: Proceedings of the 2010 International Conference on Advances in Social Networks Analysis and Mining, ASONAM 2010, pp. 301–305 (2010)
32. Orman, G.K., Orman, G.K., Labatut, V., Labatut, V., Cherifi, H., Cherifi, H.: Qualitative comparison of community detection algorithms. In: Cherifi, H., Cherifi, H., Zain, J.M., Zain, J.M., El-Qawasmeh, E., El-Qawasmeh, E. (eds.) DICTAP 2011 Part II. CCIS, vol. 167, pp. 265–279. Springer, Heidelberg (2011)
33. Palla, G., Derényi, I., Farkas, I., Vicsek, T.: Uncovering the overlapping community structure of complex networks in nature and society. Nature **435**(7043), 814–818 (2005)
34. Latapy, M., Latapy, M., Pons, P., Pons, P.: Computing communities in large networks using random walks. In: Yolum, I., Yolum, I., Özturan, C., Özturan, C., Gürgen, F., Gürgen, F., Güngör, T., Güngör, T. (eds.) ISCIS 2005. LNCS, vol. 3733, pp. 284–293. Springer, Heidelberg (2005)
35. Rabbany, R., Takaffoli, M., Fagnan, J., Zaiane, O., Campello, R.: Relative validity criteria for community mining algorithms. In: 2012 International Conference on Advances in Social Networks Analysis and Mining (ASONAM), August 2012
36. Rabbany, R., Chen, J., Zaïane, O.R.: Top leaders community detection approach in information networks. In: Proceedings of the 4th Workshop on Social Network Mining and Analysis (2010)
37. Rabbany, R., Chen, J., Zaïane, O.R.: Top leaders community detection approach in information networks. In: SNA-KDD Workshop on Social Network Mining and Analysis (2010)
38. Rabbany, R., Takaffoli, M., Fagnan, J., Zaïane, O.R., Campello, R.: Relative validity criteria for community mining algorithms. In: Social Networks Analysis and Mining (SNAM) (2013)
39. Rabbany, R., Zaïane, O.R.: A diffusion of innovation-based closeness measure for network associations. In: IEEE International Conference on Data Mining Workshops, pp. 381–388 (2011)
40. Rabbany, R., Zaïane, O.R.: Generalization of clustering agreements and distances for overlapping clusters and network communities. CoRR abs/1412.2601 (2014)
41. Rosvall, M., Bergstrom, C.T.: An information-theoretic framework for resolving community structure in complex networks. Proc. Nat. Acad. Sci. **104**(18), 7327–7331 (2007)
42. Rosvall, M., Bergstrom, C.T.: Maps of random walks on complex networks reveal community structure. Proc. Nat. Acad. Sci. **105**(4), 1118–1123 (2008)
43. Rosvall, M., Bergstrom, C.T.: Mapping change in large networks. PLoS One **5**(1), e8694 (2010)
44. Spirin, V., Mirny, L.A.: Protein complexes and functional modules in molecular networks. Proc. Nat. Acad. Sci. **100**(21), 12123–12128 (2003)

45. Traud, A.L., Kelsic, E.D., Mucha, P.J., Porter, M.A.: Comparing community structure to characteristics in online collegiate social networks. SIAM Rev. **53**(3), 526–543 (2011)
46. Traud, A.L., Mucha, P.J., Porter, M.A.: Social structure of facebook networks. Phys. A: Statis. Mech. Appl. **391**(16), 4165–4180 (2012)
47. Wagner, A., Fell, D.A.: The small world inside large metabolic networks. Proc. Royal Soc. Lond. Ser. B: Biol. Sci. **268**(1478), 1803–1810 (2001)
48. Xu, X., Yuruk, N., Feng, Z., Schweiger, T.A.: Scan: a structural clustering algorithm for networks. In: Proceedings of the 13th ACM SIGKDD International Conference on Knowledge Discovery and Data Mining, pp. 824–833. ACM (2007)
49. Yang, J., Leskovec, J.: Defining and evaluating network communities based on ground-truth. In: Proceedings of the ACM SIGKDD Workshop on Mining Data Semantics, p. 3. ACM (2012)
50. Yang, T., Jin, R., Chi, Y., Zhu, S.: Combining link and content for community detection: a discriminative approach. In: Proceedings of the 15th ACM SIGKDD International Conference on Knowledge Discovery and Data Mining, pp. 927–936. ACM (2009)
51. Yang, Y., Sun, Y., Pandit, S., Chawla, N.V., Han, J.: Perspective on measurement metrics for community detection algorithms. In: Mining Social Networks and Security Informatics, pp. 227–242. Springer (2013)
52. Zhou, Y., Cheng, H., Yu, J.X.: Graph clustering based on structural/attribute similarities. Proc. VLDB Endowment **2**(1), 718–729 (2009)

# Leveraging the Common Cause of Errors for Constraint-Based Data Cleansing

Ayako Hoshino[1]([⊠]), Hiroki Nakayama[3], Chihiro Ito[2], Kyota Kanno[1],
and Kenshi Nishimura[2]

[1] Knowledge Discovery Research Laboratories, NEC Corporation, 1753,
Shimonumabe Nakahara-ku, Kawasaki, Kanagawa 211-8666, Japan
a-hoshino@cj.jp.nec.com, k-kanno@ah.jp.nec.com
[2] System Integration, Services and Engineering Operations Unit, NEC Corporation,
1753, Shimonumabe Nakahara-ku, Kawasaki, Kanagawa 211-8666, Japan
{c-ito,k-nishimura}@az.jp.nec.com
[3] NEC Informatec Systems, Ltd., 1753, Shimonumabe Nakahara-ku, Kawasaki,
Kanagawa 211-8666, Japan
h-nakayama@cj.jp.nec.com

**Abstract.** This study describes a statistically motivated approach to constraint-based data cleansing that derives the cause of errors from a distribution of conflicting tuples. In real-world dirty data, errors are often not randomly distributed. Rather, they often occur only under certain conditions, such as when the transaction is handled by a certain operator, or the weather is rainy. Leveraging such common conditions, or "cause conditions", the algorithm resolves multi-tuple conflicts with high speed, as well as high accuracy in realistic settings where the distribution of errors is skewed. We present complexity analyses of the problem, pointing out two subproblems that are NP-complete. We then introduce, for each subproblem, heuristics that work in sub-polynomial time. The algorithms are tested with three sets of data and rules. The experiments show that, compared to the state-of-the-art methods for Conditional Functional Dependencies (CFD)-based and FD-based data cleansing, the proposed algorithm scales better with respect to the data size, is the only method that outputs complete repairs, and is more accurate when the error distribution is skewed.

**Keywords:** Data cleansing · Conditional functional dependencies

## 1 Introduction

Data cleansing is a crucial step in data integration. As more data are made available, this task has gained a considerable attention both in business and research. One promising approach is constraint-based data cleansing, which is based on traditional Functional Dependencies (FDs) or recently proposed Conditional Functional Dependencies (CFDs) [1]. Below are examples of an FD, a variable CFD and a constant CFD.

© Springer International Publishing Switzerland 2015
X.-L. Li et al. (Eds.): PAKDD 2015, LNCS 9441, pp. 164–176, 2015.
DOI: 10.1007/978-3-319-25660-3_14

Each constraint expresses regularity in the data. The first constraint $\phi_1$ is an example of FD, indicating "the company ID and employee ID determine individual names". The second constraint $\phi_2$ is an example of CFD, indicating "when company ID is 001, desk address determines employee ID". The third constraint designates "when the company ID is 001 and the person name is Alice B., the desk address is F12-S-123". Such constraints can be used to detect errors in the data, as well as to determine the correct values.

$\phi_1$: company ID, employee ID $\rightarrow$ person name
$\phi_2$: company ID, desk address $\rightarrow$ employee ID, (001, _ || _)
$\phi_3$: company ID, person name $\rightarrow$ desk address, (001, "Alice B." || "F12-S-123")

Data can have multi-tuple conflicts with an FD or a variable CFD. For example, an erroneous tuple $t_k$: (company ID, employee ID, person name) = (001, A123, "John") will cause a *conflict*, when there is another tuple $t_1$: (001, A123, "Paul") and thus, the two tuples *violate* constraint $\phi_1$. Also, an erroneous tuple $t_k$: (company ID, desk address, employee ID) = (001, F12-North345, A123) will cause a *conflict*, when there is another tuple $t_2$: (001, F12-North345, A456) and thus, the two tuples *violate* constraint $\phi_2$.

We propose a data-cleansing method that addresses the problem of discovering a common cause of errors. By discovering such a condition, we can both cut down the search space and obtain a more accurate repair. While CFD is an addition to FD in that it specifies the subset of data where a constraint holds, our proposed "cause condition" specifies the subset of the data that contains conflict-causing errors. The discovery of cause condition is much more difficult as we will prove, but often needed in realistic data-cleansing settings.

This paper is organized as follows. Section 2 summarizes the previous research on constraint-based data cleansing. Section 3 describes our method for discovering error conditions and generating a repair. Section 4 presents our experimental evaluation. Section 4.2 provides analyses on the results. Finally, Sect. 5 concludes our paper.

## 2    Related Work

With the recent appearance of Conditional Functional Dependencies (CFD) [1], constraint-based data cleansing is experiencing a revival. Numerous methods have already been proposed on CFD-based data cleansing [2–8]. Prior to CFD, there had been data cleansing with FDs [9–12], and Association Rules (ARs) [13], but here we focus on the methods that have been applied to CFD.

The cleansing algorithm of Cong et al.'s BatchRepair and IncRepair is, just like their predecessor [14], a cost-based algorithm where the optimal repair is chosen based on the editing cost from the original data [2], measured in Levenstein's edit distance [15], or measured by the number of tuples to be removed [16]. Note that all cost-based methods follow "majority policy". Beskales et al. proposed a sampling-based method that generates repairs from among repairs with minimal changes [7], which can also be categorized as a cost-based method.

Chiang and Miller [3] proposed a method for deriving CFDs that almost hold (i.e. X → A holds on $D$, allowing some exception tuples), filtering these *approximate CFDs* using an interest measure, and then detecting dirty data values. In their definition, dirty values are infrequent Right Hand Side (RHS) values within the set of Left Hand Side (LHS) matched tuples, which makes them also follow the "majority policy". Notably, only values on RHS are the target of detection.

Fan et al. [4,5] proposed a highly accurate method that uses hand-crafted editing rules and human-validated certain region of the table. The correction may not always follow the majority policy, but preparing editing rules and a certain region requires a human input, which is often not available in reality.

Stoyanovich et al. tried to learn the generative process of the data, not with CFDs but with their proposed model Meta-Rule Semi Lattices (MRSL). Although their method has an assumption model for the data, they had no assumption for how errors occur [17]. Also, they dealt with only completion of missing values, while wider variations of data errors can be dealt with by using FDs or CFDs.

In our study, we develop a method called CondRepair that identifies erroneous tuples when there are conflicts with FD or CFD rules. It relies on neither the majority RHS nor edit distance-based cost metrics, which do not work when the differences (in frequency or in cost) among candidate fixes are not significant. It determines the wrong values based on the common cause of errors. Although the idea of leveraging the patterns among errors has been explored for other types of data cleansing [18], to the best of our knowledge, the idea has never been applied with (C)FDs or ARs. In the experimental evaluation, we use error injection with both uniform and skewed error distribution whose design is based on our qualitative study on the real errors.

## 3    Data Cleansing Based on Error Conditions

In this section, we first introduce the problem of CFD-based data cleansing, and highlight some of its difficulties by showing the class of problems its subproblems belong to. We then describe our proposed method, which consists of two steps: (1) finding the cause conditions and (2) generating a repair.

### 3.1    Problem Description

The problem of CFD-based data cleansing is defined as follows. Let $D$ be the input relation and $\Sigma$ be a set of CFD rules. We assume $D$ consists of one table. Let $D_{\text{repr}}$ be an output relation of the cleansing process. It is required that $D_{\text{repr}} \models \Sigma$, which is, there is no violation in $D$ w.r.t. any rules in $\Sigma$. Let $A$, $B$, and $C$ denote attributes, and $X$, $Y$ and $Z$ denote sets of attributes. Each tuple in $D$ has a tuple ID so that $D = \{t_1, t_2, ..., t_N\}$, where $N$ is the total number of tuples in $D$. We refer to a cell in a tuple as $c$. Figure 1 shows an illustrative example of an input rule set (consisting of one rule) and data with conflicts and possible outputs of previous methods and ours.

**Input:**

Constraint : Category, Price -> Tax, ( _ , _ || _ )

|  | Category | Operator | Product | Price | Tax |
|---|---|---|---|---|---|
| t1: | CD | Operator A | my songs | 15 | 3 |
| t2: | CD | Operator A | ... | 20 | 2 |
| t3: | CD | Operator B | ... | 20 | 0 |
| t4: | Book | Operator B | ... | 15 | 1 |
|  | ... | Operator B | ... | ... | ... |
| tN: | Book | Operator B | ... | 15 | 0 |

**Output of Inconsistency Detection:**
t2, t3, t4, tN

**Output of Previous Work's Data Cleansing:**
(t2, Tax) = 0, (t4, Category) = <OTHER>

**Output of This work's Data Cleansing:**
possible cause of errors: Operator="Operator B"
(t3, Tax) = 2, (t4, Category) = <OTHER>

**Fig. 1.** Example constraint, data, and outputs of cleansing algorithms. Arrows on the right side of the table show conflicting tuples.

We now examine two subproblems that belong to the class of problems that are known to be difficult to solve.

**Theorem 1.** *The problem of selecting the tuples to be corrected among the ones in conflicts includes an NP-complete problem.*

*Proof.* Here, we try to solve the conflicts with more tuples first, i.e. we do not take a naive approach such as modifying all tuples that are involved in a conflict. Let the set of tuples that are involved in multi-tuple conflicts be $D_{\text{doubt}}$, and the set of conflicts between tuples $t_i, t_j \in D_{\text{doubt}}$ be $f_{ij}$. The problem of finding tuples to be corrected is selecting the subset $D'_{\text{doubt}}$ of $D_{\text{doubt}}$ at least one of whose members have conflict with all the remaining tuples in set $D_{\text{doubt}} \backslash D'_{\text{doubt}}$. There is a polynomial time projection from the set $D_{\text{doubt}}$ to the set of vertices $V$ and from conflicts $f_{ij}$ to the set of edges $E$ of a graph $(V, E)$. The problem can be reduced to the dominating set problem of a graph $(V, E)$, which is known to be NP-complete. A naive solution for this problem takes computation order of $O(2^n n)$ and will be intractable as the number of tuples in $D_{\text{doubt}}$ increases.

Note that there are some exceptional cases where conflicts between two tuples remain. These conflicts should be solved after resolving the ones with more tuples. Also note that we have not yet mentioned which cells of the tuples to be corrected. Still, the problem of selecting tuples to be corrected is already NP-hard.

Secondly, we show that, even after we select $D'_{\text{doubt}}$, the problem of finding a common condition among those tuples is difficult.

**Theorem 2.** *The problem of discovering a common condition among the tuples in $D'_{\text{doubt}}$ is NP-complete.*

*Proof.* As pointed out by Zaki and Ogihara, the problem of finding a common itemset among the tuples is NP-complete, since it can be reduced to the problem of finding a clique in a bipartite graph [19]. Similarly, the problem of finding a common set of attribute values among a set of tuples can be reduced to a bipartite clique problem as follows. Assume we have a graph $G = (U, V, E)$, where $G$ is a bipartite graph consisting of parts $U$ and $V$, and edges $E$. A set of tuples can be projected to $U$ and a set of attribute values to $V$, and the existence of a tuple containing a set of attribute values to an edge in $E$. A clique in a bipartite graph is equivalent of a set of attribute values that is common in a set of tuples. Then, the problem of finding a common attribute values is reduced to the problem of finding a clique in a bipartite graph $G$. This problem is known to be NP-complete and, for instance, finding the largest clique requires computation $O(|U||V|)$.

Here, we introduce some key concepts.

**Definition 1.** *An LHS value sets $\{S_{\phi,1}, S_{\phi,2}, ..., S_{\phi,k}\}$ is defined for a CFD rule $\phi \in \Sigma$, which is a set of tuple sets $S_\phi = \{\{t_{1,1}, t_{1,2}, ..t_{1,N1}\}, \{t_{2,1}, t_{2,2}, ..t_{2,N2}\}, ..\}$ where each tuple within each set (or, LHS value set) matches the condition of the rule $\phi$, and has the same values on the LHS of the rule $\phi$, namely $t_{k,i}[\phi.LHS] = t_{k,j}[\phi.LHS]$ holds for all $i, j \in \{1, 2, ..., N_k\}$ for all $k$ tuple sets. (We denote the LHS attribute set as $\phi.LHS$, and the values of attribute set $A$ as $t[A]$).*

**Definition 2.** *A doubt tuple is a tuple in conflict w.r.t. a rule in $\Sigma$, namely $\{t \mid \exists t' \in D \wedge t, t' \in S_{\phi,k} \wedge t[\phi.RHS] \neq t'[\phi.RHS]\}$. We call a set of doubt tuples $D_{\text{disagree},\phi,k}$, which is the kth tuple set in $S_\phi$ where any pair of the member tuples disagree on the RHS of $\phi$.*

**Definition 3.** *Cause attribute $(Z, v)$ is defined as a set of attribute values that is common to the tuples to be corrected in $D$.*

**Finding the Cause Conditions.** The condition we try to discover is defined as a form of a triplet $\mathbf{Z}$, $\mathbf{v}$, $\kappa(\mathbf{Z} = \mathbf{v}, L = \text{"doubt"})$, which are a set of attributes, their values, and an agreement metrics which evaluates co-occurrence between a condition and a "doubt" label. We first identify the cause of error $\mathbf{Z}$ (hereafter called *cause attributes*) among $\texttt{attr}(D)$, using a sample of data $D_{\text{sample}}$.

We treat a tuple as a basic unit for computing probability. We label tuples in $D$ either "doubt" or "clean", using a set of labels for tuples $L = \{$"clean", "doubt"$\}$, where $L(t) = $ "clean" when tuple $t$ is not in conflict and $L(t) = $

"doubt" when in conflict with any rule in $\Sigma$. In Fig. 1, doubt tuples are $t_2$, $t_3$, $t_4$ and $t_N$, and all the rest are clean tuples.

When determining the error attributes, CondRepair uses an agreement statistics Kappa which indicates co-occurrence between the doubt tuples and candidates for the cause condition. The Kappa statistics $\kappa$ is defined as follows.

The Kappa agreement statistics: $\kappa(\mathbf{Z} = \mathbf{v}, L = \text{"doubt"}) = \dfrac{P_{\text{actual}} - P_{\text{coincidental}}}{1 - P_{\text{coincidental}}}$

where $P_{\text{actual}} = \dfrac{|\{t \mid t[\mathbf{Z}] = \mathbf{v} \wedge L(t) = \text{"doubt"}\}|}{|D_{\text{sample}}|}$

and $P_{\text{coincidental}} = \left(\dfrac{|\{t \mid t[\mathbf{Z}] = \mathbf{v}\}|}{|D_{\text{sample}}|}\right)\left(\dfrac{|\{t \mid L(t) = \text{"doubt"}\}|}{|D_{\text{sample}}|}\right).$

The meaning of Kappa index is, basically, the difference between the rate of actual co-occurrence and the rate of theoretical co-occurrence normalized by the negation of coincidental co-occurrences (when the probability of coincidental co-occurrence is higher, $\kappa$ will be higher).

We now describe a heuristics introduced in response to the subproblem described in Theorem 2. We could have discovered a common condition among a set of doubt tuples in an apriori-like manner ([20]). However, the apriori algorithm is known to be still computationally expensive especially with data of high arity. So we developed a more efficient inference method for cause discovery using the Kappa index. The virtue of Kappa index is, it evaluates different attribute values with a single viewpoint, a co-occurrence with doubt tuples. We obtain attribute values in a single list in the order of Kappa value and seek if there is a composed cause condition $(\mathbf{Z} \cup A, \mathbf{v} + v)$ that has higher Kappa than a simpler condition $(\mathbf{Z}, \mathbf{v})$.

**Generating a Repair.** When tuples to be corrected are determined, it is fairly straightforward to generate a repair. We use *equivalence classes* proposed by Bohannon et al., based on the description given by Beskales et al. [1,7]. Equivalence class is a useful data structure to repair data with multiple rules. It groups cells into sets within which all member cells should have the same value when the cleansing is completed, delaying decision on the exact value each cell in the set will have.

Use of equivalence classes assures a complete repair, i.e. a repair with no remaining violation. However, as Bohannon et al. have noted as *collision* problem, it often generates excessively large equivalence sets by applying repeated merges with multiple rules. For example, an equivalence class with cell $t[B]$ is merged with the one with cell $t'[B]$ based on $\phi_1 : A \to B$, then an equivalence class with cell $t[C]$ is merged with the one with $t'[C]$, based on another rule $\phi_2 : B \to C$, and so on. We make some modifications to Beskales et al.'s equivalence class. First, we do not make equivalence classes where there is no conflict, whereas Beskales' method first merges all cells that have the same values. Secondly, we merge equivalence classes not based on their LHS equivalence classes, but simply based on the values on the LHS attributes. In order to achieve a complete repair, we impose some limitations on the order and the involving attributes of rules in the input rule, so that $\Sigma^{<^{\text{rules}}} = \{\phi \mid \forall A \in \phi.\text{LHS}, A \notin \phi'.\text{RHS}, \forall \phi' <^{\text{rules}} \phi\}$, which means $\Sigma$ is a list of rules sorted in the order $<^{\text{rules}}$ where any attribute on LHS of rule $\phi$ is not included in the RHS of any preceding rule $\phi'$.

During the repair generation, a cell's value $t[B]$ is changed to another tuple's value $t'[B]$ where there is a cleaner tuple, which is a tuple that is assigned with the lowest probability of being errorneous among the ones in the same equivalence class, $t'$ within the equivalence class.

Equivalence classes cannot produce corrections for constant CFDs. So, constant CFDs are treated separately by changing any of the cell in LHS to a special symbol OTHER_VALUE, which indicates a value not in the domain of the attribute and defined not to match any value (thus, OTHER_VALUE $\neq$ OTHER_VALUE). The specific value will require a human to fill in the process of verification, which is out of the scope of this paper. We now provide a step by step description of the algorithm CondRepair (Algorithm 1). Detailed explanations are given in a separate publication.

## 4    Experiments

The proposed algorithm, along with two previous methods, is tested in terms of its scalability and accuracy in detecting and correcting error cells with different degrees of error skewness. The algorithms are implemented in Java$^{\text{TM}}$and all experiments are conducted on a Linux CentOS with 16-Core Xeon E5-2450 (2.1 GHz) and 128-GB memory.

### 4.1    Experimental Settings and Key Results

We describe experimental settings followed by some key results.

**Datasets.** We used three datasets, two of which are from the UCI machine learning database: (1) Wisconsin Breast Cancer (WBC) and (2) US Census dataset (Adult). WBC is a numeric data and US Census contains mostly nominal values. The third dataset is DBGen ([21]), a synthetic data set obtained from the authors of a previous algorithm [7].

**The Previous Algorithms.** Two previous algorithms were used for comparison, which are IncRepair by Cong et al. [2] and FDRepair by Beskales et al. [7]. IncRepair is an incremental algorithm that cleans $\Delta D$ when $\Delta D$ has been added to a dataset $D$ so $\Delta D \cup D$ satisfies $\Sigma$. Note that it performs with a better scalability than its batch counterpart (BatchRepair) without loss of accuracy. We used IncRepair so that it treated all the data as $\Delta D$ as Cong et al. did in their experiment. IncRepair was re-implemented using the same basic utility classes as CondRepair for data IO and for CFD validations.

**Algorithm 1.** CondRepair

---

**Input:** $D, \Sigma, n(sample size), m(a\ threshold\ to\ limit\ the\ size\ of\ S)$
**Output:** $D_{\mathrm{repr}} \models \Sigma$
1: $D_{\mathrm{repr}} := D$
2: take $D_{\mathrm{sample}}$, a sample of size $n$ from $D_{\mathrm{repr}}$

//label each tuple
3: **for** each $\phi \in \Sigma$ **do**
4:     $D_{\mathrm{disagree},\phi} := \{S \mid t, t' \in S_{\phi,k} \wedge S_{\phi,k} \subseteq D_{\mathrm{sample}} \wedge t[\phi.RHS] \neq t'[\phi.RHS]\}$
5:     **if** $|S_{\phi,k}| \leq m$ where $S_{\phi,k}$ has a conflict **then**
6:         `label`$(t) :=$ "doubt" for all $t \in S_{\phi,k}$

//infer the cause condition
7: **for** each $(A, v) \in D_{\mathrm{disagree}}$, a set of tuples whose labels are "doubt" **do**
8:     calculate $\kappa(A = v, L =$ "doubt"$)$
9: **for** each $(A, v)$ in the descending order of kappa **do**
10:     **if** $A \notin \mathbf{Z}$ and $\kappa(\mathbf{Z}, \mathbf{v}) < \kappa(\mathbf{Z} \cup A, \mathbf{v} + v)$ **then**
11:         $(\mathbf{Z}, \mathbf{v}) := (\mathbf{Z} \cup A, \mathbf{v} + v)$ **else** break

// fix LHS of constant CFDs
12: **for** each $t \not\models \phi \in \Sigma, t \in D_{\mathrm{repr}}$, where $phi$ is a constant CFD **do**
13:     $t[B] =$ OTHER_VALUE for any attribute $B \in \phi.LHS$

// build equivalence classes
14: `BuildEquivRel`$(D_{\mathrm{repr}}, \Sigma)$

//fix values
15: **for** each $e \in E$ **do**
16:     $c^* :=$ a cell under $(\mathbf{Z}, \mathbf{v})$ which has the smallest $\kappa$ in $E$
17:     **for** each $c \in e$ **do**
18:         `val`$(c) := $ `val`$(c^*)$
19: return $D_{\mathrm{repr}}$

---

FDRepair is a repair algorithm based on Beskales et al.'s proposed notion of cardinality-set-minimal repairs. It employs the equivalence classes originally proposed by Bohannon et al. [14] and attempts to rectify the *collision* problem that we described in Sect. 3.1 by reverting the values to the original ones where it does not cause a violation. FDRepair is a sampling algorithm that produces samples from the cardinality-set-minimal repairs. We used a Java implementation of FDRepair obtained from the author.

**Input Rules.** The CFD rules we used was extracted from WBC and Adult datasets before error injection using a FastCFD algorithm with the support threshold set to 10 percent of the number of tuples in input data, where 10 percent is a popularly used value in previous work. The number of CFD rules can be excessive, and rules with a large number of attributes on LHS are often not useful in data cleansing, so we have limited the size of LHS to at most four. For FDRepair, we used FDs which were included in the result of the CFD discovery, and for the other two algorithms, we used the same number of randomly sampled CFD rules. As a result, 35 rules from WBC and Adult have been extracted. For the dataset DBGen, we used the same 18 FD rules as used in the Beskales et al.'s experiment [7].

**Injected Errors.** We injected errors by turning an attribute value of a random tuple $(t, A)$ into the value of the same attribute of another randomly chosen tuple $(t', A)$. In effect, this can cause multiple cells with originally different values to have the same value, or multiple cells with originally the same value to have different values. When $(t, A)$'s value was equal to $(t', A)$, OTHER_VALUE was inserted in the selected cell. The default error rate was set to 0.05 (i.e. the number of errors injected is 5 % of the total number of tuples).

For experiments with error skewness, we injected the errors that follow the probability $P(\mathrm{Err}_t)$, or the probability of tuple $t$ includes an error, as follows:

$$P(\mathrm{Err}_t) = \begin{cases} \epsilon s/|\{t \mid t[\mathbf{Z}] = \mathbf{v}\}| & (t[\mathbf{Z}] = \mathbf{v}) \\ \epsilon(1.0 - s)/|\{t \mid t[\mathbf{Z}] \neq \mathbf{v}\}| & (\text{otherwise}) \end{cases}$$

where $\epsilon$ is the overall error rate in the dataset and $s(0 \leq s \leq 1)$ is the skewness factor denoting the proportion of errors that occur under specified condition $(\mathbf{Z}, \mathbf{v})$. When $s \gg |\{t \mid t[\mathbf{Z}] = \mathbf{v}\}|/|\{t \mid t \in D\}|$ holds, if the cell is within the specified area $\mathbf{Z} = \mathbf{v}$, the cell is erroneous for the specified probability, otherwise the cell can still be erroneous, but for a much smaller probability.

**Scalability.** We first look at the runtime of the repair algorithms as the input data size increases. Figures 2–4 describe the results with each dataset (the average of 10 iterations). IncRepair performed the fastest and looked the most scalable with WBC, but clearly did not seem to scale well with the two larger datasets. We stopped the runs where it took too long to complete. The result

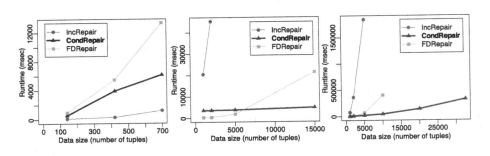

**Fig. 2.** Scalability (WBC)  **Fig. 3.** Scalability (DBGen)  **Fig. 4.** Scalability (Adult)

shows that IncRepair's exploration of all values in the domain of attribute $C$ to find a fix that satisfies $\Sigma$ is prohibitively expensive with a large dataset with unbounded attribute domains. FDRepair's runtime, as shown in the original paper, is at least quadratic, and looks sensitive even when the data consist of limited number of different values as with WBC. We think that the result is due to the algorithm's high cost for reverting and validating the candidate corrections. As opposed to the two previous algorithms, we observe that CondRepair's runtime is closer to linear with the data size (Figs. 2, 3 and 4).

**Effect of Error Skewness.** We then change the error skewness using the aforementioned error distribution model (Figs. 5, 6 and 7). Overall error rate was fixed to 0.05. A set of tuples with a predetermined condition is called "high error area" or HIGH, which is defined as HIGH = $\{t \mid t[\mathbf{Z}] = \mathbf{v}$ where $\mathbf{v}$ is a set of values selected from the domains of attributes in $\mathbf{Z}\}$. For $(\mathbf{Z}, \mathbf{v})$, we used a single attribute and $\mathbf{v}$ was selected so the number of tuples with $t[\mathbf{Z} = \mathbf{v}]$ is closest to 10 % of the input tuples. Cause conditions clump_thickness = "10" for WBC, state = NULL for DBGen, and occupation="Adm-clerical" for Adult were used throughout the iterations. The parameter $s$ varied from 0.05, 0.1 (no skew) to 1.0 (extremely skewed, where all errors occur under condition $\mathbf{Z} = \mathbf{v}$, but no errors occur in other areas).

As noted in some of the previous work, an injected error does not always violate a CFD rule, which may lead to a low recall. To separate the problem of errors' not being detected by the input rules, we measure the performances with the score metrics defined as follows:

$$\text{Precision} = \frac{\text{\# correctly detected errors}}{\text{\# detected errors}}, \text{Recall} = \frac{\text{\# correctly detected errors}}{\text{\# conflict introducing errors}}.$$

Figures 5, 6 and 7 show the accuracy (precision and recall) with different degrees of skewness (average of 20 iterations). The precision and recall scores are calculated on the cell-base count of errors.

With all datasets, CondRepair exceeded the other two algorithms both in precision and recall. CondRepair's score ranged 0.4-0.6 with all data sets with an exception for the precision for DBGen, where all the other algorithm's scores

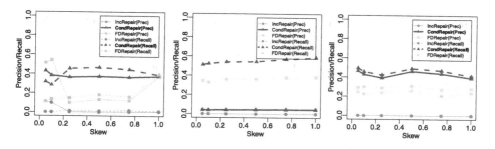

**Fig. 5.** Accuracy (WBC)      **Fig. 6.** Accuracy (DBGen)      **Fig. 7.** Accuracy (Adult)

were low as well. FDRepair performed equal to or better than CondRepair only with WBC and where there is little or no skewness. IncRepair's scores were especially low. We think this is because the type of errors used could not be correctly detected by the edit distance metrics.

In summary, CondRepair's runtime is nearly linear with the data size and its accuracy surpassed that of IncRepair and FDRepair with all tested datasets when the skewness is larger than 0.1.

## 4.2   Result Analysis

Results are examined from the aspects of (1) completeness of repairs and (2) correctness of repair values.

**Completeness of Repairs.** To test the completeness of repairs, we have used a basic function for CFD validation based on original definition of CFD described in Bohannon et al. [1], matching LHS value sets and RHS values for all pairs of tuples for all input rules. CondRepair produced repairs without a violation with WBC and Adult datasets, and left on average 43.2 tuples with violation with DBGen, because the input FD set contained rules that lead to the *collision* problem. It should be noted, that if we are allowed to impose order restriction described in Sect. 3.1 on the input rules, there should be no remaining errors also with DBGen. There were on average 308.5 tuples with remaining violations with IncRepair, 534.6 with FDRepair (WBC), 271.2 with IncRepair and 268.4 with FDRepair (1K tuples of DBGen), and 4.8 with IncRepair and 236.6 with FDRepair (1K tuples of Adult), when the error rate 0.05 and no skew.

IncRepair, when multiple rules in $\Sigma$ cannot be satisfied at once by changing the focused $k$ values within the tuple, the tuple is left with violations. In the case of FDRepair, although we could not examine it thoroughly, there is a possibility that a misconception is in their routine of building equivalence class, in that they do not create equivalence classes for singleton values. Leaving singleton values as they are can result in remaining violations because singleton values on a rule's RHS attribute can cause a conflict. In fact, FDRepair generated much less number of corrections than the number of conflict-introducing errors.

**Correctness of Repair Values.** We look at precision and recall of corrections, which are the rate of correctly fixed errors over all fixes made and the rate of correctly fixed errors over all conflict-introducing errors, respectively. Table 1 summarizes numbers of injected errors, conflict-introducing errors, and scores for tuple-wise detection, cell-wise detection (same as shown in Figs. 5-7), and scores for correction (skewness 0.25, a weak skew). Simply injecting errors to the datasets did not produce sufficient number of conflicts, so we repeated all tuples in the datasets so each tuple appears twice, which leads to sufficient number of conflicts for evaluation.

The scores of CondRepair were the highest except for tuple-wise detection with WBC and DBGen and for cell-wise detection precision with DBGen. IncRepair's

**Table 1.** Correctness of error detection and correction when s = 0.25 (ICV: injected and caused violation, TDP: tuple-wise detection precision, TDR: tuple-wise detection recall, DP: cell-wise detection precision, DR: cell-wise detection recall, CP: correction precision, CR: correction recall)

| dataset | WBC (2x699 lines) | | | | | | DBGen (2x1000 lines) | | | | | | Adult (2x1000 lines) | | | | | |
|---|---|---|---|---|---|---|---|---|---|---|---|---|---|---|---|---|---|---|
| # ICV | 38.1 for CFDs, 46.7 for FDs | | | | | | 90.5 | | | | | | 24.2 for CFDs, 33.65 for FDs | | | | | |
| Algorithm | TDP | TDR | DP | DR | CP | CR | TDP | TDR | DP | DR | CP | CR | TDP | TDR | DP | DR | CP | CR |
| IncRepair | .07 | **.57** | .00 | .01 | .00 | .00 | .14 | **.93** | .00 | .00 | .00 | .00 | .31 | .02 | .00 | .00 | .00 | .00 |
| FDRepair | .43 | .53 | .10 | .15 | .09 | .14 | .16 | .72 | **.05** | .36 | .04 | .27 | .66 | .30 | .24 | .29 | .16 | .19 |
| CondRepair | **.47** | .38 | **.36** | **.45** | **.36** | **.45** | **.18** | .63 | .04 | **.54** | **.04** | **.50** | **.69** | **.67** | **.39** | **.42** | **.22** | **.24** |

tuple-wise detection was higher with the two cases with tule-wise detection, but notably, its cell-wise detection scores and correction scores were zero or very low. FDRepair performed much better than reported in the original paper, but did not exceed in the scores for correction of CondRepair. CondRepair were able to find 67 % tuples with conflict-introducing errors with 69 % precision, which looks promising for a practical use. The scores for correction are not so high as we can leave the machine an important data to cleanse, but the algorithm can be used to suggest human users possible corrections.

## 5   Conclusions

We have proposed a data-repairing technique that discovers and leverages the common cause of errors. Our method CondRepair, achieved a nearly linear scalability and accuracy of error detection that is higher than previous methods. Further directions include (1) a closer observation of real-world data cleansing work and incorporation of observed characteristics of errors in experimental settings, (2) an incremental version of the algorithm, and (3) interaction with a human user to efficiently achieve an optimal repair.

## References

1. Bohannon, P., Fan, W., Geerts, F., Jia, X., Kementsietsidis, A.: Conditional functional dependencies for data cleaning. In: ICDE, pp. 746–755 (2007)
2. Cong, G., Fan, W., Geerts, F., Jia, X., Ma, S.: Improving data quality: consistency and accuracy. In: VLDB, pp. 315–326 (2007)
3. Chiang, F., Miller, R.J.: Discovering data quality rules. PVLDB **1**(1), 1166–1177 (2008)
4. Fan, W., Li, J., Ma, S., Tang, N., Yu, W.: Towards certain fixes with editing rules and master data. PVLDB **3**(1), 173–184 (2010)
5. Fan, W., Geerts, F.: Capturing missing tuples and missing values. In: PODS, pp. 169–178 (2010)
6. Yeh, P.Z., Puri, C.A.: Discovering conditional functional dependencies to detect data inconsistencies. In: Proceedings of the Fifth International Workshop on Quality in Databases at VLDB2010, (2010)

7. Beskales, G., Ilyas, I.F., Golab, L.: Sampling the repairs of functional dependency violations under hard constraints. VLDB Endowment **3**(1–2), 197–207 (2010)
8. Fan, W., Li, J., Ma, S., Tang, N., Yu, W.: Interaction between record matching and data repairing. In: SIGMOD Conference, pp. 469–480 (2011)
9. Bertossi, L., Bravo, L., Franconi, E., Lopatenko, A.: The complexity and approximation of fixing numerical attributes in databases under integrity constraints. Inf. Sys. **33**(4–5), 407–434 (2008)
10. Chomicki, J., Marcinkowski, J.: Minimal-change integrity maintenance using tuple deletions. Inf. Comput. **197**(1–2), 90–121 (2005)
11. Kolahi, S., Lakshmanan, L.V.S.: On approximating optimum repairs for functional dependency violations. In: Proceedings of the 12th International Conference on Database Theory, service, ICDT 2009, pp. 53–62. ACM, New York (2009)
12. Chandel, A., Koudas, N., Pu, K.Q., Srivastava, D.: Fast identification of relational constraint violations. In: Proceedings of the 2007 ICDE Conference, pp. 776–785. IEEE Computer Society, The Marmara Hotel, Istanbul (2007)
13. Weijie Wei, B.Z.X.T., Zhang, M.: A data cleaning method based on association rules. In: ISKE International Conference on Intelligent Systems and Knowledge Engineering (2007)
14. Bohannon, P., Flaster, M., Fan, W., Rastogi, R.: A cost-based model and effective heuristic for repairing constraints by value modification. In: SIGMOD Conference, pp. 143–154 (2005)
15. Damerau, F.J.: A technique for computer detection and correction of spelling errors. Commun. ACM **7**(3), 171–176 (1964)
16. Golab, L., Karloff, H.J., Korn, F., Srivastava, D., Yu, B.: On generating near-optimal tableaux for conditional functional dependencies. PVLDB **1**(1), 376–390 (2008)
17. Stoyanovich, J., Davidson, S.B., Milo, T., Tannen, V.: Deriving probabilistic databases with inference ensembles. In: ICDE, pp. 303–314 (2011)
18. Berti-Equille, L., Dasu, T., Srivastava, D.: Discovery of complex glitch patterns: A novel approach to quantitative data cleaning. In: ICDE, pp. 733–744 (2011)
19. Zaki, M.J., Ogihara, M.: Theoretical foundations of association rules. In: 3rd ACM SIGMOD Workshop on Research Issues in Data Mining and Knowledge Discovery (1998)
20. Agrawal, R., Imieliński, T., Swami, A.: Mining association rules between sets of items in large databases. SIGMOD Rec. **22**(2), 207–216 (1993)
21. Gray, J., Sundaresan, P., Englert, S., Baclawski, K., Weinberger, P. J.: Quickly generating billion-record synthetic databases. In: Proceedings of the 1994 ACM SIGMOD International Conference on Management of Data, service, SIGMOD 1994, pp. 243–252 (1994)

# Analyzing User Behaviors Based on Temporal Patterns of Sequential Pattern Evaluation Indices on Twitter

Hidenao Abe[✉]

Department of Information Systems, Bunkyo University,
1100 Namegaya, Chigasaki, Kanagawa 2538550, Japan
hidenao@shonan.bunkyo.ac.jp

**Abstract.** With social media sites, such as Twitter, providing a visual record of the daily interests and concerns of users in the form of tweets and tweeting behaviors, there is growing demand among users, such as corporations, to identify other interested users. However, accurately determining whether users who receive information (such as tweets) from enterprise users have a genuine interest in it can be difficult. In this study, the user behavior of resending information received on Twitter (retweeting) is analyzed with the aim of developing a method for constructing a model for predicting retweeting behavior using the content of past tweeting history via evaluation indices of words and phrases in the users' tweets. This paper analyzes the tweets sent by large online retail websites and by the followers who receive them, comparing the feature words obtained from the retweets with those in the tweets sent by the followers. This paper also discusses the feasibility of constructing a behavior prediction model by extracting temporal patterns of evaluation indices that are created from the usage frequencies of feature words and phrases obtained from followers' tweets.

**Keywords:** Temporal text mining · Sequential pattern evaluation index · User behavior prediction

## 1 Introduction

The recent rise of social media sites, such as Twitter, provides a media-based visual record of the speech and behavior of social media users, simply called users in this paper, that reflect their routine interests and concerns. Consequently, users, such as corporations and politicians, have begun looking for more efficient ways to communicate ideas with a large number of other users who have similar interests or concerns to theirs. As a result, many approaches have been developed in order to distinguish users having similar interests, using network analysis methods or/and text mining-based analysis methods [1]. However, because accurate identification of future user behavior without considering the user's speech and behavior history is a difficult to undertaking, there is a serious need to develop methods that more accurately predict users' behavior and interests.

© Springer International Publishing Switzerland 2015
X.-L. Li et al. (Eds.): PAKDD 2015, LNCS 9441, pp. 177–188, 2015.
DOI: 10.1007/978-3-319-25660-3_15

This study focuses on the Twitter behavior known as "retweeting", in which users disseminate information by resending it, and develops a method for constructing analytic models that can predict retweeting behavior using the content of user tweeting history. Accordingly, this paper examines the differences between groups of feature words and phrases contained in retweeted text and groups of feature words contained in the tweeting history of users believed to be interested in information from particular Twitter account holders, who are known as followers. Then, follows a discussion of explicit patterns in users' tweeting history based on temporal patterns obtained for groups of evaluation indices, computed using the usage frequencies of feature words contained in the followers' past tweets. These results are used to discuss the development of a method for constructing a model that predicts information-retweeting behavior using temporal patterns of evaluation indices of the feature words in the tweeting history.

This paper is organized as follows. Section 2 describes the proposed method. Section 3 presents evaluation index group definitions used for feature word selection. In Sect. 4, the feature words and phrases extraction is performed to three online retail website Twitter accounts that had a substantial number of followers in Japan. The method extracts feature word groups contained in retweeted text and in the tweet histories of retweeting followers. It also generates temporal patterns of the indices that are used as keyword evaluation indices for the followers' tweeting histories of one Twitter account. Finally, a conclusion is offered in Sect. 5.

## 2  Construction of a Model for Predicting Retweeting Behavior Using Temporal Patterns in Tweeting History

In this method, we assume that users' targeted tweeting behavior by an analyst is affected not only by the content of received tweets but also their history of tweets. In order to construct a model for predicting such targeted tweeting behavior of followers, we should set up more proper features for considering the history of their tweets, which are obtained from past tweeted content.

In the text analysis, feature word extraction from a text corpus is a well-known method for obtaining the features from text in previously posted content. Then, huge number of the feature words and phrases are often selected by the conventional methods, which are depended on one particular evaluation index. However, it is very difficult to develop universal evaluation index on various context. In various situation, there is no trivial answer for evaluating usefulness of the feature words. In addition, feature word groups that are obtained using feature word extraction do not indicate when the information was obtained or their temporal trends. Therefore, we focus on patterns of change over time (temporal patterns), and developed a method for constructing a model that predicts the appearance of phrases using the temporal patterns of the evaluation indices of multiple phrases [2].

From the point of view that use more various features enable more explicit descriptions of hidden dependent variable relationships, it is not trivial that conventional features based on the appearance of feature sequential patterns may or may not be better predictors than temporal patterns [3]. Therefore, an improved method should use both the appearance of feature words and the phrases' temporal patterns, which were obtained from the user tweet history, as features in order to more accurately characterize the content history. Moreover, this method could also identify behaviors by similarly linking temporal patterns of the tweet counts and intervals.

In order to develop this method, we firstly used actual data to extract feature word groups that represent the tweet content of users who performed specific behaviors and the temporal patterns indicating changes in usage trends of the feature words. The overview of this process is illustrated in Fig. 1.

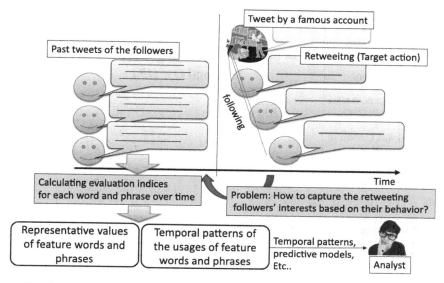

**Fig. 1.** Overview for capturing users' past behavior for detecting a target action.

## 3  Evaluation Indices Based on Appearance Frequency of Words and Sequential Patterns

In the text, words and phrases[1] are represented by a series of one or more words. Given words $w_i$ and $w_j$ in a sequential relationship, the order relation $i < j$ is always true, and a term $term_x$ that is formed from these two words is expressed as $term_x = <w_i, w_j>$. Because of this phrase property, all sentences can be considered sequential data, having an ordered sequential relationship, and terms can be considered to be subsequences. With considering the common ordered relations of items in each data of the dataset, both of a natural language processing-based phrase importance indices and sequential pattern evaluation indices can be used to evaluate phrases. The definitions of these indices are shown in Table 1.

---

[1] Hereafter, words and phrases are called 'term'. Each term consists of one or more words.

**Table 1.** Importance evaluation indices and sequential pattern indices for each appearance frequency measurement standard for a term.

| | Frequency Measurement Standard | |
|---|---|---|
| | Document Frequency $DF = \mid D_{\in term_i} \mid$ | Term Frequency $TF = \sum_j freq(term_i, d_j)$ |
| Support | $DF / \mid D \mid$ | $TF / \sum TF_{term_i}$ |
| Odds | $DF / (\mid D \mid - DF)$ | $TF / (\sum TF_{term_i} - TF)$ |
| Self-Information | $(DF / \mid D \mid) \log_2(DF / \mid D \mid)$ | $(TF / \sum TF_{term_i}) \log(TF / \sum TF_{term_i})$ |
| Jaccard Coefficient | $\dfrac{DF}{DF(w_1 \cup ... \cup w_L)}$ | $\dfrac{TF}{TF(w_1 \cup ... \cup w_L)}$ |
| TFIDF | $TF * \log(\mid D \mid / DF)$ | |
| Head Confidence (H-Conf) | $\dfrac{DF}{DF(w_1, D)}$ | $\dfrac{TF}{TF(w_1, D)}$ |
| Max Confidence (MaxConf) | $\max\left(\dfrac{DF}{DF(w_l, D)}\right)$ | $\max\left(\dfrac{TF}{TF(w_l, D)}\right)$ |
| All Confidence (AllConf) | $\dfrac{DF}{\max(DF(w_l, D))}$ | $\dfrac{TF}{\max(TF(w_l, D))}$ |
| Sequential All Confidence (SeqAllConf) | $\dfrac{DF}{\max(DF(\beta_{\subseteq term_i}, D))}$ | $\dfrac{TF}{\max(TF(\beta_{\subseteq term_i}, D))}$ |

### 3.1  Importance Evaluation Indices for Words and Phrases

Multiple importance evaluation indices have been developed for natural language processing and text mining in order to measure the importance of words and phrases for extracting features. The primary standard these indices use is the appearance frequency of the word or phrases. Two appearance measurement references are commonly used for term appearance frequency: the term frequency (TF), which counts the number of times a term is repeated in one or more documents, and the document frequency (DF), which counts the number of documents in which the term appears.

Table 1 displays the typical evaluation indices for a term consisting of $L$ words ($L \geq 1$), i.e., $term_i = <w_1, ..., w_L>$. The term frequency and inverse document frequency (TFIDF) method is most commonly used to evaluate the importance of the words and phrases for keyword extraction. It considers both the TF and DF and uses the ratio between the entire target document $\mid D \mid$ and the DF as a weight. A simple ratio that compares every pair of appearance frequency measurement standards can be used to index measuring properties based on appearance frequency.

## 3.2  Phrase Evaluation Indices Using Sequential Pattern Evaluation Indices

Sequential pattern evaluation indices are indices that quantify multiple properties of sequential patterns using the appearance frequency $freq(\alpha, D)$ of partial sequence $\alpha$ in sequential data set $D = \{s_i\}$, containing sequential data $s_i = <i_1, ..., i_m>$, which are strings of items $i \in I$ that belong to item set $I$. Similar to the method used to determine keyword evaluation indices, two appearance frequency standards are typically used in order to count the appearance frequency of partial sequence $a = <i_1, ..., i_j> (j \leq m)$ in sequential data set $D$.

Applying the TF frequency standard, which considers repetitions in each document, and the DF frequency standard, which does not consider repetitions, a confidence-based index is defined using an evaluation index group for the non-sequential item set [4] and an evaluation index group that considers the items in a sequential pattern [5]. I consider a sequence $\alpha$ to be the term $term_i$ and each item to be word $w_l$ within $term_i$.

As is also displayed in Table 1, when the sequential relationships between the items of a phrase's sequential pattern are considered, more than eight indices can be defined for the various confidences, which are the combined ratio of the appearance frequency of $\alpha$ and the appearance frequency of $\beta$, a subsequence of $\alpha$.

## 4  Tweeting Behavior Analysis of Online Retail Twitter Accounts and Their Followers

This section examines user-sent texts (tweets), which contain 140 characters or less, obtained from a Twitter application programming interface (API) [6]. By gathering tweets both from some prominent account holders and from their followers tweets over the time, the relationships between the users' interests and concerns are analyzed as the features of resent tweets (retweets) that originate from the well-known Twitter accounts and of tweets sent by the retweeting users during a previous time period. In order to provide a broader analysis of general user interests, we define retweeting as the action of tweeting a feature word contained in a retweeted tweet.

The analysis procedure is as follows.

1. The feature words contained in tweets that were retweeted by some followers from a well-known Twitter account during a given period are extracted.
2. The followers that retweeted tweets including the feature words in (1) are listed.
3. The tweets sent by the followers in (2) during a time period prior to that of (1) are gathered.
4. The feature words contained in the tweets gathered in (3) and the temporal patterns of evaluation index groups based on their appearance frequencies are extracted.

The goal of this study is to develop a method for constructing a model that predicts information-based retweeting behavior using the temporal patterns of the tweeting history. Thus, the following analysis was performed as an application of this method using the procedure described above.

In order to obtain candidate phrases (phrases that could be characteristic phrases) from the gathered text, the test applied an automatic terminology extraction method, which is used in natural language processing, to each document set. Additionally, in order to extract the phrases serving as feature word candidates, we used the FLR score-based automatic terminology extraction method [7] developed by Nakagawa. The nouns used in the FLR score calculation were identified from morphological analysis results using MeCab [8] and the IPA[2] dictionary (mecab-ipadic-2.7.0-20070801) distributed with it. Applying the FLR score calculation results, feature word candidates were selected from the phrases having *FLR(term$_i$, D) > 1.0.*

## 4.1   Extraction of Feature Words Contained in Retweeted Text

Our test extracted feature words from sets of retweeted text (retweets) that were sent from the official Twitter accounts of 7 Net Shopping (7_netshopping), Amazon.co.jp (AmazonJP), and Rakuten Ichiba (RakutenJP).

The covered tweets were sent from these Twitter accounts between January 15, 2015, and January 20, 2015. Table 3 shows the number of retweeted tweets and the number of FLR score-based feature word candidate phrases in the tweets sent from the Twitter accounts (Table 2).

**Table 2.** Number of retweeted tweets and number of FLR score-based candidate phrases in tweets sent from three major retail Twitter accounts between January 15 and 20, 2015

| Retailer | |D| | FLR score-based candidate phrases |
|---|---|---|
| 7 Net Shopping | 76 | 369 |
| Amazon.co.jp | 193 | 857 |
| Rakuten Ichiba | 127 | 540 |

Table 4 shows the top ten phrases for the Twitter accounts based on their TFIDF values, along with the support and the head confidence (H-Conf) measures for these phrases. The support and the head confidence were calculated using a standard for counting frequencies based on document frequency (DF).

The results in Table 4 provide characteristic phrase groups for the tweets that the followers retweeted. These feature word groups are phrases contained in the tweets sent by the Twitter accounts and can be considered to align with some of the followers' interests.

However, these feature words and phrases do not reflect the followers' interests directly. The issue is to capture more implicit interests and concerns of the followers from their behavioral history. Therefore, in order to obtain term groups that corresponded to a broader set of follower interests, the historic tweet content of followers who retweeted the tweets containing the original phrases must be examined. This will result in changes in the usage frequency of feature words and phrases.

---

[2] This IPA dictionary is a Japanese morpheme dictionary made by the project run by the Information-Technology Promoting Agency in Japan.

**Table 3.** Top ten phrases for Twitter accounts based on TFIDF values and the support and the head confidence levels for these phrases (document frequency standard).

| Terms | 7 Net Shopping | | | Term | Amazon.co.jp | | | Term | Rakuten Ichiba | | |
|---|---|---|---|---|---|---|---|---|---|---|---|
| | TFIDF | Support(DF) | H-Conf(DF) | | TFIDF | Support(DF) | H-Conf(DF) | | TFIDF | Support(DF) | H-Conf(DF) |
| 限定 (Limited) | 41.39 | 0.26 | 1.00 | タイム セール (Time Sales) | 73.57 | 0.22 | 1.00 | 楽天 ポイント ("Rakuten" Points) | 84.18 | 0.23 | 0.58 |
| セブン(Seven) | 33.47 | 0.29 | 1.00 | OFF | 63.38 | 0.20 | 1.00 | 楽天 ("Rakuten") | 74.57 | 0.39 | 1.00 |
| 特典 (Special-gift) | 32.95 | 0.22 | 1.00 | 人気(Popular) | 53.11 | 0.14 | 1.00 | 応募 (Application) | 51.21 | 0.26 | 1.00 |
| 予約 (Reservation) | 32.53 | 0.43 | 1.00 | PC | 52.78 | 0.06 | 1.00 | フォロワー (Follower) | 51.21 | 0.26 | 1.00 |
| 予約 受付 (Reservation Accepting) | 31.95 | 0.37 | 0.85 | 限定(Limited) | 52.14 | 0.10 | 1.00 | ♪ | 46.70 | 0.38 | 1.00 |
| 月 (Month) | 30.02 | 0.17 | 1.00 | 受付 (Accepting) | 52.12 | 0.12 | 1.00 | フォロー 解除 (Unfollow) | 44.47 | 0.26 | 1.00 |
| 発売(For-sale) | 29.21 | 0.20 | 1.00 | チェック (Check-it) | 51.10 | 0.13 | 1.00 | 当選 確率 (Winning Probability) | 44.47 | 0.26 | 1.00 |
| アカチャンホンポ ("Akachan-honpo") | 27.06 | 0.14 | 1.00 | 予約 受付 (Reservation Accepting) | 50.03 | 0.12 | 0.89 | 完了 (Finished) | 44.47 | 0.26 | 1.00 |
| セブン ネット ("Seven Net") | 26.96 | 0.22 | 0.77 | % OFF | 48.80 | 0.11 | 0.75 | 下 (Under) | 44.31 | 0.23 | 1.00 |
| DVD | 26.49 | 0.21 | 1.00 | 最大 (Maximum) | 45.34 | 0.10 | 1.00 | RT | 43.29 | 0.24 | 1.00 |

## 4.2 Feature Words and Temporal Patterns of Text Retweeted by Users

Twitter accounts can attract followers, who will receive all the information sent from the account. Tweets sent from followers contain various phrases, which are determined by their interests and most likely reflect those interests. Thus, this method hypothesized that when users retweeted tweets sent from the three well-known Twitter accounts, these retweets would contain feature words that relate to their previously sent tweets.

This section describes our process for testing this hypothesis by examining the content of tweets sent from the followers of our three well-known online retail Twitter accounts before the retweets were sent. In order to obtain the temporal patterns of the evaluation indices, we extracted feature words and the patterns of temporal change from these previous tweets. For followers who retweeted tweets sent from the three well-known Twitter accounts between January 15 and 20, 2015, we gathered the tweets sent between January 1 and 20, 2015, by the followers[3] of each of the well-known accounts. Then, the tweets gathered between January 1 and 14 are used to obtain the following temporal patterns of each evaluation index on each well-known retailer followers's tweets. For all of the terms, the 18 evaluation indices values were calcluated in each timestamped dataset. Then, the values of each term consists of each data of the term.

---

[3] Due to restrictions in the Twitter API, these users were the users who met the criteria from the randomly acquired 5,000 users.

**Table 4.** Number of tweets between January 1 and 14 sent by the retweeting followers.

| | Following Accunt | | |
|---|---|---|---|
| | 7 Net Shopping | Amazon.co.jp | Rakute Ichba |
| 1st Januray | 19,577 | 130 | 0 |
| 2nd January | 20,906 | 55 | 15 |
| 3rd January | 21,571 | 37 | 67 |
| 4th January | 22,103 | 2,303 | 27 |
| 5th January | 22,773 | 10,899 | 0 |
| 6th January | 25,776 | 18,012 | 0 |
| 7th January | 24,636 | 19,734 | 109 |
| 8th January | 23,771 | 24,189 | 96 |
| 9th January | 25,467 | 22,746 | 16 |
| 10th January | 26,956 | 23,358 | 13 |
| 11th January | 27,542 | 24,815 | 100 |
| 12th January | 27,902 | 25,817 | 107 |
| 13th January | 36,810 | 33,992 | 5,073 |
| 14th January | 35,835 | 30,273 | 22,651 |
| Total | 361,625 | 236,360 | 28,274 |

Table 5 shows the number of gathered tweetes between January 1 and 14, 2015[4] of the followers who sent tweets containing one of the phrases listed in Table 3 between January 15 and 20, 2015 for each account.

After applying the FLR scores to extract feature terms from these user tweets, the candidate terms were extracted as shown in Table 6. For each top 1000 terms with the FLR score, the importance evaluation indices and sequential pattern evaluation indices are calculated in each daily set of documents. Then, for each evaluation index, the values for each timepoint, every daily set, of each term was converted into one temporal data. So, the dataset of one particular evaluation index for temporal pattern extraction contains up to 1000 instances with the values on each timepoint in this experiment.

Subsequently, a clustering method was then applied to the conveted temporal datasets to obtain the temporal patterns of each index, reflecting the followers' activities before retweeting the tweets from the well-known account. For the clustering method, a simple $k$-means implementation in Weka [9] was applied to the datasets in this analysis. The value of $k$ was set to 10, which is the upper limit for the obtaining clusters, since null clusters were allowed in this execution. For calculating the similarity between two instances, the Euclidean distance with normilization on each variable, which is correspond to each timepoint, was employed.

---

[4] Considering more realistic situation, the gathered tweets are not re-retrieved in the prior period after listing the followers who tweeted the tweets containing the feature words and phrases listed in Table 3.

**Table 5.** Number of candidate feature words and phrases based on the FLR score in the entire dataset of tweets counted in Table 5 for each well-known account.

| Retailer | |D| | FLR score-based candidate phrases |
|---|---|---|
| 7 Net Shopping | 361,625 | 271,234 |
| Amazon.co.jp | 236,360 | 211,730 |
| Rakuten Ichiba | 28,274 | 40,080 |

**Table 6.** Description of the clusters obtained for each evaluation index on each account dataset.

| | Following Account | | | | | |
|---|---|---|---|---|---|---|
| | 7 Net Shopping | | Amazon.co.jp | | Rakuten Ichiba | |
| | # Clusters | s.s.e | # Clusters | s.s.e | # Clusters | s.s.e |
| TFIDF | 10 | 4.07 | 10 | 9.95 | 10 | 15.62 |
| Support(DF) | 10 | 3.62 | 10 | 5.02 | 10 | 6.38 |
| Support(TF) | 10 | 1.34 | 10 | 6.77 | 10 | 9.14 |
| MaxConf(DF) | 6 | 105.31 | 7 | 126.30 | 7 | 17.87 |
| MaxConf(TF) | 7 | 115.95 | 7 | 148.77 | 7 | 20.50 |

Table 6 shows the numbers of temporal clusters obtained and their sum of squared errors (s.s.e) values within the clusters on each dataset from the five evaluation indices. As shown in Table 6, TFIDF and Support achieved small s.s.e values compared with those of MaxConf datasets. Figure 1 shows the temporal patterns of the indices of 7 Net Shopping followers who retweeted its tweets between January 15 and 20. Since the clusters are obtained by using the Euclidean distance, the lines, the centroids of each cluster, are calculated as the averages of each cluster.

Most of the patterns represents the differences of the averages of each evaluation index based on their temporal values in Fig. 2. As shown in Fig. 2(a), the temporal patterns represent the levels of the averaged values of the member of each cluster. This means that the averaged value of this evaluation index is suitable than the menbership to each temporal cluster.

However, the Cluster#6 of MaxConf(DF) shows significant difference from the other patterns.

Figure 3 shows those contained words and phrases included in the temporal patterns as the temporal clusters that have the evaluation index scores in the top ten in each cluster. By examining the temporal values of these words and phrases in the Cluster#6, most of these phrases appeared after 5th January for promoting new popular games on smart-phones such as Android terminals. The pattern includes changings of the promotion targets of the retweeting followers.

These results demonstrate that we can capture different aspects of the historical behaviors of users by obtaining the temporal clusters of the different types of evaluation indices. These patterns will reveal more about the followers' concerns from the viewpoint of the enterprise users. This will help analysts for promoting their sales items to adequate followers by selecting the temporal patterns and the term groups included

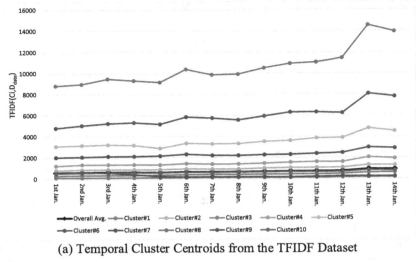

(a) Temporal Cluster Centroids from the TFIDF Dataset

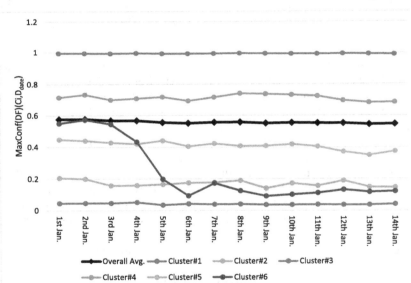

(b) Temporal Cluster Centroids from the MaxConf(DF) Dataset

**Fig. 2.** Temporal patterns of TFIDF(a) and MaxConf(DF)(b) in 7 Net Shopping's retweeting followers' tweets.

in the selected temporal pattern. By targeting the follower's action to promotions of false rumors, it will be able to detect demagogues more quickly based on the values of the evaluation indices of the temporal pattern, which is not necessary to include each particular word itself.

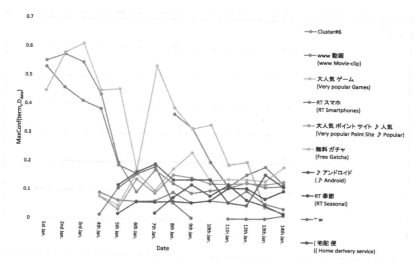

**Fig. 3.** Representative words and phrases of Cluster#6 of MaxConf(DF) in 7 Net Shopping retweeting followers' tweets.

In addition to the above effect, these behaviors also include mechanical accounts (called "bots") as well as human accounts; however. Among the viral marketing and social media mining field, it is one of the important issue to distinguish such mechanical bots as spam. So, the different behaviors reflected by the temporal patterns will also help in distinguishing the spam accounts.

## 5 Conclusion

In this paper, we examined the Twitter behavior known as retweeting, which refers to the dissemination of information that occurs when users resend tweets. We examined the differences between the feature word groups that are contained in retweeted text and the feature word groups contained in the tweet history of the followers. We assume that these users have an interest in the information sent from specific Twitter accounts. In our assessment of three well-known retailers' Twitter accounts, the method discovered the significant terms that the terms contained in retweets differed from those of the users' previous tweets. I further concluded that using different dates produced changes in the combinations of the same phrase and that the resulting evaluation index differed not only in value but also in relative ranking.

Our future goal is to use this study to construct a predictive model using the presence or absence of these temporal patterns as an explanatory variable for retweeting behavior. In addition to the patterns of phrase usage frequency changes, we will also acquire the temporal patterns of behavior changes, such as tweeting intervals, for the purpose of developing a method of constructing a predictive model that can be combined with conventional feature word-based characterization.

**Acknowledgement.** This work was supported by JSPS KAKENHI Grant Numbers 24500175 and 26240036.

# References

1. Goonetilleke, O., Sellis, T., Zhang, X., Sathe, S.: Twitter analytics: a big data management perspective. SIGKDD Explor. Newsl. **16**(1), 11–20 (2014)
2. Abe, H.: Analysis for finding innovative concepts based on temporal patterns of terms in documents. In: Sakurai, S. (ed.) Theory and Applications for Advanced Text Mining, pp. 37–50. InTech, Osaka (2012). doi: 10.5772/52210. https://www.intechopen.com/books/theory-and-applications-for-advanced-text-mining/analysis-forfinding-innovative-concepts-based-on-temporal-patterns-of-terms-in-documents
3. Abe, H., Tsumoto, S.: Mining classification rules for detecting medication order changes by using characteristic CPOE subsequences. In: Kryszkiewicz, M., Rybinski, H., Skowron, A., Raś, Z.W. (eds.) ISMIS 2011. LNCS, vol. 6804, pp. 80–89. Springer, Heidelberg (2011)
4. Wu, T., Chen, Y., Han, J.: Association mining in large databases: a re-examination of its measures. In: Proceedings of the 11th European Conference on Principles and Practice of Knowledge Discovery in Databases, pp. 621–628 (2007)
5. Lin, C.X., Ji, M., Danilevsky, M., Han, J.: Efficient mining of correlated sequential patterns based on null hypothesis. In: Proceedings of the 2012 International Workshop on Web-Scale Knowledge Representation, Retrieval and Reasoning (Web-KR 2012), pp. 17–24 (2012)
6. Twitter Web API 1.1. https://dev.twitter.com/docs/api/1.1
7. Nakagawa, H.: Automatic term recognition based on statistics of compound nouns. Terminology **6**(2), 195–210 (2000)
8. MeCab: Yet Another Part-of-Speech and Morphological Analyzer. https://code.google.com/p/mecab/
9. Witten, I.H., Frank, E.: Data Mining: Practical Machine Learning Tools and Techniques with Java Implementations. Morgan Kaufmann, San Francisco (2000)

# Model Selection of Symbolic Regression to Improve the Accuracy of PM$_{2.5}$ Concentration Prediction

Guangfei Yang[✉] and Jian Huang

School of Management Science and Engineering, Dalian University of Technology,
Dalian, China
gfyang@dlut.edu.cn

**Abstract.** As one of the main components of haze, topics with respect to PM$_{2.5}$ are coming into people's sight recently in China. In this paper, we try to predict PM$_{2.5}$ concentrations in Dalian, China via symbolic regression (SR) based on genetic programming (GP). During predicting, the key problem is how to select accurate models by proper interestingness measures. In addition to the commonly used measures, such as R-squared value, mean squared error, number of parameters, etc., we also study the effectiveness of a set of potentially useful measures, such as AIC, BIC, HQC, AICc and EDC. Besides, a new interestingness measure, namely Interestingness Elasticity (IE), is proposed in this paper. From the experimental results, we find that the new measure gains the best performance on selecting candidate models and shows promising extrapolative capability.

**Keywords:** PM$_{2.5}$ · Symbolic regression · Model selection · Interestingness measures

## 1 Introduction

The atmospheric environment has been seriously polluted in recent years, and the lives of people are disturbed. Especially in China, PM$_{2.5}$ is the primary pollutant that should be controlled. PM$_{2.5}$ is also called fine particulate matter, whose diameter is 2.5 micrometers or less, about one twentieth the diameter of human hair. PM$_{2.5}$ contains a lot of harmful substances, which can enter the body through breathing, causing respiratory disease, lung cancer and other diseases. The research of Chan and Yao (2008) suggests that the air pollution in mega cities is highlighted gradually in the last a few years, restricting China's economic development seriously [1]. Pope and Dockery (2006) find that particulate matter (PM) air pollution has adverse effects on cardiopulmonary health, and is one of the sources of cardiopulmonary morbidity and mortality [2]. Therefore, the timely prevention and treatment of PM$_{2.5}$ is extremely important.

In this article, we attempt to forecast the value of PM$_{2.5}$ concentrations during the upcoming day in Dalian, China. The method we use is symbolic regression based on genetic programming. One of the important issues that affect the performance of SR is model selection. A model with a high accuracy usually means a large complexity. To construct an unknown function in a high-dimensional space from a finite number of

© Springer International Publishing Switzerland 2015
X.-L. Li et al. (Eds.): PAKDD 2015, LNCS 9441, pp. 189–197, 2015.
DOI: 10.1007/978-3-319-25660-3_16

samples bears the risk of overfitting [3]. Among the expressions SR produced, how to choose an appropriate interestingness measure or criterion to select the right model from the candidates fitting the data occupies an important position. Up to now, there have been some measures being applied to find the optimal solution, such as Akaike's information criterion (AIC), corrected AIC (AICc), Bayesian information criterion (BIC), Hannan-Quinn criterion (HQC), the efficient detection criterion (EDC), and so on. Besides these, we put forward a new kind of measure named Interestingness Elasticity to compare with the above-mentioned measures. Our results show that IE outperforms the other interestingness measures, which means to choose a better model and to give a more accurate result at the same time.

So far, many interestingness measures have been proposed and verified by researchers in various data sets, but the conclusions are inconsistent. Most of the measures were used in model selection for linear equations. Cherkassky and Ma (2003) compared three approaches namely AIC, BIC and the structural risk minimization (SRM). The results demonstrated that SRM and BIC showed similar predictive performance, and is better than AIC [4]. Wagenmakers and Farrell (2004) transformed AIC values to so-called Akaike weights, and proved that these weights could reveal the conditional probabilities for each model and promote the interpretation [5]. Chen and Huang (2005) evaluated the performance of seven criteria on different size of samples. They found that the conditional model estimator (CME) can select the best model and fuse multiple models for prediction [6]. Garg and Sriram (2013) studied the effect of three model selection criteria via GP while modeling the stock, two data transformations were also tested. It is discovered that PE is superior to the other methods [7]. Posada and Buckley (2004) discussed some fundamental concepts and techniques of model selection in the context of phylogenetics. They claimed that AIC and BIC have advantages to compare multiple nested or non-nested models [8].

## 2  Methodology

### 2.1  Symbolic Regression Based on GP

Genetic programming is a breakthrough algorithm first proposed by American professor Koza in 1992. As a new heuristic method, the emergence of GP has brought forth a great revolution to evolutionary computation field all over the world. And until now the implantation of GP can also be seen everywhere. In the design of GP, the individual adopts a tree structure, which is more flexible to express the arithmetic or logic relationship between variables. Through reproduction, crossover and mutation, GP produces new offspring by iteration based upon the current population. The algorithm stops until the termination condition reaches. GP has been used in many areas successfully, for example, financial markets, industrial processes, chemical and biological processes, mechanical models, and so on [9, 10].

Symbolic regression is one of the earliest applications of GP. The purpose of SR is to explore mathematical patterns hidden in the data and to construct symbolic expressions of functions between the input and the output variables. GP-trees were regarded as the evolving structures that represent symbolic expressions or models. The regression task can be thought as a supervised learning problem if the functionals and the terminals have been selected [11]. As is well known, a fundamental difficulty in symbolic regression is the choice of an appropriate model. A good interestingness measure can always pick the most appropriate model fitting the existing data.

## 2.2 Interestingness Measures for Model Selection

Interestingness measure is a way to solve model selection problems. The main idea of existing interestingness measures is to calculate a measure index value of each model, and then rank the models in ascending order according to the corresponding values. We usually select the best expression to achieve the prediction. Generally speaking, the optimal candidate is the one with the minimum or maximum index value (Depends on the definition of the indicator), which can be seen as follows:

$$V(k) = \{V(1), V(2), V(3), \ldots, V(n)\}_{MIN|MAX} \tag{1}$$

Here, $n$ is the number of models generated by GP and $V(k)$ denotes the index value of the optimal model.

Up to now, although model selection occupies a decisive position in symbolic regression, there is not a unified view to judge the most outstanding method, especially for nonlinear models. In the earliest years, people select a model from a set of individuals SR generated mainly according to the model accuracy, such as R-squared, prediction error (PE). The PE used in our experiment is defined below.

$$PE = \frac{SSE}{N} \tag{2}$$

$N$ indicates the number of experimental data points, and $SSE$ is the residual sum of squares.

With the in-depth study on GP, researchers found that model selection should be based not only on goodness-of-fit, but must also consider model complexity [12]. An expression that best captures the potential information of data always suffers the risk of overfitting, which causing a bad generalization ability of model. Based on this, many measures have been put forward to solve the problem, and most of them originated in statistics and econometrics. The measures used in this article are AIC [13–15], AICc [16, 17], BIC [18], HQC [19] and EDC [20]. The measures mentioned above were proposed to deal with selection of linear equations, however, nonlinear model must also weigh against the complexity and precision, so they may be applied in this case.

The Akaike's information criterion was proposed by Akaike in 1973. It is a common interestingness measure being applied in model selection for linear regression. AIC makes a tradeoff between accuracy and model complexity, it looks for the equation that can best explain the data but contains the fewest free parameters. Another advantage of AIC is that it can compare very different models. The definition of AIC is shown in Eq. 3 and $k$ stands for the total number of parameters in an estimated equation.

$$AIC = N \ln(SSE/N) + 2k \tag{3}$$

Corrected AIC is a corrected form of AIC. Unlike AIC, AICc evaluates the accuracy and complexity, and it considers the size of sample as well. Sample size is an important index, especially for small sample data. Equation 4 displays the formula of AICc.

$$AICc = AIC + \frac{2k(k+1)}{N-k-1} \tag{4}$$

The Bayesian information criterion is another famous measure in model selection. The formula of AIC and BIC is very similar, but the principles of them are different. The perspective of AIC is the population perspective, whereas that of BIC is the sample perspective. BIC follows the formula below.

$$BIC = N \ln(SSE/N) + k \log(N) \tag{5}$$

Equation 6 presents the content of Hannan-Quinn criterion. HQC can also be seen in articles, but it seems that the second term is not so practical, since this latter number is small even for a very large $N$.

$$HQC = N \ln(SSE/N) + 2k \log(\log(N)) \tag{6}$$

In addition, the last measure being adopted in the experiment is the efficient detection criterion, Kundu and Murali (1996) done a simulation study to choose the proper penalty function of EDC, which is shown in Eq. 7.

$$EDC = N \ln(SSE/N) + k N^{0.5} \tag{7}$$

### 2.3   Interestingness Elasticity

In this part, we put forward a new measure namely Interestingness Elasticity. Based upon our experiments, we find that IE has a more outstanding performance than the other methods. IE is inspired from the concept of elasticity in economics, it refers to the property that a variable occurs a certain percentage of change with respect to another variable. Elasticity could be applied between all variables which have a causal relationship. Usually, a model which has a lower error means more parameters to be estimated at the same time. Under the background of model selection, one should balance the relationship between prediction precision and the size of the model. Therefore, IE may be used to solve the current problem. When the equations are sorted in ascending order of complexity, IE can be defined in formula 8.

$$IE = \left| \frac{(E_1 - E_2)/E_1}{(C_2 - C_1)/C_2} \right| \tag{8}$$

$E$ is the mean squared error of an expression obtained from the training sets. $C$ stands for the number of nodes in the tree structure, which reflects the complexity of a model in another aspect. IE aims to find models that possess an excellent fitting degree but don't at the expense of complexity because that a simpler equation is easier to understand. Therefore, a smaller IE value represents that the magnitude of change of precision is smaller than the change of complexity.

Above all, the interestingness measures fall into three categories. The first class is composed by the approaches that solely consider the accuracy. The second class includes the measures raised by other researchers, and all the members of this class take the factor of complexity into account. The last one is the new measure we proposed. In the next section, a detailed comparison of these measures will be elaborated.

## 3 Experiment and Result

### 3.1 Experiment and Data

Our aim is to make a prediction of the $PM_{2.5}$ concentration. The independent variables are the concentration of other pollutants in the atmosphere and weather condition indicators. The experiment is divided into 24 groups to predict the concentration of $PM_{2.5}$ in the next 1–24 h respectively. In each group, 10 different training and test sets are applied and we choose each of the last ten days as a test set, and all the data before the day as the training set.

In the experiment, the data consists of two parts: The pollutant concentration data per hour and corresponding weather condition data of the same time. The scope of the data is from May $4^{th}$ 18:00 to September $4^{th}$ 23:00 in 2014. The pollutant data was collected from the website: http://www.pm25.in/, and the weather data got from the network station of Central Meteorological Station. To predict the value of $PM_{2.5}$ concentration, 20 variables are used to form the independent space, including $CO$, $SO_2$, $NO_2$, $O_3$, $PM_{10}$, mean value of various pollutants within 24 h, temperature, wind speed, relative humidity, pressure, and so on. By the statistics, there are a total of 2231 points of data collected, and in order to ensure the validity and applicability of data, we impute the missing values using the interpolation method in SPSS. A linear conversion is used to avoid the impact of different dimensions of variables, which can also speed up the convergence.

The prediction process can be divided into two stages. In the first stage, we run the program using the existing data. In the second phase, we select the models via interestingness measures and evaluate the result.

### 3.2 Experimental Results and Analysis

The tool used in the experiment is named Eureqa. In order to determine which measure performs better than the other measures when selecting a model from a few candidates being produced, we compare each type of measure separately. Figure 1 represents the result of comparison between IE and the approaches of the first category. The vertical axis indicates the average error of each method when selecting the optimal models and applied on the test sets. Each error in the figure is modified by subtracting the average value of three measures. An error smaller than zero implies the accuracy is higher than the average level, whereas the opposite. From the figure, we can discovery that in most of the groups, IE outperforms the other methods. In fact, in more than half of the groups, it shows an apparent lower error. We could conclude that the models IE selected have better generalization ability when faced with a new data.

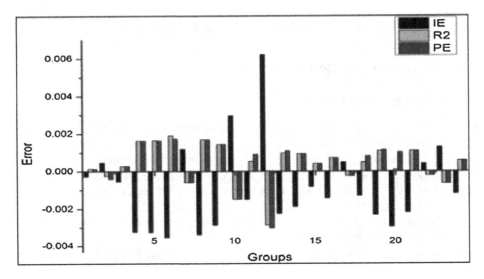

**Fig. 1.** Comparison of IE with the first category measures (Each error is modified by subtracting the average value of three measures. A smaller error indicates a higher accuracy)

Figure 2 is draw following the same way as Fig. 1. To avoid confusion, we show the circumstances of each group separately. In the figure, an intuitive contrasting result of IE and the other model selection measures is shown. 17 of the groups illustrate that IE holds a lower prediction error than the mean level. Actually, the error of IE is the least in 15 groups. We can also find that in almost all groups, AIC and AICc have the same features, which might imply that the sample size does not have a significant influence for our data. The difference between AIC, BIC and HQC is not obvious. Sometimes they even choose the same equation, and we guess this may because that these three measures have the similar structure. They all mainly contain two items, one term assesses the accuracy and the other is a penalty term of model size. The former terms of the measures are the same, only a change on the latter term seems to cause no remarkable effect on the selection.

Besides, Table 1 shows the statistical analysis of mean absolute errors in all the test sets. The standard deviation illustrates that IE has a better robustness. And the maximum error and the average error occur in IE are lower than other methods. IE tends to generate a model with smaller error, which means a better extrapolative capability.

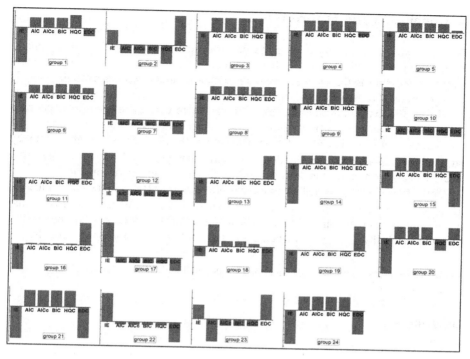

**Fig. 2.** Comparison of IE with the second category measures (Each error is modified by subtracting the average value of six measures.)

**Table 1.** Statistical analysis of errors in all the test sets (SD is short for standard deviation and Num is the number of test sets.)

|        | Max        | Min          | Avg          | SD           | Num |
|--------|------------|--------------|--------------|--------------|-----|
| $R^2$  | 0.0062     | 0.270585     | 0.057712     | 0.044861     | 240 |
| PE     | **0.006193** | 0.270585   | 0.057722     | 0.044872     | 240 |
| AIC    | 0.0062     | 0.270585     | 0.057842     | 0.045251     | 240 |
| AICc   | 0.0062     | 0.270585     | 0.057842     | 0.045251     | 240 |
| BIC    | 0.0062     | 0.270585     | 0.05781      | 0.045356     | 240 |
| HQC    | 0.006193   | 0.270585     | 0.057865     | 0.045315     | 240 |
| EDC    | 0.00524    | **0.239281** | 0.057662     | 0.044123     | 240 |
| IE     | **0.006193** | **0.239281** | **0.056412** | **0.042954** | 240 |

## 4    Conclusion and Future Work

Model selection plays a very important role for symbolic regression based on genetic programming. In previous studies, there is no consistent conclusion that which interestingness measure is the most appropriate to choose an expression from the models being generated. From the analysis in the previous section, we could get the consequence as follows. Firstly, among the above-mentioned three classes of measures, the new measure Interestingness Elasticity shows a more outstanding performance to predict the concentrations of $PM_{2.5}$ in Dalian, China. The models IE selected have a higher accuracy and a relative smaller size. Secondly, the approaches proposed previously by other researchers do not achieve the desired result in this non-linear environment.

For the future work, we will try to forecast the values of $PM_{2.5}$ in the major cities of China. An in-depth study on IE will be carried out to explore the underlying reasons that why IE outperforms the others. And more interestingness measures would be used to check the capability of measures when being applied to choose non-linear models.

**Acknowledgements.** This work is supported by the National Natural Science Foundation of China (71001016).

## References

1. Chan, C.K., Yao, X.: Air pollution in mega cities in China. Atmos. Environ. **42**(1), 1–42 (2008)
2. Pope III, C.A., Dockery, D.W.: Health effects of fine particulate air pollution: lines that connect. J. Air Waste Manage. Assoc. **56**(6), 709–742 (2006)
3. Vladislavleva, E.J., Smits, G.F., Den Hertog, D.: Order of nonlinearity as a complexity measure for models generated by symbolic regression via pareto genetic programming. Trans. Evol. Comput. IEEE **13**(2), 333–349 (2009)
4. Cherkassky, V., Ma, Y.: Comparison of model selection for regression. Neural Comput. **15**(7), 1691–1714 (2003)
5. Wagenmakers, E.J., Farrell, S.: AIC model selection using Akaike weights. Psychon. Bull. Rev. **11**(1), 192–196 (2004)
6. Chen, H., Huang, S.: A comparative study on model selection and multiple model fusion. In: 2005 8th International Conference on Information Fusion, pp. 820–826. IEEE (2005)
7. Garg, A., Sriram, S., Tai, K.: Empirical analysis of model selection criteria for genetic programming in modeling of time series system. In: Conference on Computational Intelligence for Financial Engineering and Economics (CIFEr), pp. 90–94. IEEE (2013)
8. Posada, D., Buckley, T.R.: Model selection and model averaging in phylogenetics: advantages of Akaike information criterion and Bayesian approaches over likelihood ratio tests. Syst. Biol. **53**(5), 793–808 (2004)
9. Koza, J.R., Rice, J.P.: Genetic programming II: automatic discovery of reusable programs. MIT Press, Cambridge (1994)
10. Kaboudan, M.A.: A measure of time series' predictability using genetic programming applied to stock returns. J. Forecast. **18**(5), 345–357 (1999)

11. Montaña, J.L., Alonso, C.L., Borges, C.E., de la Dehesa, J.: Penalty functions for genetic programming algorithms. In: Murgante, B., Gervasi, O., Iglesias, A., Taniar, D., Apduhan, B.O. (eds.) ICCSA 2011, Part I. LNCS, vol. 6782, pp. 550–562. Springer, Heidelberg (2011)
12. Myung, I.J.: The importance of complexity in model selection. J. Math. Psychol. **44**(1), 190–204 (2000)
13. Akaike, H.: An information criterion (AIC). Math. Sci. **14**(153), 5–9 (1976)
14. Yamaoka, K., Nakagawa, T., Uno, T.: Application of Akaike's information criterion (AIC) in the evaluation of linear pharmacokinetic equations. J. Pharmacokinet. Biopharm. **6**(2), 165–175 (1978)
15. Bozdogan, H.: Model selection and Akaike's information criterion (AIC): the general theory and its analytical extensions. Psychometrika **52**(3), 345–370 (1987)
16. Seghouane, A.K., Bekara, M.: A small sample model selection criterion based on Kullback's symmetric divergence. Trans. Signal Process. IEEE **52**(12), 3314–3323 (2004)
17. Hurvich, C.M., Tsai, C.L.: Regression and time series model selection in small samples. Biometrika **76**(2), 297–307 (1989)
18. Burnham, K.P., Anderson, D.R.: Multimodel inference understanding AIC and BIC in model selection. Sociol. Methods Res. **33**(2), 261–304 (2004)
19. Hannan, E.J., Quinn, B.G.: The determination of the order of an autoregression. J. R. Stat. Soc. Ser. B (Methodol.), 190–195 (1979)
20. Kundu, D., Murali, G.: Model selection in linear regression. Comput. Stat. Data Anal. **22**(5), 461–469 (1996)

# Internal Clustering Evaluation of Data Streams

Marwan Hassani[✉] and Thomas Seidl

Data Management and Data Exploration Group,
RWTH Aachen University, Aachen, Germany
{hassani,seidl}@cs.rwth-aachen.de

**Abstract.** Clustering validation is a crucial part of choosing a clustering algorithm which performs best for an input data. Internal clustering
validation is efficient and realistic, whereas external validation requires a
ground truth which is not provided in most applications. In this paper,
we analyze the properties and performances of eleven internal clustering measures. In particular, as the importance of streaming data grows,
we apply these measures to carefully synthesized stream scenarios to
reveal how they react to clusterings on evolving data streams. A series of
experimental results show that different from the case with static data,
the *Calinski-Harabasz index* performs the best in coping with common
aspects and errors of stream clustering.

## 1 Motivation

Clustering validation is necessary for most applications and is regarded as much
important as the clustering itself [20]. There are two types of clustering validation [19]. The *external* validation, which compares the clustering result to
a reference result which is considered as the truth. If the result is somehow
similar to the reference, we regard the result as a "good" clustering. This validation is straightforward when the similarity between two clusterings has been
well-defined, however, it has fundamental caveat that the reference result is not
provided in most real applications. Therefore, external evaluation is largely used
for synthetic data and mostly for tuning clustering algorithms.

The other type is *internal* validation where the evaluation of the clustering
is compared only with the result itself, i.e. the structure of found clusters and
their relations to each other. This is much more realistic and efficient in many
real-world scenarios as it does not refer to any references from outside which is
not always feasible to obtain. Particularly, with the huge increase of the data
size and dimensionality as in recent applications with streaming data output,
one can hardly claim that a complete knowledge of the ground truth is available
or always valid. For the previous reasons, we focus in this paper on the internal
clustering validation and study its usability for drifting streaming data.

The remainder of this paper is organized as follows: Sect. 2 examines some
popular criteria of deciding whether found clusters are valid, and the general
procedure we used in this paper to evaluate stream clustering. In Sect. 3 we list
eleven different mostly used internal evaluation measures and shortly show how

© Springer International Publishing Switzerland 2015
X.-L. Li et al. (Eds.): PAKDD 2015, LNCS 9441, pp. 198–209, 2015.
DOI: 10.1007/978-3-319-25660-3_17

they are actually exploited in clustering evaluation. In Sect. 4, we introduce a set of thorough experiments on different kinds of data streams with different errors to show the behaviors of these internal measures in practice. In addition, we investigate more concretely how the internal measures react to stream-specific properties of data. In order to do this, several common error scenarios in stream clusterings are simulated and also evaluated with internal clustering validation. Finally, in Sect. 5, we summarize the contents of this paper.

## 2   Internal Clustering Validation

In this section we describe the main idea of internal clustering validation scheme and how they are realized in existing internal validation measures. Additionally, we will show a general procedure to make use of these measures in streaming environments in practice.

### 2.1   Validation Criteria

Contrary to external validation, internal clustering validation is based on the information intrinsic to the data alone. Since we can only refer to the input dataset itself, internal validation needs assumptions about a "good" structure of found clusters which are normally given by reference result in external validation. Two main concepts, the compactness and the separation, are the most popular ones. Many other methods are actually variations of these two [22].

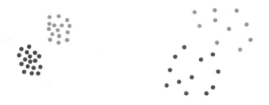

**Fig. 1.** Clusters on the left have better compactness than the ones on the right.

The *Compactness* measures how closely data points are grouped in a cluster. Grouped points in a cluster are supposed to be related to each other, by sharing a common feature which is called a meaningful pattern in practice. Compactness is normally based on distances between in-cluster points. The very popular example is variance, i.e. average distance to the mean, to estimate how objects are bonded together with its mean as its center. A lower variance indicates a high compactness (cf. Fig. 1). Alternatively, maximum or average pairwise distance, and maximum or average center based-distance are used.

The *Separation* measures how different found clusters are from each other. People using clustering algorithms do not want similar and vague patterns, which means clusters are not well-separated (cf. Fig. 2). A distinct cluster that is far

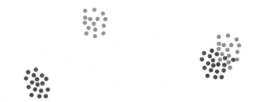

**Fig. 2.** Clusters on the left have better separation than the ones on the right.

from the others corresponds to a unique pattern. Similar to the compactness, distances between objects are widely used to measure separation, e.g. pairwise distances between cluster centers, or pairwise minimum distances between objects in different clusters. Separation is an inter-cluster criterion in the sense of relation between clusters.

### 2.2    General Procedure

Using the internal validation measures, we can determine the best partition and the optimal parameter settings for clustering tasks in streaming applications. A general procedure of this process is listed in Algorithm 1 which was used similarly for static data in [16, 17]:

---

**Algorithm 1.** InternalValidationProcedure()

---

1: Prepare the current stream batch from the dataset and initialize a list of clustering algorithms;
2: Run the clustering algorithms with different set of parameters;
3: Compute the corresponding internal validation index of each partition obtained in 2:;
4: Choose the best partition and the optimal cluster number according to the criteria;
5: At the end of the stream, average all the results from all batches;

---

## 3    Discussed Internal Evaluation Measures

In this section, we briefly review the most used eleven internal clustering measures in recent works. One can easily figure out of each measure which design criteria is chosen and how they are realized in mathematical form. We will first introduce important notations used in the formula of these measures: $D$ is input dataset, $n$ is the number of points in $D$, $g$ is the center of whole dataset $D$, $P$ is the number of dimensions of $D$, $NC$ is the number of clusters, $Ci$ is the $i$-th cluster, $n_i$ is the number of data points in $C_i$, $c_i$ is the center of cluster $C_i$, $\sigma(C_i)$ is the variance vector of $C_i$, and $d(x, y)$ is the distance between points $x$ and $y$.

For the convenience, we will put an abbreviation for each measure and use it through the rest of this paper.

First, some measures are designed to evaluate either only one of compactness or separation. The simplest one is *Root-mean-square standard deviation (RMSSTD)*:

$$RMSSTD = \left( \frac{\sum_i \sum_{x \in C_i} \|x - c_i\|^2}{P \sum_i (n_i - 1)} \right)^{1/2} \tag{1}$$

Which is the square root of the pooled sample variance of all the attributes, which measures only the compactness of found clusters [7]. A measure which considers only the separation between clusters is *R-squared (RS)* [7]:

$$RS = \frac{\sum_{x \in D} \|x - g\|^2 - \sum_i \sum_{x \in C_i} \|x - c_i\|^2}{\sum_{x \in D} \|x - g\|^2} \tag{2}$$

Which is the ratio of sum of squared distances between objects in different clusters to the total sum of squares. It is intuitive and simple formulation of measuring difference between clusters. Another measure considering only separation is *Modified Hubert $\Gamma$ statistic ($\Gamma$)* [14]:

$$\Gamma = \frac{2}{n(n-1)} \sum_{x \in D} \sum_{y \in D} d(x, y) d_{x \in C_i, y \in C_j}(c_i, c_j) \tag{3}$$

Which counts the number of data point pairs which has disagreement in cluster assignments, and sums up all the distances between those pairs.

The following measures are designed to reflect both compactness and separation at the same time. Naturally, considering only one of the two criteria is not enough to evaluate complex clusterings. We will introduce first the *Calinski-Harabasz index (CH)* [3]:

$$CH = \frac{\sum_i d^2(c_i, g)/(NC - 1)}{\sum_i \sum_{x \in C_i} d^2(x, c_i)/(n - NC)} \tag{4}$$

*CH* measures the two criteria simultaneously with a help of average between and within cluster sum of squares. The numerator means the degree of separation in the way of how much the cluster centers are spread, and the denominator corresponds to compactness, to reflect how close the in-cluster objects are gathered around the cluster center. The following two measures also share this type of formulation, i.e. numerator-separation/denominator-compactness. First, *I index(I)* [18]:

$$I = \left( \frac{1}{NC} \frac{\sum_{x \in D} d(x, g)}{\sum_i \sum_{x \in C_i} d(x, c_i)} \max_{i,j} d(c_i, c_j) \right)^P \tag{5}$$

In order to measure separation, *I* adopts the maximum distance between cluster centers. For compactness, distance from a data point to its cluster center is used like *CH*. Another famous measure is the *Dunn's indices (D)* [6]:

$$D = \min_i \min_j \left( \frac{\min_{x \in C_i, y \in C_j} d(x,y)}{\max_k \left( \max_{x,y \in C_k} d(x,y) \right)} \right) \tag{6}$$

$D$ uses the minimum pairwise distance between points in different clusters as the inter-cluster separation and the maximum diameter among all clusters as the intra-cluster compactness. As mentioned above, $CH$, $I$, and $D$ follow the form $(Separation)/(Compactness)$, though they use different distances and different weights to the two factors. The optimal cluster number can be achieved by maximizing these three indices.

Another commonly used measure is *Silhouette index (S)* [21]:

$$S = \frac{1}{NC} \sum_i \left( \frac{1}{n_i} \sum_{x \in C_i} \frac{b(x) - a(x)}{max[b(x), a(x)]} \right) \tag{7}$$

where $a(x) = \frac{1}{n_i - 1} \sum_{y \in C_i, y \neq x} d(x,y)$ and $b(x) = \min_{j \neq i} \left[ \frac{1}{n_j} \sum_{y \in C_j} d(x,y) \right]$. $S$ does not take $c_i$ or $g$ into account and uses pairwise distance between all the objects in a cluster for numerating compactness ($a(x)$). $b(x)$ measures separation with the average distance of objects to alternative cluster, i.e. second closest cluster. *Davies-Bouldin index (DB)* [5] is an old but still widely used internal validation measure:

$$DB = \frac{1}{NC} \sum_i \max_{j \neq i} \frac{\frac{1}{n_i} \sum_{x \in C_i} d(x, c_i) + \frac{1}{n_j} \sum_{x \in C_j} d(x, c_j)}{d(c_i, c_j)} \tag{8}$$

$DB$ uses intra-cluster variance and inter-cluster center distance to find the worst partner cluster, i.e. close and scattered, for each cluster. Thus, minimizing DB gives us the optimal number of clusters. Later, the *Xie-Beni index (XB)* was published in [23] and is defined as:

$$XB = \frac{\sum_i \sum_{x \in C_i} d^2(x, c_i)}{n \cdot \min_{i \neq j} d^2(c_i, c_j)} \tag{9}$$

Along with $DB$, $XB$ has a form of $(Compactness)/(Separation)$ which is the opposite of $CH$, $I$, and $D$. Therefore, it reaches the optimum clustering by being minimized. It defines the inter-cluster separation as the minimum square distance between cluster centers, and the intra-cluster compactness as the mean square distance between each data object and it cluster center.

In the following we present more recent clustering validation measures. The *SD validity index (SD)* [9]:

$$SD = Dis(NCmax) \cdot Scat(NC) + Dis(NC) \tag{10}$$

- $Scat(NC) = \frac{1}{NC} \sum_i \frac{\|\sigma(C_i)\|}{\|\sigma(D)\|}$
- $Dis(NC) = \frac{\max_{i,j} d(c_i, c_j)}{\min_{i,j} d(c_i, c_j)} \sum_i \left( \sum_j d(c_i, c_j) \right)^{-1}$

$SD$ is composed of two terms; $Scat(NC)$ stands for "scattering" within clusters and $Dis(NC)$ means "dispersion" between clusters. Like $DB$ and $XB$, $SD$ measures compactness with variance of clustered objects and separation with distance between cluster centers, but by using them in a different way. A revised version of $SD$ is $S\_Dbw$ [8]:

$$S\_Dbw = Scat(NC) + Dens\_bw(NC) \tag{11}$$

$$- Dens\_bw(NC) = \frac{1}{NC(NC-1)} \sum_i \left( \sum_{j \neq i} \frac{\sum_{x \in C_i \cup C_j} f(x, u_{ij})}{\max\left( \sum_{x \in C_i} f(x, c_i), \sum_{x \in C_j} f(x, c_j) \right)} \right)$$

$$- f(x, y) = \begin{cases} 0 & \text{if } d(x, y) > \tau, \\ 1 & \text{otherwise.} \end{cases}$$

where $u_{ij}$ is a middle point of $c_i$ and $c_j$, $\tau$ is a threshold to determine the neighbors, and $Scat(NC)$ is the same as that of $SD$. $S\_Dbw$ takes the density into account to measure separation between clusters. It assumes that for each pair of cluster centers, at least one of their densities should be larger than the density of their midpoint to be a "good" clustering. Both $SD$ and $S\_Dbw$ indicate the optimal clustering when they are minimized.

# 4    Internal Validation of Stream Clusterings

In this section, we evaluate the result of stream clustering algorithms with internal validation measures.

## 4.1    Robustness to Conventional Clustering Aspects

The results on using internal evaluation measures for clustering static data with simple errors in [16] prove that the performance of the internal measures is affected by various aspects of input data, i.e. noise, density of clusters, skewness, and subclusters. Each measure of the discussed 11 evaluation measures reacts differently to those aspects. We perform more complex experiments than the ones in [16], this time on stream clusterings to see how the internal measures behave in real-time continuous data. We run the clustering algorithm with different parameters, choose the optimal number of clusters according to the evaluation results, and compare it to the true number of clusters.

Streaming data fundamentally have usually complex properties that are happening at the same time. The experiments in [16], however, are limited to very simple toy datasets reflecting only one clustering aspect at a time. To make it more realistic, we use a single data stream reflecting five conventional clustering aspects at the same time.

**Experimental Settings.** In order to simulate streaming scenarios, we use *MOA (Massive Online Analysis)* [2] framework. We have chosen *RandomRBFGenerator*, which emits data instances continuously from a set of circular clusters, as the input stream generator (cf. Fig. 3). In this stream, we can specify the size, density, and moving speed of the instance-generating clusters, from which we can simulate the skewness, different density, and the subcluster aspect. We set the parameters as follows: number of generating clusters = 5, radius of clusters = 0.11, their dimensionality = 10, varying range of cluster radius = 0.07, varying range of cluster density = 1, cluster speed = 0.01 *per* 200 *points*, noise level = 0.1, noise does not appear inside clusters. The parameters which are not mentioned are not directly related to this experiment and are set by default of MOA. For clustering algorithm, we have chosen *CluStream* [1] with *k-means* as its macro-clusterer. We vary the parameter $k$ from 2 to 9, where the optimal number of clusters is 5. We set the evaluation frequency to 1000 points and run our stream generator till 30000 points, which gives 30 evaluation results.

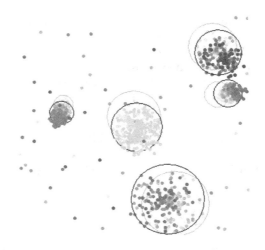

**Fig. 3.** A screenshot of the Dimensions 1 and 2 of the synthetic data stream used in the experiment. Colored points represent the incoming instances, and the colors are faded out as the processing time passes. Ground truth cluster boundaries are drawn in black circle. Gray circles indicate the former state, expressing that the clusters are moving. Black (faded out to gray) points represent noise points (Color figure online).

**Results.** Table 1 contains the mean value of 30 evaluation results which we obtained in the whole streaming interval. It shows that *RMSSTD*, *RS*, *CH*, *I*, and *S_Dbw* correctly reach their optimal number of clusters, while others do not. According to the results in [16], the optimal value of each of *RMSSTD*, *RS*, and *Γ* is difficult to determine. For this reason, we do not accept their results even if some of them show a good performance.

In the static case in [16], *CH* and *I* were unable to find the right optimal number of clusters. *CH* is shown to be vulnerable to noise, since the noise inclusion (in cases when $k < 5$) makes the found clusters larger and less compact. However, in the streaming case, most clustering algorithms follow the online-offline-phases model. The online phase removes a lot of noise when summarizing

**Table 1.** Evaluation results of internal validation on the stream clusterings. The optimum values (not necessarily the maximum or the minimum) are in bold.

| k | RMSSTD | RS | Γ | CH | I | D | S | DB | XB | SD | S_Dbw |
|---|--------|-----|-----|-----|-----|-----|-----|-----|-----|-----|-----|
| 2 | 0.0998 | 0.7992 | 0.3522 | 3196 | 0.4980 | 0.1921 | **0.6535** | **0.5528** | 0.1065 | **4.5086** | 0.2284 |
| 3 | 0.0763 | 0.8593 | 0.3724 | 3619 | 0.5564 | **0.2208** | 0.6003 | 0.5782 | 0.1561 | 6.1623 | 0.1601 |
| 4 | 0.0621 | 0.9117 | 0.3834 | 3860 | 0.5840 | 0.0936 | 0.6143 | 0.5531 | **0.0932** | 6.7154 | 0.1251 |
| 5 | **0.0538** | **0.9330** | 0.3967 | **4157** | **0.6134** | 0.0669 | 0.5855 | 0.5656 | 0.1143 | 8.6382 | **0.1087** |
| 6 | 0.0528 | 0.9355 | **0.4007** | 3510 | 0.4945 | 0.0309 | 0.5200 | 0.6360 | 0.1845 | 11.1729 | 0.1319 |
| 7 | 0.0481 | 0.9464 | 0.4002 | 3435 | 0.4697 | 0.0042 | 0.4861 | 0.6610 | 0.2580 | 14.7443 | 0.1192 |
| 8 | 0.0463 | 0.9512 | 0.4007 | 3095 | 0.4001 | 0.0099 | 0.4617 | 0.6853 | 0.2977 | 16.8715 | 0.1338 |
| 9 | 0.0430 | 0.9580 | 0.4026 | 3154 | 0.3943 | 0.0000 | 0.4544 | 0.6913 | 0.3085 | 19.5362 | 0.1355 |

the data into microclusters, and the offline phase ($k$-means in the case of CluStream [1]) deals only with these "cleaned" summaries. Of course, there will be always a chance to get a summary that is completely formed of noise points, but those will have less impact over the final clustering than the static case. Thus, since not all the noise points are integrated into the clusters, the amount of cluster expansion is a bit smaller than the static case. Therefore, the effect of noise to $CH$ is less in the streaming case than the static one.

In the static case, $I$ was slightly affected by different density of clusters, and the reasons were not well revealed. Therefore, it is not surprising that $I$ performs well as we take average of its evaluation results for the whole streaming interval.

$D$ shows a poor performance, since it gives unconditional zero values in most evaluation points (before they are averaged as in Table 1). This is because the numerator of Eq. (6) could be zero when at least one pair of $x$ and $y$ happens to be equal to each other, i.e. the distance between $x$ and $y$ is zero. This case rises when $C_i$ and $C_j$ are overlapped and the pair $(x, y)$ is elected from the overlapped region. Streaming data has high possibility to have overlapped clusters, and so does the input of this experiment. This drives $D$ to produce zero, making it an unstable measure in streaming environments.

Similar to the static data case, $S$, $DB$, $XB$, and $SD$ perform bad in the streaming settings. The main reason also lies in the overlapping of clusters. Overlapping clusters are the extreme case of subclusters in the experiments of the static case discussed in [16].

## 4.2    Sensitivity to Common Errors of Stream Clustering

In this section, we perform a more detailed study on the behaviors of internal measures in streaming environments. The previous experiment is more or less a general test on a single data stream, so we use here the internal clustering indices on a series of elaborately designed experiments which well reflects the stream clustering scenarios. *MOA* framework has an interesting tool called *ClusterGenerator*, which can produce a found clustering by manipulating ground truth clusters with a certain error level. It can simulate different kinds of error types and even combine them to construct complicated clustering error scenarios.

It is very useful since we can test the sensitivity of evaluation measures to specific errors [15].

Evaluating a variation of the ground truth seems a bit awkward in the sense of internal validation since it actually refers to the predefined result, however, this kind of experiment is absolutely meaningful, because we can watch reactions of internal measures errors of interest. [15] used this tool to show the behavior of internal measures, e.g. $S$, *Sum of Squares (SSQ)*, and *C-index*. Although the error types exploited in [15] are limited, those measures are not of our interest or already proved to be bad in the previous experiments.

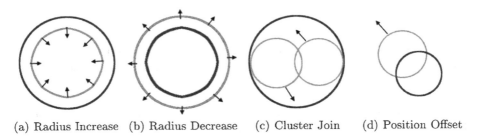

(a) Radius Increase    (b) Radius Decrease    (c) Cluster Join    (d) Position Offset

**Fig. 4.** Common errors of stream clusterings. A green circle represents a true cluster, and a blue circle indicates the corresponding found cluster (error). The cause of the error is the fast evolution of the stream in the direction of the arrows (Color figure online).

**Experimental Settings.** *ClusterGenerator* has six error types as its parameters, and they effectively reflect common errors of stream clusterings. "Radius increase" and "Radius decrease" change the radius of clusters (Fig. 4(a) and (b)), which normally happens in the stream clustering since data points keep fading in and out. "Cluster add" and "Cluster remove" change the number of found clusters, which are caused by grouping noise points or falsely detecting meaningful patterns as a noise cloud. "Cluster join" merges two overlapping clusters as one cluster (Fig. 4(c)), which is a crucial error in streaming scenarios. Finally, "Position offset" changes the cluster position, and this commonly happens due to the movement of clusters in data streams (Fig. 4(d)).

We perform the experiments on all the above error types. We increase the level of one error at a time and evaluate its output with $CH$, $I$ and $S\_Dbw$, which performed well in the previous experiment. For the input stream, we use the same stream settings as in Sect. 4.2.

**Results.** In Fig. 5, the evaluation values are plotted on the $y$-axis according to the corresponding error level on the $x$-axis. From Fig. 5(a), we can see that $CH$ value decreases as the level of "Radius increase", "Cluster add", "Cluster join", and "Position offset" errors increases. $CH$ correctly and constantly penalizes the four errors, since smaller $CH$ value corresponds to worse clustering. However, it shows completely reversed curves in "Radius decrease" and "Cluster remove" errors.

The reason for wrong rewarding of the "Radius decrease" error, is that the reduction of the size of clusters increases their compactness and thus both $CH$ and $I$ increase. The "Cluster remove" error detection is a general problem for all internal measures as they compare their clustering result only to its self. Regardless of the "Radius decrease" and the "Cluster remove" errors, $CH$ has generally the best performance on streaming data compared to the other measures.

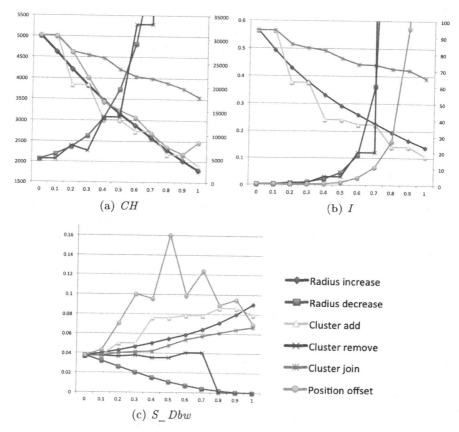

(a) $CH$                    (b) $I$

(c) $S\_Dbw$

**Fig. 5.** Experimental results for each error type. Evaluation values (y-axis) are plotted according to each error level (x-axis). Some error curves are drawn on a secondary axis due to its range: (a) "Radius decrease" and "Cluster remove", (b) "Radius decrease", "Cluster remove", and "Position offset".

We can see in Fig. 5(b) that $I$ also misinterprets the "Radius decrease" and "Cluster remove" error situations. The reason for it is similar to that of $CH$, since $I$ also adopts the distance between objects within clusters as the intra-cluster compactness and the distance between cluster centers as the inter-cluster separation. In addition, $I$ wrongly favorites the "Position offset" error instead of penalizing it. If the boundary of found clusters are moved besides the truth, they often miss the data points, which produces similar situation as "Radius decrease" which $I$ is vulnerable to.

$S\_Dbw$ produces high values when it regards a clustering as a bad result, which is opposite to the previous two measures. In Fig. 5(c), we can see that it correctly penalizes the three error types "Radius increase", "Cluster add", and "Cluster join". For "Position offset" error, one can say that the value is somehow increasing but the curve is actually fluctuating too much. It also fails to penalize "Cluster remove" correctly.

From these results, we can determine that, among the discussed internal evaluation measures, $CH$ is the best internal evaluation one which can well handle many stream clustering errors. Even though $S\_Dbw$ performs very well on the static data (cf. [16]) and on the streaming data in the previous experiments (cf. Sect. 4.2), but it is shown that it has weak capability to capture common errors of stream clustering.

## 5   Conclusion

Evaluating clustering results is very important to the success of clustering tasks. In this paper, we discussed the internal clustering validation scheme, which is much more efficient and much more widely used than the external validation. We explained fundamental theories of internal validation measures and its examples. Furthermore, we performed a set of clustering validation experiments that well reflect the properties of streaming environment with five common clustering aspects at the same time. These aspects reflect monotonicity, noise, different densities of clusters, skewness and the existence of subclusters in the underlying streaming data. The three winners from the first experimental evaluation were then further evaluated in the second phase of experiments. The sensitivity of each of those three measures was tested w.r.t. four stream clustering errors. Different to the results gained in a recent work on static data, our final experimental results on streaming data showed that *Calinski-Harabasz index (CH)* [3] has, in general, the best performance in streaming environments. It is robust to the combination of the five conventional aspects of clustering, and also correctly penalizes the common errors in stream clustering.

In the future, we want to test those measures on different categories of stream clustering algorithms like density-based ones (e.g. DenStream [4] and HAStream [13]) of projected/subspace ones (e.g. PreDeConStream [12] and SubClusTree [11]). Additionally, we want to evaluate the measures when streams of unbalanced clusters of different sizes, of varying densities, of non-convex shapes and within subspaces [10], are processed by the above algorithms.

## References

1. Aggarwal, C.C., Han, J., Wang, J., Yu, P.S.: A framework for clustering evolving data streams. In: VLDB, pp. 81–92 (2003)
2. Bifet, A., Holmes, G., Pfahringer, B., Kranen, P., Kremer, H., Jansen, T., Seidl, T.: MOA: massive online analysis, a framework for stream classification and clustering. JMLR **11**, 44–50 (2010)

3. Calinski, T., Harabasz, J.: A dendrite method for cluster analysis. Commun. Stat. **3**(1), 1–27 (1974)
4. Cao, F., Ester, M., Qian, W., Zhou, A.: Density-based clustering over an evolving data stream with noise. In: SIAM SDM, pp. 328–339 (2006)
5. Davies, D., Bouldin, D.: A cluster separation measure. IEEE PAMI **1**(2), 224–227 (1979)
6. Dunn, J.: Well separated clusters and optimal fuzzy partitions. J. Cybern. **4**(1), 95–104 (1974)
7. Halkidi, M., Batistakis, Y., Vazirgiannis, M.: On clustering validation techniques. J. Intell. Inf. Syst. **17**(2), 107–145 (2001)
8. Halkidi, M., Vazirgiannis, M.: Clustering validity assessment: finding the optimal partitioning of a data set. In IEEE ICDM, pp. 187–194 (2001)
9. Vazirgiannis, M., Halkidi, M., Batistakis, Y.: Quality scheme assessment in the clustering process. In: Żytkow, J.M., Zighed, D.A., Komorowski, J. (eds.) PKDD 2000. LNCS (LNAI), vol. 1910, pp. 265–276. Springer, Heidelberg (2000)
10. Hassani, M., Kim, Y., Seidl, T.: Subspace MOA: subspace stream clustering evaluation using the MOA framework. In: DASFAA, pp. 446–449 (2013)
11. Hassani, M., Kranen, P., Saini, R., Seidl, T.: Subspace anytime stream clustering. In: SSDBM, p. 37 (2014)
12. Hassani, M., Spaus, P., Gaber, M.M., Seidl, T.: Density-based projected clustering of data streams. In: Link, S., Fober, T., Seeger, B., Hüllermeier, E. (eds.) SUM 2012. LNCS, vol. 7520, pp. 311–324. Springer, Heidelberg (2012)
13. Hassani, M., Spaus, P., Seidl, T.: Adaptive multiple-resolution stream clustering. In: Perner, P. (ed.) MLDM 2014. LNCS, vol. 8556, pp. 134–148. Springer, Heidelberg (2014)
14. Hubert, L., Arabie, P.: Comparing partitions. J. Intell. Inf. Syst. **2**(1), 193–218 (1985)
15. Kremer, H., Kranen, P., Jansen, T., Seidl, T., Bifet, A., Holmes, G., Pfahringer, B.: An effective evaluation measure for clustering on evolving data streams. In: ACM SIGKDD, pp. 868–876 (2011)
16. Liu, Y., Li, Z., Xiong, H., Gao, X., Wu, J.: Understanding of internal clustering validation measures. In: ICDM, pp. 911–916 (2010)
17. Liu, Y., Li, Z., Xiong, H., Gao, X., Wu, J., Wu, S.: Understanding and enhancement of internal clustering validation measures. IEEE Trans. Cybern. **43**(3), 982–994 (2013)
18. Maulik, U., Bandyopadhyay, S.: Performance evaluation of some clustering algorithms and validity indices. IEEE PAMI **24**, 1650–1654 (2002)
19. Rendón, E., Abundez, I., Arizmendi, A., Quiroz, E.M.: Internal versus external cluster validation indexes. Int. J. Comput. Commun. **5**(1), 27–34 (2011)
20. Rezaee, M.R., Lelieveldt, B.B.F., Reiber, J.H.C.: A new cluster validity index for the fuzzy c-mean. Pattern Recogn. Lett. **19**(3–4), 237–246 (1998)
21. Rousseeuw, P.: Silhouettes: a graphical aid to the interpretation and validation of cluster analysis. J. Comput. Appl. Math. **20**(1), 53–65 (1987)
22. Tan, P.-N., Steinbach, M., Kumar, V.: Introduction to Data Mining. Addison-Wesley Longman Inc., Boston (2005)
23. Xie, X.L., Beni, G.: A validity measure for fuzzy clustering. IEEE PAMI **13**(8), 841–847 (1991)

# Feature Maximization Based Clustering Quality Evaluation: A Promising Approach

Jean-Charles Lamirel[1,2]([✉]) and Shadi Al Shehabi[3]

[1] Department of Computer Science, University of Tartu,
J. Liivi 2, 50409 Tartu, Estonia
jean-charles.lamirel@ut.ee
[2] LORIA, Equipe Synalp, Bâtiment B, 54506 Vandoeuvre Cedex, France
lamirel@loria.fr
[3] Türk Hava Kurumu Üniversitesi, Anakara, Turkey
shadialshehabi@gmail.com

**Abstract.** Feature maximization is an alternative measure, as compared to usual distributional measures relying on entropy or on Chi-square metric or vector-based measures, like Euclidean distance or correlation distance. One of the key advantages of this measure is that it is operational in an incremental mode both on clustering and on traditional classification. In the classification framework, it does not presents the limitations of the aforementioned measures in the case of the processing of highly unbalanced, heterogeneous and highly multidimensional data. We present a new application of this measure in the clustering context for setting up new cluster quality indexes whose efficiency ranges for low to high dimensional data and that are tolerant to noise. We compare the behaviour of these new indexes with usual cluster quality indexes based on Euclidean distance on different kinds of test datasets for which ground truth is available. Proposed comparison clearly highlights the superior accuracy and stability of the new method.

**Keywords:** Clustering · Quality indexes · Feature maximization · Big data

## 1 Introduction

Unsupervised classification or clustering is becoming a more and more central data analysis technique with increasing areas of application. Hence, providing that the datasets to be analyzed have growing size, it becomes clearly unfeasible to get ground truth that permits to operate on them in a supervised way. A central problem that then arises in clustering is to qualify the obtained results in terms of quality: a quality index is a criterion which indeed makes it possible all together to decide which clustering method to use, to fix an optimal number of clusters, and to evaluate or to develop a new method. Many approaches have been developed for that purpose as it is pointed out in [3, 25, 26, 29]. However, even if there exist recent alternative approaches [6, 15, 17], the usual quality indexes are

© Springer International Publishing Switzerland 2015
X.-L. Li et al. (Eds.): PAKDD 2015, LNCS 9441, pp. 210–222, 2015.
DOI: 10.1007/978-3-319-25660-3_18

mostly based on the concepts of dispersion of a cluster and dissimilarity between clusters. Computation of those latter criteria are themselves relying on Euclidean distance. The most used indexes that implement in slightly different ways the above mentioned concepts are the Dunn index (DU) [10], the Davies-Bouldin index (DB) [9], the Silhouette index (SI) [27], the Calinski-Harabasz index (CH) [8] and the Xie-Beni index (XI) [30].

As stated in [14, 29] usual indexes have the defect to be sensitive to the noisy data and outliers. In [20], we also observed that the proposed indexes are not suitable to analyze clustering results in highly multidimensional space as well as they are unable to detect degenerated clustering results. Moreover, said indexes are not independent on the clustering method with is exploited. As an example, a clustering method which tends to optimize WGSS, like k-means [24], will also tend to naturally produce low value of that criteria, leading to optimize indexes output, but without guarantying coherent results, as it has been also shown in [20]. Last but not least, as Forest also pointed out in [13], the experiments on these indexes in the literature are often performed on unrealistic test corpora constituted of low dimensional data and embedding a small number of "well-shaped" virtual clusters. As an example, in their reference paper, Milligan and Cooper [25] compared 30 different methods for estimating the number of clusters relying only on simulated data described in a low dimensional Euclidean space. Same remark can be done on the comparison performed in [29]. Nonetheless, using Reuters test collection, it has been shown by Kassab and Lamirel [18] that aforementioned indexes are often properly unable to identify an optimal clustering model whenever the dataset is constituted by complex data that must be represented in a both highly multidimensional and sparse description space, obviously embedding non-Gaussian clusters, as it is often the case with textual data. Silhouette index is known to be one of the more reliable of the above mentioned indexes, especially in the case of multidimensional data, mainly because it is not a diameter-based index optimized for Gaussian context. However, similarly to Dunn and Xie-Beni indexes, it has the main defect to be computationally expensive, which could also represents a major drawback in the case of its exploitation on large datasets of highly multidimensional data.

In order to get rid of method-index dependency problem and of their sensitivity to noise, as well to escape from computation complexity, we are proposing hereafter to exploit features of the data points attached to clusters instead of cluster centroids information and to substitute Euclidean distance by more reliable quality estimator based on feature maximization measure. This measure has been already successfully used for solving complex highly multidimensional classification problems with highly imbalanced and noisy data gathered in similar classes thanks to its very efficient feature selection and data resampling capabilities [22]. Furthermore, we show in our upcoming experimental section that cluster quality indexes relying on this measure do not have any of the defects of usual approaches, including computation complexity.

Section 2 presents feature maximization measure and our new indexes proposal. Section 3 presents our experimental context. Section 4 presents our results. Section 5 draws our conclusion and perspectives.

## 2  Feature Maximization for Feature Selection

Feature maximization is an unbiased measure with whichto estimate the quality of a classification, whatever it is supervised or unsupervised.

In unsupervised classification (i.e. clustering), this measure exploits the properties (i.e. the features) of data points that can be attached to their nearest cluster after learning without prior examination of the generated cluster profiles, like centroids. Its principal advantage is thus to be totally independent of the clustering method and of its operating mode.

Consider a partition $C$ which results from a clustering method applied to a dataset $D$ represented by a group of features $F$. The feature maximization measure favours clusters with a maximal feature F-measure. The feature F-measure $FF_c(f)$ of a feature $f$ associated with a cluster $c$ is defined as the harmonic mean of the feature recall $FR_c(f)$ and of the feature predominance $FP_c(f)$, themselves defined as follows:

$$FR_c(f) = \frac{\Sigma_{d \in c'} W_d^f}{\Sigma_{c' \in C} \Sigma_{d \in c'} W_d^f} \quad FP_c(f) = \frac{\Sigma_{d \in c} W_d^f}{\Sigma_{f' \in F_c, d \in c} W_d^{f'}} \tag{1}$$

with

$$FF_c(f) = 2 \left( \frac{FR_c(f) \times FP_c(f)}{FR_c(f) + FP_c(f)} \right) \tag{2}$$

where $W_d^f$ represents the weight[1] of the feature $f$ for the data $d$ and $F_c$ represents all the features present in the dataset associated with the cluster $C$.

Feature maximization measure can be exploited to generate a powerfull feature selection process [16]. In the clustering context, such selection process can be defined as non-parametered process based on clusters content in which a cluster feature is characterised using both its capacity to discriminate between clusters ($FP_c(f)$ index) and its ability to faithfully represent the cluster data ($FR_c(f)$ index). The set $S_c$ of features that are characteristic of a given cluster $c$ belonging to a partition $C$ is translated by:

$$S_c = \left\{ f \in F_c \mid FF_c(f) > \overline{FF}(f) \text{ and } FF_c(f) > \overline{FF}_D \right\} \text{ where} \tag{3}$$

$$\overline{FF}(f) = \Sigma_{c' \in C} \frac{FF_{c'}(f)}{|C_{/f}|} \text{ and } \overline{FF}_D = \Sigma_{f \in F} \frac{\overline{FF}(f)}{|F|} \tag{4}$$

where $C_{/f}$ represents the subset of $C$ in which the feature $f$ occurs.

---

[1] The weight figures out the influence of a feature for a given data. It could be either Boolean or real-valued. An example of weighting is given in Figs. 1 to 3.

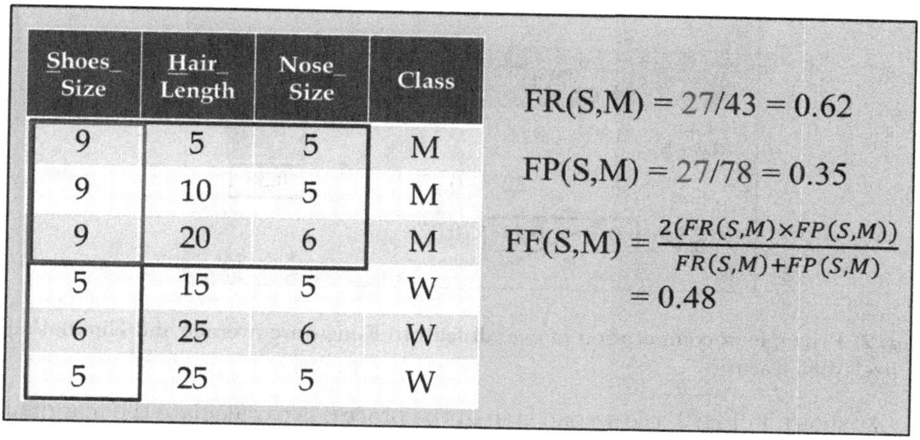

| Shoes_ Size | Hair_ Length | Nose_ Size | Class |
|:-----------:|:------------:|:----------:|:-----:|
| 9 | 5 | 5 | M |
| 9 | 10 | 5 | M |
| 9 | 20 | 6 | M |
| 5 | 15 | 5 | W |
| 6 | 25 | 6 | W |
| 5 | 25 | 5 | W |

$$FR(S,M) = 27/43 = 0.62$$

$$FP(S,M) = 27/78 = 0.35$$

$$FF(S,M) = \frac{2(FR(S,M) \times FP(S,M))}{FR(S,M) + FP(S,M)}$$
$$= 0.48$$

**Fig. 1.** Principle of computation of feature F-measure on example data.

Finally, the set of all selected features $S_C$ is the subset of $F$ defined by:

$$S_C = \cup_{c \in C} S_C. \tag{5}$$

In other words, the features that are judged relevant for a given cluster are those whose representations are better than average in this cluster, and better than the average representation of all the features in the partition, in terms of feature F-measure. Features that never respect the second condition in any cluster are discarded.

A specific concept of contrast $G_c(f)$ can be defined to figure out the performance of a retained feature $f$ for a given cluster $c$. It is an indicator value which is proportional to the ratio between the F-measure $FF_c(f)$ of a feature in the cluster $c$ and the average F-measure $\overline{FF}$ of this feature for the whole partition [23][2]. It can be expressed as:

$$G_c(f) = FF_c(f)/\overline{FF}(f) \tag{6}$$

The active features of a cluster are those for which the contrast is greater than 1. Moreover, the higher is the contrast of a feature for one cluster, the better is its performance for describing the cluster content.

We give below an example of operating mode of the method on a basis of a toy dataset including two predefined categories (i.e. classes) (*Men (M), Women (F)*) described with 3 features: *Nose_Size Hair_Length, Feet_Size*. Figure 1 shows the source data and also shows how does operate the calculation of F-measure of the *Feet_Size* feature in the *Men* class.

---

[2] Using p-value highligting the signifance of a feature for a cluster by comparing its contrast to unity constrast would be a potential alternative. However, this method would introduce unexpected Gaussian smoothing in the process.

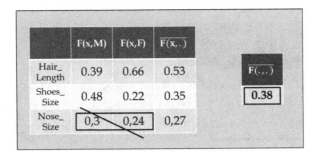

**Fig. 2.** Principle of computation of overall feature F-measure average and elimination of irrelevant features.

As shown in Fig. 2, the second step in the process is to calculate the marginal average of F-measure for each feature and the overall average of F-measure for the combination of all features and all classes. Feature with a F-measure that is systematically lower than the overall average are eliminated. The *Nose_Size* feature is thus removed.

Remaining features (i.e. selected features) are considered active in the classes in which their F-measure is above marginal average:

1. *Feet_Size* is active in the *Men* class,
2. *Hair_Length* is active in the *Women* class[3].

Contrast ratio highlights the degree of activity/passivity of the selected features as regards to their F-measure marginal average in different classes. Figure 3 illustrates how contrast is calculated on the presented example. In the context of this example, the contrast may thus be considered as a function that will virtually have the following effects:

1. Increase the length of womens' hairs,
2. Increase the size of the mens' feet,
3. Decrease the length of the mens' hairs,
4. Reduce the size of womens' feet.

As already mentioned before, active (or positive) features in a cluster are those for which the contrast is greater than 1 in that cluster. Conversely, passive (or negative) features in a cluster are those present in the cluster data for which contrast is less than 1[4]. A simple way to exploit obtained features is to use positive features and their associated contrast for cluster labelling [19,21]. A more sophisticated way, as we propose hereafter, is to exploit active and passive extracted features for defining clustering quality indexing identifying an optimal partition. Such partition is expected to maximize the contrast described by Eq. 6. This approach leads to the definition of two different indexes:

---

[3] Method has been shown in [22] to have a low sensitvity to feature scaling.

[4] As regards to the principle of the method, negative features that have not been removed are necessarily selected with a constrast greater than 1 in other clusters.

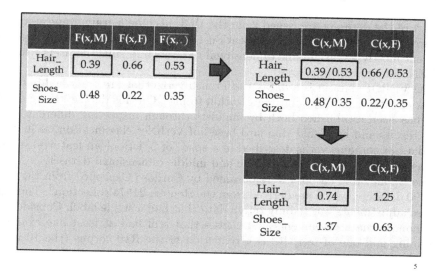

**Fig. 3.** Principle of computation of contrast on selected features.

The PC index, whose principle corresponds by analogy to that of intra-cluster inertia in the usual models, is a macro-measure based on the maximization of the average positive weighted contrast for optimal partition. For a partition comprising $k$ clusters, it can be expressed as:

$$PC_k = \frac{1}{k} \sum_{i=1}^{k} \frac{1}{n_i} \sum_{f \in S_i} G_i(f) \tag{7}$$

The EC index, whose principle corresponds by analogy to that of the combination between intra-cluster inertia and inter-cluster inertia in the usual models, is based on the maximization of the average compromise between positive weighted contrast and the inverse of the negative weighted constrast for optimal partition:

$$EC_k = \frac{1}{k} \sum_{i=1}^{k} \left( \frac{\frac{|s_i|}{n_i} \sum_{f \in S_i} G_i(f) + \frac{|\overline{s_i}|}{n_i} \sum_{h \in S_i} \frac{1}{G_i(h)}}{|s_i| + |\overline{s_i}|} \right) \tag{8}$$

where $n_i$ is the number of data associated with the cluster $i$, $|s_i|$ represents the number of active features in $i$, and $|\overline{s_i}|$, the number of passive features in the same cluster.

## 3    Experimental Data and Process

To objectively figure out the accuracy of our new indexes, we use several different datasets with various dimensionality and various sizes for which the optimal number of clusters (i.e. ground truth) is known in advance.

Part of the datasets are issued from the UCI machine learning repository [2] and are usually exploited for classification tasks. The 4 selected UCI datasets represent mostly low to middle dimensional datasets and small datasets (except for PEN dataset which is large).

The VERBF dataset is a dataset of French verbs that are described both by semantic features and by subcategorization frames. On this dataset, the ground truth has been established both by linguists through inspecting different clustering results and by a gold standard based of VerbNet classification, as in [28]. This dataset contains verbs described in a space of 231 Boolean features. It can be considered as a typical middle size and middle dimensional dataset.

The R8 and R52 corpora were obtained by Cardoso Cachopo[5] from the R10 and R90 datasets, which are derived from the Reuters 21578 collection[6]. The aim of these adjustments was to only retain data that had a single label. Considering only monothematic documents and classes that still had at least one example of training and one of test, R8 is a reduction of the R10 corpus (the 10 most frequent classes) to 8 classes and R52 is a reduction of the R90 corpus (90 classes) to 52 classes. The R8 and R52 are large and multidimensional datasets with respective size of 7674 and 9100 and associated bag of words description spaces of 1187 and 2618 words. This datasets can be considered as large and high dimensional datasets. The summary of datasets overall characteristics is provided in Table 1.

**Table 1.** Datasets overall characteristics.

|            | IRIS | WINE | PEN   | ZOO | VRBF  | R8   | R52  |
|------------|------|------|-------|-----|-------|------|------|
| Nbr. class | 3    | 3    | 12    | 7   | 12-16 | 8    | 52   |
| Nbr data   | 150  | 178  | 10992 | 101 | 2183  | 7674 | 9100 |
| Nbr feat   | 4    | 13   | 16    | 114 | 231   | 3497 | 7369 |

We exploited 2 different usual clustering methods that are, k-means [24], a winner-take-all method, and GNG [12], a winner-take-most method with Hebbian learning. For text or linguistic features datasets we specifically use the IGNGF neural clustering method [20] that has already been proven to outperform other clustering methods, including spectral methods, on this kind of data [28]. We usually report the method that produced the best results in the following experiments.

As soon a class labels are provided in all datasets and considering that clustering method could only produce approximate results as compared to reference categorization, we make a complementary use of purity measures to estimate the quality of the partition generated by the method as regards to category ground truth. Following [28], we use modified purity (mPUR) to evaluate the clusterings

---

[5] http://web.ist.utl.pt/~acardoso/datasets/.

[6] http://www.research.att.com/~lewis/reuters21578.html.

produced. It is computed as follows. Each induced cluster $c$ is assigned the gold class (its *prevalent class*, $\text{prev}(c)$) to which most of its member data belong. A data $d$ is then said to be correctly affected if the gold associates it with the prevalent class of the cluster it is in. Given this, purity is the ratio between the number of correctly affected data in the clustering and the total number of data in the clustering[7]:

$$mPUR = \frac{|P|}{|D|} \tag{9}$$

where $P = \{d \in D \mid \text{prec}(c(d)) = g(d) \wedge |c(d)| > 1\}$ with $D$ being the set of exploited data points, $c(d)$ a function that provides the cluster associated to data $d$ and $g(d)$ a function that provides the gold class associated to data $d$.

For the same reason, we also vary the number of clusters in a range up to 3 times that determined by the ground truth. An index which gives no indication of optimum in the expected range is considered as out-of-range or diverging index (- out-).

Lastly, we end up with a process that consists in generating perturbation in the clustering results by migrating data from one cluster to another to a fixed extend. This process, which simulates noisy clustering results, aims at estimating the robustness of the proposed estimators.

# 4   Results

The results are presented in Tables 2 and 3. Some complementary remarks must be done on validation process. In the tables, MaxP represents the number of clusters of the partition with highest mPur value (Eq. 9), or in some cases, the interval of partition sizes with highest stable mPur value. When a quality index identifies an optimal model with MaxP clusters and MaxP differs from the number of categories established by ground truth, its estimation is still considered as valid. This approach takes into account the fact that clustering would quite systematically produce sub-optimal results as compared to ground truth. Such situation happens when clustering identifies categories subparts as separate clusters, or conversely, merge different categories into a single one. It might thus leads to an optimal number of clusters which is greater or lower than the expected number of categories. In our datasets sample, it might be the case with IRIS dataset which is known to contain 2 overlapping categories. Partitions with highest purity values are thus considered for dealing with such situation, as well as skip of one or two single values in prediction as compared to the optimal $k$ value is tolerated. When indexes are still increasing and decreasing (depending on they are maximizers or minimizers) when the number of clusters is more than 3 times the number of expected classes, there are considered as out-of-range (-out- symbol in Tables 2 and 3).

When considering the results presented in Table 2, it is firstly possible to remark that some of experimented indexes never provides any correct answer,

---

[7] Clusters for which the prevalent class has only one element are considered as marginal and are thus ignored.

**Table 2.** Overview of the indexes estimation results.

|        | IRIS | WINE | PEN | ZOO | VRBF | R8 | R52 | Number of correct matches |
|--------|------|------|------|------|------|------|------|------|
| DB     | 5    | 2    | -out- | -out- | -out- | 4 | -out- | 1/7 |
| CH     | -out- | -out- | -out- | -out- | -out- | -out- | -out- | 0/7 |
| DU     | 2    | -out- | 17 | -out- | 2 | -out- | -out- | 1/7 |
| SI     | 4    | -out- | 12 | 16 | -out- | -out- | 54 | 3/7 |
| XB     | -out- | -out- | 19 | -out- | 23 | -out- | -out- | 0/7 |
| EC     | 3    | 5    | 9 | 6 | 18 | -out- | -out- | 4/7 |
| PC     | 2    | 5    | 9 | 7 | -15 | 6 | 52 | 7/7 |
| MaxP   | 3    | 5    | 12 | 10 | 12-16 | 6-10 | 45-55 | |
| Method | GNG  | GNG  | K-means | GNG | IGNGF | IGNGF | IGNGF | |

**Table 3.** Indexes estimation results in the presence of noise (UCI ZOO dataset).

|        | ZOO | ZOO Noise 10 % | ZOO Noise 20 % | ZOO Noise 30 % | Number of correct matches |
|--------|------|------|------|------|------|
| DB     | -out- | -out- | -out- | -out- | 0/4 |
| CH     | -out- | -out- | -out- | -out- | 0/4 |
| DU     | -out- | -out- | -out- | -out- | 0/4 |
| SI     | 16   | 16   | -out- | -out- | 0/4 |
| XB     | -out- | -out- | -out- | -out- | 0/4 |
| PC     | 6    | 4    | 11 | 9 | 1/4 |
| EC     | 7    | 5    | 6 | 9 | 2/4 |
| MaxP   | 10   | 13   | 13 | 13 | |
| Method | GNG  | GNG  | GNG | GNG | |

being systematically out of range (i.e. diverging). This is the case of Calinski-Harabasz (CH) index. This phenomenon has already been observed in some of our former experiments [11]. Some other indexes provides answers (i.e. maximum or minimum value depending on their core behaviour, maximizers or minimizers) in the range of the variation of $k$, but this answer is too far from ground truth or even too far from optimal purity among the set of generated clustering models. This is the case of Dunn (DU), Davis-Bouldin (DB) and Xie-Beni (XB) indexes. Some indexes are in the low mid-range of correctness and provide unstable answers. This is the case of Silhouette (SI) index. On its own side, our PC index performs slightly better than average but it is obviously a better low dimensional problem estimator than a high dimensional one. The help of negative features seems somehow mandatory for estimating optimal model in high

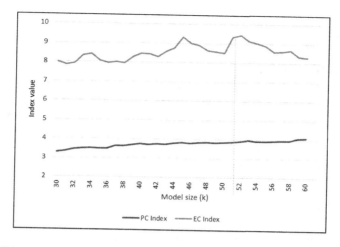

**Fig. 4.** Trends of PC and EC indexes on Reuters R52 dataset.

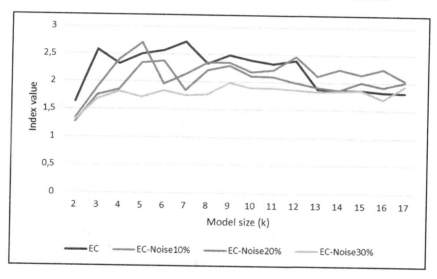

**Fig. 5.** Trends of EC indexes on UCI ZOO dataset with and without noise.

dimensional problems. Yet, in our experimental context, EC index that exploits negative feature never fails in its estimation[8], whatever it faced with low or high dimensional estimation problem.

The Fig. 4 draws the trends of evolution of EC and PC indexes in the case of the R52 dataset. It highlights what is a suitable index behaviour (EC index) and

---

[8] Taking into account purity tolerance criteria due to imperfect behaviour of clustering methods.

in a parallel way what represents the out-of-range index behaviour we mentioned before (PC index).

Interestingly, on the UCI ZOO dataset, the results of noise sensitivity analysis presented in Table 3 highlight that noise has relatively limited effect on the operation of PC and EC indexes. The Fig. 5 presents a parallel view of the different trends of EC value on non noisy and noisy clustering environment, respectively. It shows that noise tends to lower the index value in an overall way and to soften the trends related to its behaviour relatively to changes in $k$ value (see Fig. 3). However, EC index has again the most stable behaviour in that context. On its own side, the Silhouette index firstly delivers wrong optimal $k$ values on this dataset before getting out of range when the noise reaches 20 % on clustering results.

In all your experiments, we observed that the quality estimation weekly depends on the clustering method. Morever, we remarked that the computation time of your index is one of the lowest of studied indexes. As an example, on R52 dataset, EC index computation time is 125 s as compared to 43000 s for Silhouette index using a standard laptop with 2,2 GHz processor and 8 GB memory.

## 5  Conclusion

We have proposed a new set of indexes for clustering quality evaluation relying on feature maximization measure. This method exploits the information carried out by the features that could be associated to clusters by the means of their associated data. Our experiments highlighted that most of the usual quality estimators are not producing satisfying results in realistic data context and that they are additionally sensitive to noise. Conversely to usual quality estimators, one of the main interest of our proposed indexes is that they produce stable results in cases ranging from low dimensional to high dimensional context with additional advantage to have low computation time. Their stable operating mode with clustering methods that could produce results that are both different and imperfect is also a determinant advantage. However, some complementary experiments must certainly be done to confirm this promising behaviour.

Additionally, we plan to test the hability of our indexes to discriminate between correct and degenerated clustering results in the context of large and heterogeneous datasets.

This research was supported by the European Union through the European Regional Development Fund.

## References

1. Aha, D., Kibler, D., Albert, M.: Instance-based learning algorithms. Mach. Learn. **6**, 37–66 (1991)
2. Alphonse, E.'E., Amrani, A., Azé, J., Heitz, T., Mezaour, A.-D.,Roche, M.: Préparation des donnés et analyse des résultats de DEFT05. In: TALN 2005- Atelier DEFT 2005, pp. 99–111 (2005)

3. Angel Latha Mary, S., Sivagami, A.N., Usha Rani, M.: Cluster validity measures dynamic clustering algorithms. ARPN J. Eng. Appl. Sci. 10(9) (2015)
4. Attik, M., Lamirel, J.-C., Al Sheabi, S.: Clustering analysis for data with multiple labels. In: Proceedings of the IASTED International Conference on Databases and Applications (DBA), Innsbruck, Austria (2006)
5. Bache, K., Lichman, M.: UCI Machine learning repository, University of California, School of Information and Computer Science, Irvine, CA, USA (2013). http://archive.ics.uci.edu/ml
6. Bock, H.-H.: Probability model and hypothese testing in partitionning cluster analysis. In: Arabie, P., Hubert, L.J., De Soete, G. (eds.) Clustering and Classification, pp. 377–453. World Scientific, Singapore (1996)
7. Bolón-Canedo, V., Sánchez-Maroño, N., Alonso-Betanzos, A.: A review of feature selection methods on synthetic data. Knowl. Inf. Syst. 34(3), 483–519 (2013)
8. Calinsky, T., Harabasz, J.: A dendrite method for cluster analysis. Commun. Statis. 3(1), 1–27 (1974)
9. Davies, D.L., Bouldin, D.W.: A cluster separation measure. IEEE Trans. Pattern Anal. Mach. Intel., PAMI 1(2), 224–227 (1979)
10. Dunn, J.: Well separated clusters and optimal fuzzy partitions. J. Cybern. 4, 95–104 (1974)
11. Falk, I., Lamirel, J.-C., Gardent, C.: Classifying french verbs using french and english lexical resources. In: Proccedings of ACL, Jeju Island, Korea (2012)
12. Fritzke, B.: A growing neural gas network learns topologies. In: Tesauro, G., Touretzky, D.S., Leen, T.K. (ed.) Advances in Neural Information Processing Systems 7, pp. 625–632 (1995)
13. Forest, D.: Application de techniques de forage de textes de nature prédictive et exploratoire à des fins de gestion et dnalyse thématique de documents textuels non structurés, Ph.D. thesis, Quebec University, Montreal, Canada (2007)
14. Guerra, L., Robles, V., Bielza, C., Larrañaga, P.: A comparison of clustering quality indices using outliers and noise. Intel. Data Anal. 16, 703–715 (2012)
15. Gordon, A.D.: External validation in cluster analysis. Bull. Int. Statis. Inst. 51(2), 353–356 (1998). Response to comments. Bulletin of the International Statistical Institute 51(3), 414–415 (1998)
16. Guyon, I., Elisseeff, A.: An introduction to variable and feature selection. J. Mach. Learn. Res. 3, 1157–1182 (2003)
17. Halkidi, M., Batistakis, Y., Vazirgiannis, M.: On clustering validation techniques. J. Intel. Inf. Syst. 17(2/3), 147–155 (2001)
18. Kassab, R., Lamirel, J.-C.: Feature based cluster validation for high dimensional data. In: IASTED International Conference on Artificial Intelligence and Applications (AIA), Innsbruck, Austria, pp. 97–103, February 2008
19. Lamirel, J.C., Ta, A.P.: Combination of hyperbolic visualization and graph-based approach for organizing data analysis results: an application to social network analysis. In: Proceedings of the 4th International Conference on Webometrics, Informetrics and Scientometrics and 9th COLLNET Meetings, Berlin, 2012 Germany (2008)
20. Lamirel, J.C., Mall, R., Cuxac, P., Safi, G.: Variations to incremental growing neural gas algorithm based on label maximization. In: Proceedings of IJCNN 2011, San Jose, CA, USA, pp. 956–965 (2011)
21. Lamirel, J.C.: A new approach for automatizing the analysis of research topics dynamics: application to optoelectronics research. Scientometrics 93(1), 151–166 (2012)

22. Lamirel, J.-C., Cuxac, P., Chivukula, A.S., Hajlaoui, K.: Optimizing text classification through efficient feature selection based on quality metric. J. Intel. Inf. Syst., Special issue on PAKDD-QIMIE **2013**, 1–18 (2014)

23. Lamirel, J.-C., Falk, I., Gardent, C.: Federating clustering and cluster labeling capabilities with a single approach based on feature maximization: French verb classes identification with IGNGF neural clustering. In: Neurocomputing, Special issue on 9th Workshop on Self-Organizing Maps (WSOM 2012), vol. 147, pp. 136–146 (2014)

24. MacQueen, J.B.: Some methods for classification and analysis of multivariate observations. In: Proceedings of 5th Berkeley Symposium on Mathematical Statistics and Probability 1, pp. 281–297. University of California Press (1967)

25. Milligan, G.W., Cooper, M.C.: An examination of procedures for determining the number of clusters in a dataset. Psychometrika **50**(2), 159–179 (1985)

26. Rendón, E., Abundez, I., Arizmendi, A., Quiroz, E.M.: Internal versus external cluster validation indexes. Int. J. Comput. Commun. **5**(1), 27–34 (2011)

27. Rousseeuw, P.J.: Silhouettes: a graphical aid to the interpretation and validation of cluster analysis. J. Comput. Appl. Math. **20**, 53–65 (1987)

28. Sun, L., Korhonen, A., Poibeau, T., Messiant, C.: Investigating the cross-linguistic potential of VerbNet-style classification. In: Proceedings of ACL, Beijing, China, pp. 1056–1064 (2010)

29. Yanchi, L., Zhongmou, L., Xiong, H., Gao, X., Wu, J.: Understanding of internal clustering validation measures. In: Proceedings of the 2010 IEEE International Conference on Data Mining, ICDM 2010, pp. 911–916 (2010)

30. Xie, X.L., Beni, G.: A validity measure for fuzzy clustering. IEEE Trans. Pattern Anal. Mach. Intel. **13**(8), 841–847 (1991)

# Data Analytics for Evidence-based Healthcare

# Integrating Content Centric Networking and Web Content Mining: A Future Efficient Internet Architecture for Healthcare

Rabia Bashir[1(✉)] and Sajjad Akbar[2]

[1] Department of Computer Science, Federal Urdu University of Arts, Science and Technology, Islamabad, Pakistan
rabia.bashir@gmail.com
[2] Faculty of Science and Technology, Bournemouth University, Bournemouth, UK
makbar@bournemouth.ac.uk

**Abstract.** Healthcare Information Systems are indispensible and require more collaboration nowadays. Network Infrastructure for communication requires extreme bandwidth for doctors' diagnosis reports and medical images in order to interchange between various hospitals. The recent Internet architecture is a host-centric network that is less appropriate for healthcare applications in terms of patient monitoring and emergency services. With an emergent use of various interactive healthcare applications, the host-centric networking approach is supposed to be less proficient as it relies on the physical location. Therefore, a new approach to networking architecture called Content-Centric Network (CCN) is considered as the prospective Internet architecture for future. It uses name of data to access the contents rather than location. It reduces the network congestion and traffic by improving the delivery speed. CCN is still less efficient due to unavailability of appropriate content in Content Servers. For this purpose, Web Content Mining (WCM) techniques can facilitate to efficiently perform the data management of CCN. Therefore, this paper contributes: Firstly, by identifying the challenges of WCM such as language independency, structure flexibility, performance, dynamicity, redundancy handling, intelligence and relevant content retrieval. Secondly, it maps identified challenges on WCM techniques to adopt most suitable WCM approach for CCN. Finally, this paper introduces an innovative Internet architecture for healthcare by integrating CCN and WCM to deal the data management issues. From Information Centric Networks (ICN), we have opted CCN for our proposed architecture. While from WCM, Agent-based approach is selected in order to locate most relevant healthcare data.

**Keywords:** Content centric networking · Web content mining · Agent-based web content mining · Healthcare · Information centric networking

© Springer International Publishing Switzerland 2015
X.-L. Li et al. (Eds.): PAKDD 2015, LNCS 9441, pp. 225–236, 2015.
DOI: 10.1007/978-3-319-25660-3_19

# 1    Introduction

Healthcare information technology should support in delivering the new medical data in patient-centric model [1, 2]. Many ill people are treated in various countries around the world which means they need to access this medical data on various locations. Therefore, the aim of healthcare information technology is to transform the data from paper based systems to electronic systems; allow this data to interoperate between various healthcare service providers [3, 4].

However, the Internet is facing dozens of issues to satisfy the current application requirements. The main reason for these issues is the basic design of the Internet, as the requirement of the network was different. The basic requirements were the communication between a limited numbers of hosts, sharing network resources among nodes that were considered precious at that time. They have considered some main design principals like Scalability [5], Heterogeneity [6], Robustness Principle [7, 8] and Loose Coupling etc. These design principles are necessary for any network architecture. The addressing scheme of the Internet was designed by considering the dependency of host IP address to its network location. In the current host-centric architecture for mobility support, Mobile IP patch [9] is used. Similarly, different patches have been included to support multiple services for the Internet. Although the added patches satisfied these requirements temporarily but also increased the complexity of the overall architecture [10]. Thus, we have two solutions to handle above issue, either we continue to keep patching or we work towards a new architecture design approach which can contain these requirements in its core design.

In this aspect, a novice network infrastructure known as Content Centric Network is supposed an impending Internet architecture [11]. It uses name of data to access the contents rather than location. It reduces the network congestion and traffic by improving the delivery speed. Moreover, it is ideal network architecture as it does not depend on conventional client-server model [12]. It uses the receiver oriented approach rather than sender oriented. It introduces the naming base information system at the network layer. Further, it uses different caching mechanisms in routers, which eliminate the dependency of users on the destination host. Hence, a node will be searching for contents rather than end hosts. Such design aspects will also support the mobility of nodes, as now nodes are concerned with the content rather than host's location. It will provide an improved efficiency in terms of scalability, bandwidth and robustness etc.

Web is the biggest source for information. With the increase of web documents, the searching is becoming time consuming process. In this regard, Data mining (DM) is domain of computer science that is used for extracting information from huge data. Web mining is application of DM and is further divided into three categories: Web Usage Mining, Web Content Mining and Web Structure Mining [13]. Web Content Mining utilizes the ideas of knowledge discovery and data mining to get more exact data. The purpose of WCM is extraction and analysis of relevant information from the web contents by using various approaches such as machine learning, statistics, assumptions, wrapper induction and using templates etc. [14].

However, the information extraction from the web is difficult task because web contents can be unstructured such as text, semi-structured (HTML documents) or structured (e.g. extracted data from database in dynamic web pages). There is also redundancy in web data; multiple web pages have the similar information. Moreover web is also noisy as the web pages contain mixture of information such as advertisements, navigation bars, main content and copyright.

Therefore, in this paper we have identified the challenges of WCM and mapped those on various WCM techniques in order to investigate that WCM approach which can outperform the other approaches. Moreover, we have proposed future efficient internet architecture for healthcare by integrating the proficient WCM approach (Agent-based) with CCN which is ICN architecture. The objective of this new healthcare network based on CCN and WCM is to efficiently handle the healthcare data in healthcare information systems by providing the useful healthcare contents (Electronic Healthcare Record) from web.

## 2    Analyzing the Web Content Mining Techniques

We have studied various approaches of WCM. The comparative study of these approaches and their limitations are discussed in this section.

### 2.1    Agent-Based Web Content Mining

In Agent-based WCM, Artificial Intelligence system is developed that autonomously or semi-autonomously performs function for specific user on its behalf. Agents intelligently search the relevant web contents by using characteristics of particular domain and profiles of users [15]. However, this technique requires training to learn from data. It highly relies on training. Therefore, it may not perform well if contents or structure of web pages is altered.

### 2.2    Template Detection-Based Web Content Mining

This technique uses already prepared master HTML shell page (Template) for creating the new web page. In templates, to show the similar look and feel the contents of new web pages are plugged into shell page. They are created by using a master HTML page which is shared among all the web pages which are linked to that website [16]. This technique robustly depends on structure or template of web pages as the template of web pages keeps changing that is why this approach is supposed unreliable.

### 2.3    Assumption-Based Web Content Mining

Assumptions and cues are made on the content nodes, tags, web page's structure and main content place. These techniques make generalization for the web pages and this tends towards less efficiency [17]. As a result, it is supposed unrealistic and not applicable for all kind of web pages.

### 2.4  Statistics-Based Web Content Mining

Statistics-based WCM involves often weights or thresholds are used which are determined through empirical experiments. It is a simple technique and has better generality [17]. On the other hand, it is difficult to find out a common set of weights or threshold values to satisfy all web pages from different websites. Therefore, it has less accuracy. Moreover, those documents having very large or short contents, this technique does not outperform the other techniques.

### 2.5  Wrapper-Based Web Content Mining

In data mining, wrapper is a program in which the contents from specific information source are extracted and then translated into a form. In wrapper generation, there are two approaches: Induction of Wrapper and Automated Data Extraction. In Wrapper Induction, learning is involved in which the rules for data extraction are learned from training examples which are labeled manually [18]. In order to make wrapper, an expert is needed to write extraction rules. Further, manual labeling is required to extract the data from large website to make the wrapper to learn. Therefore, it is time consuming and less efficient. Another issue with wrapper is its maintenance that is hard because when web page is altered then one needs to make new wrapper for it.

### 2.6  Machine Learning-Based Web Content Mining

These approaches rely on training sessions and during these trainings, system gets the domain expertise. Moreover, they focus on prediction on the basis of properties which they learn from training data. Clustering and Classification are examples. By using word assorting and classifying, it provides high accuracy but it little bit complicates the solution [17]. In this technique, human intervention is high as web pages are manually labeled. Moreover, whenever contents or structure of web pages is changed then needs to train the data.

## 3  Challenging Facets of Web Content Mining

After thorough study of WCM, we have identified seven challenging factors that any WCM technique requires to deal. Figure 1 describes the identified challenges.

## Challenge # 1
## Language Independency

The content mining strategy should be self-sufficient so that it could be applicable on web data in any language. Many WCM systems have been proposed but still they are dialect dependent.

## Challenge # 2
## Performance

The data extraction techniques should be capable to handle colossal data in a short timeframe. Therefore, extraction mechanisms must be agile to work irrespective of data size.

## Challenge # 3
## Dynamicity

Web is dynamic as its information is constantly updated. It is a big challenge to introduce such mining technique which can cope with dynamic nature of web.

## Challenge # 4
## Intelligence

The web is noisy. A web page typically contains main content, advertisements, navigation panels and copyright notices. In any application only part of the information is useful and the rest are noises. As a matter of fact, it is challenging to only identify the main contents.

## Challenge # 5
## Structure Flexibility

WCM techniques should be independent of particular structure or template.
If extraction technique depends on website templates and structure then it will be unreliable.
As time to time updation of particular web pages or websites will also force to change extraction algorithms according to template or structure.

## Challenge # 6
## Redundancy Handling

Information on the web is redundant. Multiple web pages may present the same or similar information using completely different formats or syntaxes.
Same type of information can be found on various pages of same website or even on different websites.

## Challenge # 7
## Relevant Content Retrieval

There is a large variety of data available on web such as images, audios, videos and text.
It is important to extract only that information which is more fascinating for the particular user.

**Fig. 1.** Challenges of web content mining

# 4    Mapping of WCM Challenging on Extraction Techniques

In this section, we have mapped the challenges of WCM with web content extraction approaches. The identified challenges are on the left side of the table while the extraction techniques are depicted horizontally. Moreover, we have assigned various verdicts such as Yes, No, Low, Medium and High to these challenges on the basis of limitations of WCM techniques. In Table 1, first challenge is Language Independency. On mapping this challenge on six extraction techniques, it is observed that wrapper and machine learning techniques are dependent on language. As their implementation is learning dependent on a particular language. Contrary to these, agent-based, template detection, assumption and statistic-based techniques are language independent because of their basic feature. Such as, agent-based WCM depends on some fuzzy logic and we can apply it in any language.

**Table 1.** Mapping of challenges

| Challenges | Extraction Techniques | | | | | |
|---|---|---|---|---|---|---|
| | Agent-based | Template Detection -based | Assumption -based | Statistics-based | Wrapper -based | Machine Learning -based |
| Language Independency | Yes | Yes | Yes | Yes | No | No |
| Structure Flexibility | Medium | Low | High | High | Low | Low |
| Performance | High | Medium | Low | Medium | Low | Medium |
| Dynamicity | No | No | No | No | No | No |
| Redundancy Handling | High | Medium | Low | Medium | Medium | High |
| Intelligence | High | Medium | Low | Medium | Medium | Medium |
| Relevant Content Retrieval | High | Medium | Low | Low | Medium | Medium |

Second challenge is Structure Flexibility. Template, wrapper and machine learning approaches are less flexible. So, we have written low because in case of template detection-based techniques, we strongly depend on the template of the web page. Since the web pages change from time to time, it surely affects the template and needs to update it accordingly. Similarly, for wrapper we need to build new wrapper when page is changed. In machine learning, the situation is same. Whenever, web page contents and structure changes, every time we need to train the dataset. However, for assumption and statistics-based techniques, structure flexibility is high because these techniques are independent of any peculiar structure or template. For agent-based WCM, though this approach also depends on training like machine learning. Any change in structure of web pages needs training. But it is medium because agents are intelligent to adopt changes efficiently. Third indispensable challenge is Performance, which is medium for template, statistics and machine learning approaches. All three approaches involve little overhead in terms of learning the particular environment. Whereas, for wrapper and assumption-based techniques, it is low because manual labeling is involved for wrapper learning which slows down the performance and time consuming. Likewise, assumption-based technique is also low in performance because we make assumptions and use cues which do not guarantee the high performance. Contrary to this, agent-based approach is supposed better than others. They search more intelligently and no manual work is involved.

Fourth challenge is Dynamicity, by deep study of literature we have concluded that all available approaches lack this feature and cannot cope with dynamic nature of web. They do not alert the users about the updation of contents on the web pages.

Fifth challenge which is identified in table is Redundancy Handling; it is medium for template, statistics and wrapper-based techniques. Wrapper-based technique is less efficient. It is assumed that it cannot outperform for redundant data. Similarly, it is already discussed that statistics-based approach is less accurate. So as a matter of fact it will provide less accurate results in case of redundant data. Template detection performs medium in terms of handling redundant data. As on a similar template, there can be common content which will create confusion for selection of appropriate data.

Sixth challenge is Intelligence. Template, statistics, wrapper and machine learning techniques have medium intelligence. Because these approaches depend on some specific structure (template), weights, thresholds and extraction rules which vary depending on page contents and nodes etc. It makes these techniques less intelligent. On the other hand, assumption-based technique is least intelligent. Because it is based on assumptions and cues that makes it unrealistic and less accurate. However, agent-based approach is highly intelligent because agents perform intelligent searching.

Relevant Content Retrieval is seventh challenge. Template, wrapper and machine learning have medium level of content retrieval. Because for template it is supposed unreliable approach as it totally depends on template of the web pages. The change in the template may affect the relevancy of content retrieval. As discussed earlier that wrappers are less efficient so their content retrieval relevancy will be medium. The reason for medium relevant content retrieval in machine learning approach is the focus of this technique on prediction on the basis of properties which it learns from training data. Moreover, if it fails to predict well then relevant content is not retrieved properly. So highly depends on the learning for good prediction. On the other hand, for assumption and statistics, it is low as assumption-based technique purely depends on assumption and cues. It makes it unreliable and provide poor guarantee for retrieval of related contents. Equivalently, lower accuracy of statistical approach makes the relevant content retrieval dubious. Therefore, it is also low in case of statistics but agents have high content retrieval ability because of being intelligent.

# 5  Information Centric Network Architectures

We have discussed different ICN approaches below so that we can find the most suitable ICN approach for our proposed Internet architecture.

## 5.1  Flat-Based ICN Architectures

Following architectures are included under flat-based ICN architecture:

### A.  Data Oriented Network Architecture (DONA): Data Oriented Network

DONA [19] is assumed to be the first ICN architecture that replaces hierarchical URLs with flat names. So it eliminates the dependency of a host to a specific location. It increases the data availability by caching it at network layer. DONA uses flat name of the data where each data element is associated with a principal. Principal is considered to be the owner of the data. These names are identified by the cryptographic hash of principal's public key P and a label L uniquely identified the data with respect to the principal.

### B.  Publish Subscribe Internet Technology (PURSUIT)

PURSUIT [20] is another potential candidate that replaces the TCP/IP architecture. For naming, it follows the flat addresses like DONA. Data object is identified by the unique pair of IDs called the scope ID and the rendezvous ID. The scope ID contains the information of a specific group whereas rendezvous ID exactly points to the required information in the group. The data objects can belong to multiple scopes but at least they must belong to one scope. Similar to NDN, PURSUIT architecture contains three functions i.e. rendezvous, topology management and forwarding functions. Rendezvous functions to create the route between subscriber and publisher.

### C.  Scalable and Adaptive Internet Solution (SAIL)

The SAIL [21] architecture combines the different elements of NDN and PURSUIT architectures. It is flexible as it allows convergence layers to use different routing and forwarding technologies. SAIL uses flat naming as well as hierarchical naming for identification of the data information. If it is using hierarchical naming schemes then it follows the basic rule of CCN for separation of naming with the location. For data object matching it uses the flat name as in PURSUIT and for the routing it can use hierarchical naming like NDN. In SAIL, name resolution and data routing can be coupled as well as decoupled.

### D.  Mobility First

The primary goal of Mobility First architecture [22] is to provide the mobility support to the node in ICN. It's a clean slate approach that provides separation of name of entity with its network name. It uses a global unique name for all the entities. These global unique names can be translated to one or the more than one network addresses. Further, it also provides the support for the mechanisms like multicast, multi homing, caching and security. In this architecture, each node is assigned a Global Unique Identifier (GUID) with the help of global naming service. These flat GUIDs are 160 bit long. These GUIDs may use self certifying hashes of data objects. If GUID (a video file name) is available at multiple locations then its GUID will be the same.

### 5.2    Hierarchical-Based ICN Architectures

#### A.    Named-Data Networking (NDN)/Content-Centric Networking (CCN)

NDN/CCN [23] is considered to be a complete architecture for ICN. To achieve the scalability, NDN approach uses hierarchical-based naming scheme. NDN uses the concept of strategy layer which makes the NDN more flexible.

## 6    Web Content Mining and Content Centric-Based Network Architecture for Healthcare

Figure 2 shows a topological diagram of the emerged architectures, where Information-Centric Networking is working combined with WCM. For such a combined Internet architecture, CCN approach is selected from ICN, whereas, for WCM, Agent-based approach is selected. The selection of these approaches is made because of their comprehensive design and easy to deploy factor as explained in the previous sections.

As NDN/CCN is assumed to be receiver driven architecture, so physicians will initiate healthcare content request. In Fig. 1: R1, R2, R3, R4 and R5 are the Content Routers. User will request R3 for healthcare data content; if R3 does not have the content then it will forward the request to R2 and R5. If R3 have the required healthcare data in its Content Store, then it will directly send to the user. Similarly, if the requested data is not available on the Content Routers, then alternatively, request will forward to the Content Server. The functionality of the Content Server is to store data and keep advertising the content availability to the Content Routers. When Content Server does not have the required healthcare data, it will search it from the Internet by applying Agent-based WCM approach. As Agent-based approach uses the artificial intelligence techniques, so, Content Server will find the most suitable and appropriate healthcare content for the request and transfer it to the Content Routers.

Similarly, later, if Physician B sends request for the same healthcare content, it will be transferred through R3-R5-Physician B as R3 have the data in its Content Store (CS).

Figure 3 is a flow diagram of the proposed architecture. Physicians initiate request by sending an Interest Message (containing required content name) to the Content Router. Content Router (CR) contains three data structures i.e. Content Store, Pending Information Table (PIT) and Forwarding Information Base (FIB).

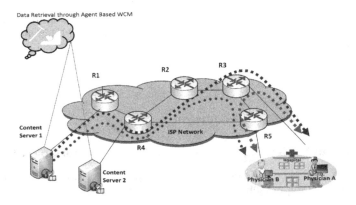

**Fig. 2.** Topological diagram of future efficient internet architecture for healthcare

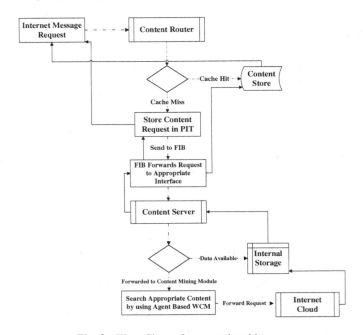

**Fig. 3.** Flow Chart of proposed architecture

Hence, CR will check either the requested healthcare content is available in CS or not. If content is available in CS, Cache Hit occurs and data is transferred to the physicians. In case of Cache Miss (data is not available in CS), request is sent to PIT, that stores it as pending request and sends to the FIB which finds the appropriate interface to forward the request to other CR or to designated Content Server. Content Server will check its local database that either requested healthcare content is available or not. In case of availability it will transfer data to the CR. CR will receive data through FIB, checks the PIT and sends data to the physicians. Further, it will store data in Content

Store (CS). When data is not available in Content Server, It will search and download data from Internet with the help of Agent-based approach and transfer to the physicians with similar procedure as described.

## 7 Conclusion and Future Work

The current Internet architecture is a host-centric networking approach, which is less appropriate for healthcare applications in terms of patient monitoring and emergency services. It is less efficient as it depends on the physical location, therefore, a new approach to networking architecture called Content-Centric Network (CCN) is considered as the impending future Internet architecture. CCN is still considered to be less efficient due to unavailability of appropriate content in Content Servers. So, we have used Agent-based WCM to store data on Content Servers.

In this paper, we have proposed efficient network architecture for healthcare by integrating ICN (CCN) and WCM (Agent-based) approach. After mapping the challenges of WCM with web content extraction approaches, we have concluded that Agent-based WCM approach is preferably better than other approaches on the basis of high performance, redundancy handling, intelligence and relevant content retrieval. The use of Agent-based WCM is significant in healthcare industry because it facilitates physicians to collect quick information. Moreover, after processing this information physicians can easily make decisions regarding patients' diagnosis and treatment. The future aspect of our research is to implement the proposed architecture in healthcare domain and provide the detailed analysis in terms of its usability and performance.

## References

1. Jayadevappa, R., Chhatre, S.: Patient centered care – a conceptual model and review of the state of the art. Open Health Serv. Policy J. **4**, 15–25 (2011)
2. Diamond, C.C., Mostashari, F., Shirky, C.: Collecting and sharing data for population health: a new paradigm. Health Aff. **28**(2), 454–466 (2009)
3. Agrawal, R., Grandison, T., Johnson, C., Kiernan, J.: Enabling the 21st century health care information technology revolution. Commun. ACM **50**(2), 34–42 (2007)
4. Vest, J.R., Gamm, L.D.: Health information exchange: persistent challenges and new strategies. JAMIA J. Am. Med. Inform. Assoc. **17**(3), 288–294 (2010)
5. Clark, D., Braden, R., Chapin, L., Hobby, R., Cerf, V.: Towards the future internet architecture (1991)
6. Carpenter, B.E.: Architectural principles of the internet (1996)
7. Postel, J.: Internet RFC760: Dod standard internet protocol. Network Working Group (1980)
8. RFC 791: Internet protocol (1981)
9. Choi, S., Kim, K., Kim, S., Roh, B.-H.: Threat of dos by interest flooding attack in content-centric networking. In: 2013 International Conference on Information Networking (ICOIN), pp. 315–319. IEEE (2013)
10. Xylomenos, G., Ververidis, C., Siris, V., Fotiou, N., Tsilopoulos, C., Vasilakos, X., Katsaros, K., Polyzos, G.: A survey of information-centric networking research (2013)

11. Akbar, M.S., Khaliq, K.A., Bin Rais, R.N., Qayyum, A.: Information-centric networks: categorizations, challenges, and classifications. In: Wireless and Optical Communication Conference, pp. 1–5 (2014)
12. Tantatsanawong, P.: Healthcare information sharing system through content-centric network: a prototype of content discovery gateway. J. Convergence Inf. Technol. **8**(5), 1145–1153 (2013)
13. Kaur, R., Kaur, K.: A review of various techniques of web content mining for HTML and XML contents. IJRCCT **3**(6), 669–672 (2014)
14. Yoon, S., Elhadad, N., Bakken, S.: A practical approach for content mining of Tweets. Am. J. Prev. Med. **45**, 122–129 (2013)
15. Bedi, P., Chawla, S.: Agent based information retrieval system using information scent. J. Artif. Intell. **3**(4), 220–238 (2010)
16. Bar-Yossef, Z., Rajagopalan, S.: Template detection via data mining and its applications. In: Proceedings of the 11th International Conference on World Wide Web (2002)
17. Al-Ghuribi, S.M., Alshomrani, S.: A comprehensive survey on web content extraction algorithms and techniques. In: International Conference on Information Science and Applications (2013)
18. Ferrara, E., et al.: Web data extraction, applications and techniques: a survey (2012). arXiv: 1207.0246
19. Stanford University Triad Project. http://wwwdsg.stanford.edu/triad/
20. Fp7 Pursuit Project. http://www.fp7-pursuit.eu/pursuitweb/
21. Fp7 Sail Project. http://www.sail-project.eu/
22. Nsf Mobility First Project. http://mobilityfirst.winlab.rutgers.edu/
23. Nsf Named Data Networking Project. http://www.named-data.net/

# Citation Enrichment Improves Deduplication of Primary Evidence

Miew Keen Choong[1,2(✉)], Sarah Thorning[3], and Guy Tsafnat[1]

[1] Centre for Health Informatics, Australian Institute of Health Innovation,
Faculty of Medicine and Health Sciences,
Macquarie University, Sydney, Australia
{miewkeen.choong, guy.tsafnat}@mq.edu.au
[2] Australian Institute of Health Innovation, Macquarie University,
Level 6, 75 Talavera Road, North Ryde, NSW 2113, Australia
[3] Faculty of Health Sciences and Medicine,
Bond University, Gold Coast, QLD, Australia
sthornin@bond.edu.au

**Abstract.** Objective: To automatically detect duplicate citations in a bibliographical database.

Background: Citations retrieved from multiple search databases have different forms making manual and automatic detection of duplicates difficult. Existing methods rely on fuzzy-similarity measures which are error-prone.

Methods: We analysed four pairs of original search results from MEDLINE and EMBASE that were used to create systematic reviews. An automatic tool deduplicated citations by first enriching citations with Digital Object Identifiers (DOI), and/or other unique identifiers. Duplication of records was then determined by comparing these unique identifiers. We compared our method with the duplicate detection function of a popular citation management desktop application in several configurations.

Results: Citation Enrichment identified 93 % (range 86 %–100 %) of the duplicates indexed online and erroneously marked 3 % (range 0 %–6 %) documents as duplicates. The citation management application found 68 % (range 64 %–72 %) without error using default setting. When set for highest deduplication, the citation management application found 94 % of duplicates (range 77 %–100 %) and 4 % error (range 0 %–8 %).

Conclusion: Citation enrichment using unique identifiers enhances automatic deduplication. On its own, the approach seems slightly superior to tools that compare citations without enrichment. Methods that combine citation enrichment with existing fuzzy-matching may substantially reduce resource requirements of evidence synthesis.

**Keywords:** Evidence · Information retrieval · Citation de-duplication

**Abbreviations**

| | |
|---|---|
| DOI | Digital Object Identifiers |
| FN | False Negatives |
| FP | False Positives |
| HTML | HyperText Markup Language |

© Springer International Publishing Switzerland 2015
X.-L. Li et al. (Eds.): PAKDD 2015, LNCS 9441, pp. 237–244, 2015.
DOI: 10.1007/978-3-319-25660-3_20

MAS       Microsoft Academic Search
MASID     MAS unique identifiers
P         Precision
PDF       Portable Document Format
R         Recall
SR        Systematic Reviews
TP        True Positives

# 1  Background

Systematic reviews (SR) and other evidence summaries typically begin with comprehensive literature retrieval that should include all relevant evidence. The Cochrane Handbook explicitly stipulates that searching MEDLINE alone is insufficient and that it is necessary to search additional databases [1]. Searching multiple databases usually leads to additional workload due to differences in databases. Citations are considered duplicates if they refer to the same article. Differences in citations are typically caused by spelling variations, abbreviations and truncations [2]. Box 1 show exemplar pairs of duplicate records that appear in MEDLINE and EMBASE respectively.

The detection and removal of duplicate records (often referred to as "deduplication") is time consuming [3] and automatic and reliable deduplication remains an elusive but necessary step in automation of systematic reviews [4] and maintaining registers of clinical studies.

The duplicate finding function in most standard bibliographic database organizers (e.g. EndNote®, ProCite®, Reference Manager®) have limited effectiveness [3]. These work by comparing the citation information (i.e. titles, authors, journals, years etc.) using a distance function, and conclude that citations with a distance above a minimum similarity threshold are duplicates.

There are a number of record deduplication works [3], mostly using field matching of the citation information, either based on distance metric [5, 6] or supervised learning techniques [3, 7]. The most related work were done by Qi et al. [2] and Rathbone et al. [8]. Qi et al. showed that combining auto- (with EndNote) and hand-searching would produce better detection. The more recent method was based on multi-iteration heuristic-based approach for field matching which was shown to outperform EndNote's default setting [8].

Here we present an alternative approach that first enriches citations with global identifiers such as Digital Object Identifiers (DOI). We tested the hypothesis that deduplication using these identifiers provides a more effective comparison measure than the traditional approach. Previously, PubMed IDs and DOIs were used to deduplicate search results in a meta-search engine [9]. However the effectiveness of this approach was never measured.

Example 1: duplicates:
MEDLINE: Ramakers BP, Riksen NP, Stal TH, Heemskerk S, van den Broek P, Peters WHM, van der Hoeven JG, Smits P, Pickkers P: **Dipyridamole augments the antiinflammatory response during human endotoxemia.** *Crit Care* 2011, 15(6):R289.

EMBASE: Ramakers BPC, Riksen NP, Stal TH, Heemskerk S, van den Broek P, Peters WHM, van der Hoeven JG, Smits P, Pickkers P: **Dipyridamole augments the anti-inflammatory response during human endotoxemia.** *Critical Care* 2011:R289.

Example 2: duplicates:
MEDLINE: Kamin W, Maydannik VG, Malek FA, Kieser M: **Efficacy and tolerability of EPs 7630 in patients (aged 6-18 years old) with acute bronchitis.** *Acta Paediatrica* 2010, 99(4):537-543
EMBASE: Kamin W, Maydannik VG, Malek FA, Kieser M: **Efficacy and tolerability of EPs 7630 in patients (aged 6-18 years old) with acute bronchitis: A randomized, double-blind, placebo-controlled clinical dose-finding study.** *Acta Paediatrica, International Journal of Paediatrics* 2010, 99(4):537-543.

Example 3: not duplicates:
MEDLINE: van der Steen JT, Albers G, Licht-Strunk E, Muller MT, Ribbe MW: **A validated risk score to estimate mortality risk in patients with dementia and pneumonia: barriers to clinical impact.** *Int Psychogeriatr* 2011, 23(1):31-43.
EMBASE: Van Der Steen JT, Albers G, Licht-Strunk E, Muller MT, Ribbe MW: **A validated risk score to estimate mortality risk in patients with dementia and pneumonia: Barriers to clinical impact.** *Palliative Medicine* 2010, 24(4):S201-S202.

Example 4: not duplicates:
MEDLINE: Altamimi S, Khalil A, Khalaiwi KA, Milner R, Pusic MV, Al Othman MA: **Short versus standard duration antibiotic therapy for acute streptococcal pharyngitis in children.** *Cochrane Database Syst Rev* 2009(1):CD004872.
EMBASE: Altamimi S, Khalil A, Khalaiwi KA, Milner R, Pusic MV, Al Othman MA: **Short versus standard duration antibiotic therapy for acute streptococcal pharyngitis in children.** *Sao Paulo Medical Journal 2010*, 128(1):48.
Box 1: examples of duplicate citations from MEDLINE and EMBASE and differences in them.

## 2   Methods

### 2.1   Data

We used the original citation lists obtained in the literature search phase of four systematic reviews: "Harms from Amoxicillin: A Systematic Review and Meta-Analysis of Randomised Controlled Trials for Any Indication" [10] (Amoxicillin harm), "Fluid Therapy for Acute Bacterial Meningitis" [11] (Fluid therapy), "Short-course versus Prolonged-course Antibiotic Therapy for Hospital-acquired Pneumonia in Critically Ill Adults" [12] (Antibiotic therapy), and "Shared Decision Making for Acute Respiratory Infections in Primary Care" [13] (Shared decision). Table 1 shows summaries of the search results of the four datasets using MEDLINE and EMBASE. Each of the eight search results sets contained no duplicate citations. Duplicate records retrieved from both databases were manually checked. The manual duplicates list was used only for evaluation of the algorithm and not for its training or construction.

**Table 1.** The number of records found in MEDLINE, EMBASE and duplicated records of the four systematic reviews used.

|  | No of records found in MEDLINE | No of records found in EMBASE | Duplicated records |
|---|---|---|---|
| Amoxicillin harm [10] | 442 | 149 | 32 |
| Fluid therapy [11] | 131 | 312 | 61 |
| Antibiotic therapy [12] | 2142 | 706 | 165 |
| Share decision [13] | 745 | 444 | 80 |

### 2.2   Algorithm

We use the algorithm in [14] for automatic evidence retrieval for systematic reviews. Given the citation set, each citation is automatically converted to search engine query by removing short words, numbers and punctuation [15]. The query is submitted to Microsoft Academic Search (MAS) (http://academic.research.microsoft.com/) — a generalized scientific literature search engine that covers more than 48 million publications with weekly updates. Microsoft provides a free application programming interface to registered users for non-commercial purposes. Other search engines (e.g. Google Scholar) can also be used in this step, subject to restrictions they impose. The query results returned from MAS contain citation information including DOI and MAS unique identifiers (MAS ID). After enriching the citation with these identifiers, duplicate detection using only the identifiers is performed. DOI were preferred in the comparison and MAS ID was used if no DOI was available. If the DOI or MAS ID was found in one citation and not the other, the citations were deemed to be different. Once a DOI is matched, citations are regarded as duplicates.

## 2.3    Evaluation

We created a gold standard list of duplicate citations by manually searching all references to ascertain that they are indexed in MAS. Other references were removed. Every enriched citation from one list was compared with every enriched citation from the other. We compared the duplicates identified by the algorithm with the gold standard.

We compared the "find duplicates" function in EndNote [16] on the same data using the settings shown in Table 2. Each citation feature set was tried with (a) "Ignore spacing and punctuation" or (b) "exact match" so that in total, EndNote was run 10 times on each dataset. The default setting in EndNote is EndNote1b: comparison based on Author, Year and Title using "ignore spacing and punctuation".

**Table 2.** Bibliographic features used by EndNote to compare citations.

| Compare | Setting name | |
|---|---|---|
| | "Ignore spacing and punctuation" | "Exact match" |
| Author, year and title | EN1a (Default) | EN1b |
| Author, year, title and journal | EN2a | EN2b |
| Author and title | EN3a | EN3b |
| Title and year | EN4a | EN4b |
| Author and year | EN5a | EN5b |

We checked the duplicates detected with the gold standard. Correctly identified duplicates were counted as true positives (TP). Duplicates that were wrongly identified were counted as false positives (FP). Missed duplicates were counted as false negatives (FN). We calculated the Recall (R) and Precision (P) and $F_1$-score of each deduplication method according to the equations below.

$$Precision = \frac{TP}{TP + FP}$$

$$Recall = \frac{TP}{TP + FN}$$

$$F_1 - score = \frac{2 \times P \times R}{P + R}$$

The primary measure was a comparison of our enrichment algorithm with default setting of EndNote.

# 3   Results

The performance of the citation enrichment algorithm is shown in Table 3. Recall is more than 86 % in all cases. Four pairs of citations were wrongly detected as being duplicates. Overall, citation enrichment had recall of 37.4 % higher than EndNote default but at a cost of up to 3.5 % in precision.

Error analysis found that 62.5 % (n = 5) undetected duplicates had errors in the title recorded in MAS and 37.5 % (n = 3) were due to errors in the title indexed in the

**Table 3.** The comparisons of the performance of citation enrichment algorithm and the default settings of Endnote for detecting duplicates.

|  | Citation enrichment | | | Default settings of EndNote (EN1a) | | |
|---|---|---|---|---|---|---|
|  | Precision | Recall | $F_1$-score | Precision | Recall | $F_1$-score |
| Amoxicillin harm | 0.944 | 1.000 | 0.971 | 1.000 | 0.647 | 0.786 |
| Fluid therapy | 1.000 | 0.864 | 0.927 | 1.000 | 0.636 | 0.778 |
| Antibiotic therapy | 0.967 | 0.951 | 0.959 | 1.000 | 0.721 | 0.838 |
| Shared decision | 0.947 | 0.900 | 0.923 | 1.000 | 0.700 | 0.825 |
| Average | 0.965 | 0.929 | 0.946 | 1.000 | 0.676 | 0.806 |

**Table 4.** Deduplication performance of EndNote normalized to availability in MAS. Highlighted in bold red are the best results. AH: Amoxicillin harm, FT: Fluid therapy, AT: Antibiotic therapy, SD: Shared decision.

|  |  | EN1a (Default) | EN1 b | EN2a | EN2 b | EN3a | EN3 b | EN4a | EN4 b | EN5a | EN5 b |
|---|---|---|---|---|---|---|---|---|---|---|---|
| AH | Precision | 1.000 | 1.000 | 1.000 | 1.000 | 0.917 | 0.917 | 0.919 | 0.919 | 0.733 | 0.733 |
|  | Recall | 0.647 | 0.647 | 0.235 | 0.235 | 0.647 | 0.647 | 1.000 | 1.000 | 0.647 | 0.647 |
|  | $F_1$-score | 0.786 | 0.786 | 0.381 | 0.381 | 0.759 | 0.759 | 0.958 | 0.958 | 0.688 | 0.688 |
| FT | Precision | 1.00 | 1.000 | 1.000 | 1.000 | 0.933 | 0.929 | 0.944 | 0.941 | 0.947 | 0.944 |
|  | Recall | 0.636 | 0.591 | 0.409 | 0.318 | 0.636 | 0.591 | 0.773 | 0.727 | 0.818 | 0.773 |
|  | $F_1$-score | 0.778 | 0.743 | 0.581 | 0.483 | 0.757 | 0.722 | 0.850 | 0.821 | 0.878 | 0.850 |
| AT | Precision | 1.000 | 1.000 | 1.000 | 1.000 | 0.937 | 0.935 | 0.968 | 0.967 | 0.748 | 0.748 |
|  | Recall | 0.721 | 0.689 | 0.459 | 0.426 | 0.738 | 0.705 | 0.984 | 0.951 | 0.754 | 0.754 |
|  | $F_1$-score | 0.838 | 0.816 | 0.629 | 0.598 | 0.826 | 0.804 | 0.976 | 0.959 | 0.751 | 0.751 |
| SD | Precision | 1.000 | 1.000 | 1.000 | 1.000 | 0.811 | 0.800 | 1.000 | 1.000 | 0.560 | 0.560 |
|  | Recall | 0.700 | 0.700 | 0.450 | 0.400 | 0.750 | 0.700 | 1.000 | 0.950 | 0.700 | 0.700 |
|  | $F_1$-score | 0.824 | 0.824 | 0.621 | 0.571 | 0.779 | 0.747 | 1.000 | 0.974 | 0.622 | 0.622 |

database. Of the 4 false positives, the most common error (n = 3; 75 %) was in retrieving the wrong citation from MAS. In these cases, both documents had the same authors and titles, or the authors and titles of one citation are substrings of the other citation. In another case (n = 1, 25 %), a systematic review and its update, which have the same DOI, were erroneously detected as duplicates.

By comparison with other EndNote settings (Table 4), EndNote setting 4 (using "Title" and "Year" with "ignore spacing and punctuation") provides the best results by $F_1$-score in three systematic reviews. EndNote deduplication setting 5 using "Author" and "Year" produced the most FP (lowest in precision).

## 4  Discussion

Our citation enrichment algorithm automatically identified duplicate citations in real-world search results from systematic reviews. Enriching citations with DOI or MAS ID, allowed more duplicates to be identified compared with traditional algorithms.

A limitation of this study is that it only used MAS for citation enrichment. Other databases such as Google Scholar and Scopus can also be used but effectiveness still needs to be tested. Another limitation is that we used citation enrichment on its own. Further analysis of the results found that 5 of the 6 missed duplicates (83.3 %) in the best Endnote setting (Endnote4a) can be found in MAS which implicates that combining citation enrichment with approximate comparison may result in improved deduplication. A separate study is needed to test this hypothesis.

## 5  Conclusions

Our approach of first enriching citations with unique identifiers before detecting duplicate citations enhances automatic deduplication with good recall. Citation enrichment has the potential to substantially reduce resource requirements of evidence synthesis.

## References

1. Lefebvre, C., Manheimer, E., Glanville, J.: Chapter 6: searching for studies, in Cochrane handbook for systematic reviews of interventions. In: Higgins, J., Green, S. (eds.) The Cochrane Collaboration (2011). www.cochrane-handbook.org
2. Qi, X., et al.: Find duplicates among the PubMed, EMBASE, and Cochrane library databases in systematic review. PLoS ONE 8(8), e71838 (2013)
3. Elmagarmid, A.K., Ipeirotis, P.G., Verykios, V.S.: Duplicate record detection: a survey. IEEE Trans. Knowl. Data Eng. 19(1), 1–16 (2007)
4. Tsafnat, G., et al.: The automation of systematic reviews. BMJ Br. Med. J. 346, f139 (2013)
5. Carvalho, M.G., et al.: Replica identification using genetic programming. In: Proceedings of the 2008 ACM symposium on Applied computing. ACM (2008)

6.  Chaudhuri, S., Ganti, V., Motwani, R.: Robust identification of fuzzy duplicates. In: 21st International Conference on Data Engineering, 2005, ICDE 2005, Proceedings. IEEE (2005)

7.  Borges, E.N., et al.: A classification-based approach for bibliographic metadata deduplication. In: Proceedings of the IADIS International Conference WWW/Internet 2011 (2011)

8.  Rathbone, J., et al.: Better duplicate detection for systematic reviewers: evaluation of systematic review assistant-deduplication module. Syst. Rev. 4(1), 6 (2015)

9.  Jiang, Y., et al.: Rule-based deduplication of article records from bibliographic databases. Database 2014, bat086 (2014)

10. Gillies, M., et al.: Harms from amoxicillin: a systematic review and meta-analysis of randomised controlled trials for any indication. Unpublished raw data (2014)

11. Maconochie, I.K., Bhaumik, S.: Fluid therapy for acute bacterial meningitis. Cochrane Database Syst. Rev. 5 (2014). doi: 10.1002/14651858.CD004786.pub4

12. Pugh, R., et al.: Short-course versus prolonged-course antibiotic therapy for hospital-acquired pneumonia in critically ill adults. Cochrane Database Syst Rev 10 (2011). doi: 10.1002/14651858.CD007577.pub2

13. Coxeter, P., Hoffmann, T., Del Mar, C.B.: Shared decision making for acute respiratory infections in primary care. Cochrane Database Syst. Rev. 1, 1–11 (2014)

14. Choong, M.K., et al.: Automatic evidence retrieval for systematic reviews. J. Med. Internet Res. 16(10), e223 (2014)

15. Choong, M.K., et al.: Automatic evidence discovery for systematic reviews. J. Med. Internet Res. 16(10) (2014)

16. EndNote. http://endnote.com/. Available from: http://endnote.com/

# Learning Entry Profiles of Children with Autism from Multivariate Treatment Information Using Restricted Boltzmann Machines

Pratibha Vellanki[(✉)], Dinh Phung, Thi Duong, and Svetha Venkatesh

Pattern Recognition and Data Analytics, Deakin University, Geelong, Australia
{pvellank,dinh.phung,thi.duong,svetha.venkatesh}@deakin.edu.au

**Abstract.** Entry profiles can be generated before children with Autism Spectrum Disorders (ASD) begin to traverse an intervention program. They can help evaluate the progress of each child on the dedicated syllabus in addition to enabling narrowing down the best intervention course over time. However, the traits of ASD are expressed in different ways in every individual affected. The resulting spectrum nature of the disorder makes it challenging to discover profiles of children with ASD. Using data from 491 children, traversing the syllabus of a comprehensive intervention program on iPad called TOBY Playpad, we learn the entry profiles of the children based on their age, sex and performance on their first skills of the syllabus. Mixed-variate restricted Boltzmann machines allow us to integrate the heterogeneous data into one model making it a suitable technique. The data based discovery of entry profiles may assist in developing systems that can automatically suggest best suitable paths through the syllabus by clustering the children based on the characteristics they present at the beginning of the program. This may open the pathway for personalised intervention.

## 1 Introduction

Autism Spectrum Disorders (ASD) are pervasive neurodevelopmental disorders which result in impaired social interaction, communication and cognitive skills [1]. The disorders begin to disrupt learning at an early age and make everyday life activities arduous, increasing the dependence of individuals with ASD on others.

Children with ASD exhibit individual learning patterns. The natural way to go through this problem would be to find subgroups among the children affected by ASD in order to decide a future course of action for therapy. However, research in this direction has suggested that the disorders occur in comorbidity. Additionally, the difference between the subgroups: Asperger's, pervasive developmental disorder, and autism are not significant, suggesting a spectrum nature [2]. Based on the degree of impairment in suggested areas, the affected individuals can be described as ranging from high to low functioning on the spectrum. This poses as a significant barrier on the path to personalised administration of interventions. Research findings propose the need for profiling systems that might open the avenue for personalised interventions [3,4].

© Springer International Publishing Switzerland 2015
X.-L. Li et al. (Eds.): PAKDD 2015, LNCS 9441, pp. 245–257, 2015.
DOI: 10.1007/978-3-319-25660-3_21

In the current study, we aim to cluster the individuals with ASD based on their characteristics as a means of screening their condition before intervention is administered. Entry profiles as we define, are a set of characteristics individuals posses at the onset of intervention. For example, children within a certain age range, belonging to certain sex and expressing difficulty in similar skills. Our interest lies in technology assisted comprehensive intervention programs. Technology can be a breakthrough for collecting and analysing clusters of children with ASD. However, an initial discovery of profiles that we label as entry profiles is essential to evaluate the progress as the child traverses through the syllabus of the program. Entry profiles can be used as ground truth for any further analysis into the performance of individuals. Additionally, our future interest lies in automatic discovery of personalised intervention based on performance of the child on the syllabus of the program. Discovery of entry profiles are fundamental for the pursuit of progress evaluation and personalised intervention.

The expression of ASD in individuals has been observed to have variations based on the sex of the individual [5]. It is found that the prevalence of ASD in the male population is higher than that of female population [6]. Nevertheless, the expression of ASD in female population is found to be more severe as compared to the male [7]. Research has also shown that intensive therapy administered at an early age, as young as 2–3 years can improve the chances of faster learning [8]. On the contrary, at a later age, therapy has been observed to have fewer positive results [9]. We try to integrate these findings in order to determine if individuals with ASD can be clustered to broader entry profiles.

We use the data from TOBY Playpad, a comprehensive intervention program with structured syllabus [10]. The syllabus in TOBY covers broad areas providing over 34 skills that can be categorised to imitation, sensory, expressive language and receptive language. The skills are arranged in a tree structure with fundamental skills at the top and the complexity increases as the child progresses through the syllabus. Initially, TOBY opens up only a limited fundamental skills in each category for the children. As the children master a skill, more complex skills are opened up one after the other. This allows each child a fixed path in the syllabus to navigate with limited choice at each stage. This makes TOBY a suitable choice for our study. Additionally, the previous studies on TOBY have reported elaborate details regarding its nature that makes it useful for further analysis [11–13].

The data obtained from TOBY is mixed-variate (age, sex and performance of entry syllabus skills ) and highly correlated in nature, which makes it challenging to deal with. This creates the need for complex techniques that can integrate the data. The data consists missing elements as well. As the individuals progress through the syllabus, the data grows. If the individual chooses to continue, for example with one skill category and master the skills within the category before progressing to another one, the performance data on certain skills maybe unavailable for the time. The framework must hence address the issue of missing data.

In summary, our aims in this study are:

1. To discover entry profiles of children based on their age, sex and performance on each of the four entry skills of a technology assisted intervention program, TOBY Playpad. We use the data collected from 491 children for this purpose.
2. To apply mixed-variate restricted Boltzmann machine (MV.RBM) for modelling the heterogeneous data and clustering the children into entry profiles.
3. Qualitative analysis of the discovered entry profiles.

In the further sections, we discuss the challenges involved and literature that guided us toward the choice of modeling technique. Additionally, we describe our dataset, framework and results. We conclude by discussing the future amendments that can be made to the model in order to tune it better to the requirements of the dataset[1].

## 2  Related Background

Every patient is capable of showing a different response to standard treatment procedures even for a well defined clinical condition. Identifying patient profiles can provide a basis for comparison to monitor the progress of the patient based on their characteristics. Howard et al. discus the benefits of a patient profiling system for psychotherapy [14]. In doing so, they propose a system of profiling that accommodates individuality of the patient by including an estimate of the expected course of treatment based on their initial characteristics. Mazlan et al. develop a profiling system for depressive disorders by using their initial screening information and the dosage of medication that was suggested as treatment [15]. They aimed at replacing the manual maintenance of profiles by an automated approach that could be used to dynamically update and selectively change the course of treatment. A similar method has been approached by Payne-Murphy and Beacham [16] for profiling chronic pain patients. They identify clusters with significant differences among them and suggest the research pathway of tailoring personalised interventions based on the cluster profiles. A recent study by Garnett et al. suggests discovery of profiles among children and adolescents with Autism Spectrum Conditions using an online questionnaire [3]. Garnett et al. mention the usefulness of such profiling in administration of personalised interventions catering to individual needs. Our research aims in a similar direction, to identify entry profiles for individuals with ASD with the data from TOBY Playpad, a comprehensive intervention program on iPad for children with ASD. We use the information about the program detailed by Venkatesh et al. [10] as prior knowledge in comprehending the profiles identified.

One of the challenges with data for profiling is that it is a combination of different types of variables. For example, we use age (continuous values), sex (Boolean values for male or female), and performance on skills that we measure in Learn Units (LU) [11]. Natural integration of these data is not common

---

[1] The work presented here is a part of an ongoing study at PRaDA.

among traditional clustering techniques. On a similar problem setting, Ngyuen *et al.* [17] use mixed-variate restricted Boltzmann machine (MV.RBM) that was proposed by Tran *et al.* [18] as an efficient approach. The mixed-variate RBM discovers the latent profiles that are further used for clustering by using t-SNE. t-SNE is a stochastic neighbour embedding based method of projecting a higher dimensional data onto a lower dimensional subspace, usually a two or three dimensional space [19].

The Learn Units can be viewed as word count data in a document. Hence, a topic modelling based approach can be applied to our data to discover the latent profiles. Replicated Softmax is a generative model of word counts that was developed by Salakhutdinov and Hinton that was modelled using RBM [20]. This model is an undirected two-layered model that can be trained using Contrastive Divergence [21]. Replicated Softmax smoothly integrates with the modelling of age and sex and can be modelled altogether using the mixed-variate RBM model.

## 3   TOBY Playpad Data

TOBY Playpad is a comprehensive intervention program on iPad. It combines the fundamental teaching principles of Applied Behaviour Analysis (ABA) with a structured syllabus, allowing caretaker intervention in a regulated manner. The structure of the syllabus is constructed in a top-down tree form with the fundamental skills placed at the top and more complex skills at the bottom. The individual can attempt the complex skills only after the fundamental skills have been mastered. The criteria for mastering are predefined. Venkatesh *et al.* explain the nature and structure of the syllabus in depth [10]. This helps us in measuring the learning of the individuals whilst keeping certain variables, like the ways in which the syllabus can be navigated, fixed to a certain extent.

Within each skill, TOBY provides various stimuli and records the individual's response. If the response of the individual is incorrect, TOBY repeats the stimulus with a prompt till the correct response is learned. If the individual obtains 8 corrects out of 10 responses without any prompting then TOBY considers the skill as mastered.

The data from TOBY is uploaded to the server with the permission of the caretaker. This data is then accessed from the server and de-identified before processing it for the experiment. Data consists of 491 children in this study. Our dataset captures information about the individuals with ASD, including their age, sex and their performance on the entry skills of the syllabus of TOBY Playpad. The inter-quartile range of the children is 3.5 years to 6.7 years. There are 264 boys and 84 girls; the sex of 143 children is unknown.

The four main skill categories in the syllabus of TOBY Playpad are: imitation, sensory, expressive language and receptive language. When an individual begins the syllabus, they are presented with opening tasks in each of the four categories that we call entry skills. The number of Learn Units (LUs) required to master each of the four entry skills are determined and used along with the age and sex as features in our framework. In the next section, we will describe the data types we use for each of the features in this mixed-variate dataset and the framework of MV.RBM.

## 4   Framework

In this section start with explaining the structure of RBMs. We then expand on this foundation to explain MV.RBM as proposed by Tran *et al.* [18].

### 4.1   Restricted Boltzmann Machine

Restricted Boltzmann machines (RBM) are building blocks for generative deep learning architectures such as the deep belief network (DBN) [22], the deep RBM [23] and the deep sigmoid belief networks (DSB) [24]. In its original form, an RBM is a generative Markov random field with two binary layers [21]. Hence it induces a bipartite structure involving a visible input layer $v = [v_1, \ldots, v_N]^\mathsf{T} \in \{0,1\}^N$ and a binary hidden layer $h = [h_1, \ldots, h_K]^\mathsf{T} \in \{0,1\}^K$. The input layer is connected to binary representation layer using weighted connections, but there is no connection within each layer. Specifically, the RBM defines the following joint distribution:

$$p(v, h \mid \theta) = \frac{1}{Z(\theta)} \exp\{-E(v, h; \theta)\} \tag{1}$$

$$E(v, h; \theta) = -\left\{a^\mathsf{T} v + b^\mathsf{T} h + v^\mathsf{T} W h\right\} \tag{2}$$

$$Z(\theta) = \sum_{v,h} \exp\{-E(v, h; \theta)\} \tag{3}$$

where $E(\cdot)$ and $Z(\cdot)$ are respectively the energy and normalization functions; $a = [a_1, \ldots, a_N]^\mathsf{T}, b = [b_1, \ldots, b_K]^\mathsf{T}$ and $W = [W_{nk}]$ are the parameters. The parameter $a$ is attached to only the visible layer and hence also known as visible bias parameter. Likewise, $b$ is the hidden bias parameter and $W$ is the matrix weights that connects the two layers.

Due to its special bipartite structure, evaluating conditional distribution in an RBM is efficient:

$$p(v \mid h, \theta) = \prod_{n=1}^{N} p(v_n \mid h), \qquad p(h \mid v, \theta) = \prod_{k=1}^{K} p(h_k \mid v) \tag{4}$$

In particular, computing the posterior $p(h_k \mid v)$ involves only $N$ links from hidden unit $h_k$ to $v$, hence using Eqs. (1) and (2):

$$p(h_k \mid v) \propto \exp\left(b_k h_k + \sum_{n=1}^{N} v_n W_{nk} h_k\right)$$

Since $h_k$ is a binary variable, it is easy to derive:

$$p(h_k = 1 \mid \boldsymbol{v}) = \frac{1}{1 + \exp\left(-b_k - \sum_{n=1}^{N} v_n W_{nk}\right)} \tag{5}$$

$$= \tau\left(b_k + \sum_{n=1}^{N} v_n W_{nk}\right) \tag{6}$$

where $\tau(x) = [1 + e^{-x}]^{-1}$ is the logistic function. Hence, if the model parameter $\theta = \{\boldsymbol{a}, \boldsymbol{b}, \boldsymbol{W}\}$ is known, then the **posterior representation** for data $\boldsymbol{v}$ using the latent posterior vector $[p(h_1 = 1 \mid \boldsymbol{v}), \ldots, p(h_K = 1 \mid \boldsymbol{v})]$ is extremely efficient to compute with the help of the equation above. For binary $v_k$ the data generative probability $p(v_k \mid \boldsymbol{h})$ is computed in a similar way.

A key task with RBM is to estimate the parameter $\theta$ from the $D$ observed data $\{\boldsymbol{v}_1, \ldots, \boldsymbol{v}_D\}$. To do so, the optimization goal is to maximize the log-likelihood:

$$l(\boldsymbol{v}_{1:D}; \theta) = \frac{1}{D} \sum_{d=1}^{D} \log p(\boldsymbol{v}_d \mid \theta) = \frac{1}{D} \sum_{d=1}^{D} \log \sum_{\boldsymbol{h}} \frac{1}{Z(\theta)} \exp\{-E(\boldsymbol{v}_d, \boldsymbol{h}; \theta)\}$$

Since the RBM belongs to the general class of exponential family, the gradient of this objective function can be computed to be dependent on the expectations of the models [22,25] and can be estimated using a special form of Monte Carlo integration known as Contrastive Divergence (CD) sampling scheme [21].

When dealing with data, as mentioned, the key advantage of an RBM lies in its representation power at the latent layer $\boldsymbol{h}$ to represent data, which can also be repeatedly constructed to build deep features. It is this versatile representation of the RBM that we leverage to model the entry profiles since the hidden layer, $p(\boldsymbol{h} \mid \boldsymbol{v}, \theta)$, is now a continuous-valued probability vector which uniformly transforms data into a consistent mathematical object to deal with, such as to perform projection, computing similarity, conducting retrieval and so on. However, our data is not simply in the form of binary, it is mixed and heterogeneous with binary, Gaussian and count components.

### 4.2    Mixed-Variate Restricted Boltzmann Machine

To address these issues, we leverage on the Mixed-Variate Restricted Boltzmann machine (MV.RBM) recently proposed in [18] in this paper. An MV.RBM is technically an RBM, but with heterogeneous visible vector $\boldsymbol{v}$, each element $v_n$ has its own type. The energy function from Eq. (2) is now redefined to be:

$$E(\boldsymbol{v}, \boldsymbol{h}; \theta) = -\left\{\sum_{n=1}^{N} \beta(v_n) + \boldsymbol{a}^{\mathsf{T}}\boldsymbol{v} + \boldsymbol{b}^{\mathsf{T}}\boldsymbol{h} + \boldsymbol{v}^{\mathsf{T}}\boldsymbol{W}\boldsymbol{h}\right\}$$

where $\beta(v_n)$ is the type-specific function; $\boldsymbol{a}$ and $\boldsymbol{b}$ retain the same functionality as the biases of the visible and hidden layers and $\boldsymbol{W} = [W_{ij}]$ are the weights specified for connections between hidden and visible layers. We note that due to the heterogeneity of the visible unit $v$, the normalization function $Z(\theta)$ in Eq. (3) is now more complicated to compute due to the sum over the $v$. A general strategy is to group the visible vector into $v = (z, x)$ where $z$ is the discrete component and $x$ is a continuous component. $Z(\theta)$ can now be computed as:

$$Z(\theta) = \int_x \sum_z \exp\left\{\sum_{n=1}^{N} \beta_n(v_n) + a^\top[x, z] + b^\top h + [x, z]^\top W h\right\} dx$$

We note that this integration must be finite for the probability model of interest to be well-defined. Lastly the type-specific function $\beta(v_n)$ can tailored for different types of data as specified in [18]. While the posterior for the latent variable $h_k$ in Eq. 5 remains easy to compute regardless the type of $v_k$, the data likelihood $p(v_k \mid h)$ becomes complicated when $v_k$ is no longer a binary variable. Again using Eqs. (1) and (2) we have:

$$p(v_n \mid h) \propto \exp\left\{\beta_n(v_n) + a_n v_n + \sum_{k=1}^{K} v_n W_{nk} h_k\right\}$$

Again the MV.RBM belongs to the standard exponential family as a result of which its gradients can be computed as the expectations of the models and CD can be used to estimate the parameters from the data. In this paper, we employ the solution proposed in [18].

## 4.3   MV.RBM for Entry Profiles

The visible parameters are multivariate in our experiment. Hence we consider three types of data in this paper as specified in [18]:

- *Binary* observation $v_n$ for sex. In this case we simply set $\beta_n(v_n) = 0$, hence $p(v_n \mid h) = \tau\left(a_n + \sum_{k=1}^{K} W_{nk} h_k\right)$.
- *Continuous* observation $v_n$ for age. We use the Gaussian variable, setting $\beta_n(v_n) = -\frac{v_n^2}{2\sigma^2}$ where $\sigma^2$ is a fixed variance specified in advance. In this case, $p(v_n \mid h)$ can be shown to be a univariate Gaussian with mean $\sigma^2\left(a_n + \sum_{k=1}^{K} W_{nk} h_k\right)$ and variance $\sigma^2$.
- *Count* observation $v_n$ for LUs required to master each entry skill. We employ the replicated softmax representation [20] which allows us to represent repeated counts in an observation such as words in a documents or tasks performed repeatedly within a section. In this case $v_n$ can move beyond from scalars to count vector $v_n \in \{1, \ldots, M\}^{L_n}$ where $M$ is the dictionary size and $L_n = |v_n|$ is the size of $v_n$. Hinton and Salakhutdinov [20] employs a simple method to represent $v_n$ by 'replicating' the $v_n$ onto a vector of $L_n$-dim vector $v'_n = (v'_{n1}, \ldots, v'_{nL_n})$ in the visible layer where $v'_{nj} \in \{1, \ldots M\}$, each is specified by softmax unit and then 'ties' the parameter through them; in other words, $p(v'_{nj} = m \mid h) \propto \exp\left(a_n + \sum_{k=1}^{K} W_{nk} h_k\right)$. We note that due to this replication procedure and parameter typing, the posterior $p(h_k = 1 \mid v)$ will also be updated to account for the replicated visible units.

Our data presents itself with missing elements. This occurs when the child is yet unable to master the skill. While registering with TOBY a caretaker may render the child's information confidential and choose not to enter the age or sex of the child. This might generate instances of missing data as well. Our data is complete in age, but for the other visible variables we substitute zero where the data is missing for simplicity. The latent posterior equation of RBM consists of the product term involving $v_n$, which results in the model to account for no statistics from these missing elements.

We employ CD [21] for learning with learning rates varying based on the data type. The parameters are updated after every 100 children, which is the size of our mini-batch, and we terminate learning in 100 data sweeps. The number of hidden units (K) is determined to be 10. The reconstruction error is observed to gradually reduce.

K number of posteriors are computed for each child. Using t-SNE [19] we then project the posterior values of hidden parameters to a two dimensional space to observe the clusters of profiles. Kmeans is used on this projection to find clusters of children sharing similar entry profiles. We present the results in the next section.

## 5    Experimental Results

In this section, we observe the clusters and the entry profiles to explore their meaningfulness. The clusters obtained are shown in Fig. 1. In the projected space we use Kmeans to discover 5 clusters. The clusters represent individuals belonging to respective entry profiles. We then observe the individual properties of each cluster. We would like to note at this point that the LUs required to master each skill are proportional to the amount of difficulty the individual faced while

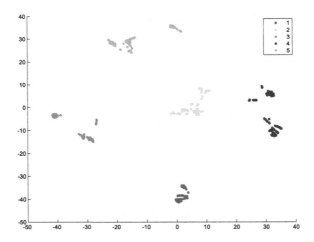

**Fig. 1.** t-SNE projection of the posterior hidden values. Clusters are obtained by Kmeans.

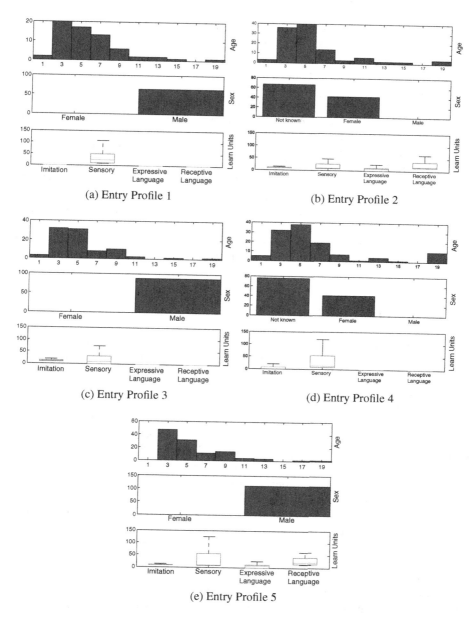

(a) Entry Profile 1

(b) Entry Profile 2

(c) Entry Profile 3

(d) Entry Profile 4

(e) Entry Profile 5

**Fig. 2.** Visualisation of clusters of individuals belonging to corresponding entry profiles. Collective properties of individuals in corresponding entry profile are shown (age, sex and learn units required to master each entry skill)

mastering it. Thus, when the LUs required to master, for example sensory, are more then those required to master imitation, we safely state that the individuals belonging to the corresponding entry profile found the sensory entry skill more difficult than imitation, and hence forth.

In the subsequent Fig. 2a to e the properties of the individuals belonging to the entry profiles 1 to 5 are collectively shown. The number of LUs required to master each entry skill are shown as a box plot.

We observe that entry profile 1 (Fig. 2a) represents male individuals who found the entry skill of sensory skill category most difficult. The entry profile 2 (Fig. 2b) includes females and the individuals whose sex is missing in the data who struggled most with the receptive language entry skill. The entry profile 3 (Fig. 2c) constitutes of male individuals who struggled with sensory more than imitation. The entry profile 4 (Fig. 2d) constitutes individuals who found sensory more difficult than imitation similar to entry profile 3. It can also be seen that these individuals collectively struggled with sensory entry skill more than their male counterparts in entry profile 3. Entry profile 5 (Fig. 2e) includes male individuals who found sensory and receptive language entry skills most difficult to master. Additionally, the age histogram is also shown for each entry profile.

# 6    Discussion and Future Work

The advantage of using technology assisted therapeutic interventions is rigorous and effortless recording of data, which allows more freedom of analysis. Nevertheless, we are often faced with challenges. Each child entering the intervention begins at a different age and a different set of abilities in terms of skills learnt, as compared with one another. It is crucial to map each child onto an entry profile at the beginning if the aim is to dynamically adapt the syllabus changing the course of intervention according to the performance and capabilities of the child. Determining the entry profile of a child can enable us to allow changes in the intervention to be made by giving the child more opportunities in areas where they are struggling. An entry profile can also be used as a ground truth for monitoring the progress of the child. The work presented in this paper is an ongoing work of exploratory analysis in an attempt to discover entry profiles that will enable comparative study of progress.

One of the main challenges that we continually face with the data is the incomplete nature of it. Missing elements in the current study were replaced with zero values for simplicity. A more accurate approach we are headed toward is to model each child as a separate MV.RBM. The model will then be a family of MV.RBMs of different sizes. This approach has also been suggested by Hinton and Salakhutdinov [26,27] as a more accurate alternative for applications where imputation of missing data is not an option. Due to the extremely random nature of skill abilities in children with ASD, imputation of the number Learn Units required to master a skill which is not yet attempted would be unjust. Additionally, due to binary assignment for sex, the individuals whose sex in currently unknown are clustered together as either male or female (in this study female). The modelling of entry profiles as a family of MV.RBMs would thus be a more accurate way of dealing with the missing data.

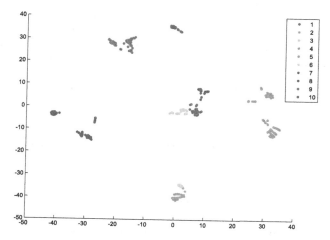

**Fig. 3.** Visualisation of the same individuals shown as 10 clusters corresponding to entry profiles.

Deciding the number of entry profiles is also an open question which ought to be explored in more depth. We present 5 broader entry profiles in this study. However, it is possible to define more number of entry profiles with finer differences between them. This is seen in Fig. 3. The same children have been clustered into 10 entry profiles in this figure. We further observed finer variations in the children's struggles with different entry skills in this clustering. This calls for further analysis.

## 7    Conclusion

The profiling of individuals with ASD is a challenging and ongoing research question. Profiling is a foundational step in determining dynamic personalisation of therapeutic interventions that can be administered based on the child's performance. Our discovery of meaningful broad entry profiles may suggest a novel approach to the problem of profiling children with ASD. We present a framework for discovery of entry profiles for children with Autism Spectrum Disorders (ASD) using mixed-variate Boltzmann machine (MV.RBM). The complexities involved with non-homogeneous data could be incorporated by using this framework. MV.RBM has the capacity of modelling data that is incomplete when it is designed as a family MV.RBMs, hence making it one of the best choices for the data at hand.

# References

1. Diagnostic and statistical manual of mental disorders, fifth edn. American Psychiatric Association, May 2013
2. Verte, S., Geurts, H.M., Roeyers, H., Oosterlaan, J., Sergeant, J.A.: Executive functioning in children with an autism spectrum disorder: can we differentiate within the spectrum? J. Autism Dev. Disord. **36**, 351–372 (2006)
3. Garnett, M.S., Attwood, T., Peterson, C., Kelly, A.B.: Autism spectrum conditions among children and adolescents: a new profiling tool. Aust. J. Psychol. **65**, 206–213 (2013)
4. Munson, J., Dawson, G., Sterling, L., Beauchaine, T., Zhou, A., Koehler, E., Lord, C., Rogers, S., Sigman, M., Estes, A., et al.: Evidence for latent classes of iq in young children with autism spectrum disorder. J. Inf. **113**, 439–452 (2008)
5. Williams, J.G., Allison, C., Scott, F.J., Bolton, P.F., Baron-Cohen, S., Matthews, F.E., Brayne, C.: The childhood autism spectrum test (cast): sex differences. J. Autism Dev. Disord. **38**, 1731–1739 (2008)
6. Bartley, J.J.: An update on autism: science, gender, and the law. Gend. Med. **3**, 73–78 (2006)
7. Dworzynski, K., Ronald, A., Bolton, P., Happé, F.: How different are girls and boys above and below the diagnostic threshold for autism spectrum disorders? J. Am. Acad. Child Adolesc. Psychiatry **51**, 788–797 (2012)
8. Dawson, G., et al.: Early behavioral intervention, brain plasticity, and the prevention of autism spectrum disorder. Dev. Psychopathol. **20**, 775 (2008)
9. Fenske, E.C., Zalenski, S., Krantz, P.J., McClannahan, L.E.: Age at intervention and treatment outcome for autistic children in a comprehensive intervention program. Anal. Interv. Dev. Disabil. **5**, 49–58 (1985)
10. Venkatesh, S., Phung, D., Duong, T., Greenhill, S., Adams, B.: Toby: early intervention in autism through technology. In: Proceedings of the SIGCHI Conference on Human Factors in Computing Systems, pp. 3187–3196. ACM (2013)
11. Vellanki, P., Duong, T., Venkatesh, S., Phung, D.: Nonparametric discovery of learning patterns and autism subgroups from therapeutic data. In: Proceedings of 22nd International Conference on Pattern Recognition (ICPR), pp. 1829–1833 (2014)
12. Venkatesh, S., Greenhill, S., Phung, D., Adams, B., Duong, T.: Pervasive multimedia for autism intervention. Pervasive Mob. Comput. **8**, 863–882 (2012)
13. Moore, D., Venkatesh, S., Anderson, A., Greenhill, S., Phung, D., Duong, T., Cairns, D., Marshall, W., Whitehouse, A.: Toby play-pad application to teach children with asd: a pilot trial. Dev. Neurorehabil. **18**, 213–217 (2013)
14. Howard, K.I., Moras, K., Brill, P.L., Martinovich, Z., Lutz, W.: Evaluation of psychotherapy: efficacy, effectiveness, and patient progress. Am. Psychol. **51**, 1059 (1996)
15. Mazalan, L., Halim, N.M., Omar, H.A., Zaini, N.M.: Profiling system for depressive disorder patient using web based approaches, pp. 207–212 (2012)
16. Payne-Murphy, J.C., Beacham, A.O.: Revisiting chronic pain patient profiling: an acceptance-based approach in an online sample. Clin. Psychol. Psychother **22**, 240–248 (2014)
17. Nguyen, T.D., Tran, T., Phung, D., Venkatesh, S.: Latent patient profile modelling and applications with mixed-variate restricted Boltzmann machine. In: Pei, J., Tseng, V.S., Cao, L., Motoda, H., Xu, G. (eds.) PAKDD 2013, Part I. LNCS, vol. 7818, pp. 123–135. Springer, Heidelberg (2013)

18. Tran, T., Phung, D., Venkatesh, S.: Mixed-variate restricted Boltzmann machines. In: ACML 2011 Proceedings of the 3rd Asian Conference on Machine Learning, [JMLR], pp. 213–229 (2011)
19. Van der Maaten, L., Hinton, G.: Visualizing data using t-sne. J. Mach. Learn. Res. **9**, 85 (2008)
20. Hinton, G.E., Salakhutdinov, R.: Replicated softmax: an undirected topic model. In: Advances in Neural Information Processing Systems, pp. 1607–1614 (2009)
21. Hinton, G.E.: Training products of experts by minimizing contrastive divergence. Neural Comput. **14**, 1771–1800 (2002)
22. Hinton, G., Osindero, S., Teh, Y.W.: A fast learning algorithm for deep belief nets. Neural Comput. **18**, 1527–1554 (2006)
23. Salakhutdinov, R., Hinton, G.E.: Deep Boltzmann machines. In: International Conference on Artificial Intelligence and Statistics, pp. 448–455 (2009)
24. Gregor, K., Danihelka, I., Mnih, A., Blundell, C., Wierstra, D.: Deep autoregressive networks (2013). arXiv preprint arXiv:1310.8499
25. Wainwright, M.J., Jordan, M.I.: Graphical models, exponential families, and variational inference. Found. Trends Mach. Learn. **1**, 1–305 (2008)
26. Hinton, G.: A practical guide to training restricted Boltzmann machines. Momentum **9**, 926 (2010)
27. Salakhutdinov, R., Mnih, A., Hinton, G.: Restricted Boltzmann machines for collaborative filtering. In: Proceedings of the 24th International Conference on Machine Learning, pp. 791–798. ACM (2007)

# Vietnamese Language
# and Speech Processing

# Fast Dependency Parsing Using Distributed Word Representations

Phuong Le-Hong[1,3]([⊠]), Thi-Minh-Huyen Nguyen[1], Thi-Luong Nguyen[2], and My-Linh Ha[1]

[1] VNU University of Science, Hanoi, Vietnam
{phuonglh,huyenntm}@vnu.edu.vn, halinh.hus@gmail.com
[2] Dalat University, Lamdong, Vietnam
luongnt@dlu.edu.vn
[3] FPT Research, Hanoi, Vietnam

**Abstract.** In this work, we propose to use distributed word representations in a greedy, transition-based dependency parsing framework. Instead of using a very large number of sparse indicator features, the multinomial logistic regression classifier employed by the parser learns and uses a small number of dense features, therefore it can work very fast. The distributed word representations are produced by a continuous skip-gram model using a neural network architecture. Experiments on a Vietnamese dependency treebank show that the parser not only works faster but also achieves better accuracy in comparison to a conventional transition-based dependency parser.

## 1 Introduction

Syntactic dependency theories use the notion of directed syntactic dependencies between the words of a natural language sentence. Figure 1 shows an example of a simple Vietnamese sentence, where each word of the sentence is labeled with its part-of-speech and each arc is labeled with a grammatical function.

In this representation, the syntactic structure of a sentence is modeled by a dependency graph, which represents each word and its syntactic modifiers through labeled directed arcs, where each arc label comes from a finite set representing possible syntactic roles. In the example above, the dependency relation from the finite verb còn (exist) to Xã (village) labeled nsubj indicates that Xã is the syntactic subject of the finite verb. An artificial word ROOT has been inserted (not shown in the figure), serving as the unique root of the graph. This is a standard device that simplifies both theoretical definitions and computational implementations.

The availability of dependency annotated corpora for multiple languages and the rise of statistical methods has led to a boom of research on data-driven dependency parsing. The use of feature-based discriminative dependency parsers has achieved much success in recent years. However, the parsers suffer from the use of a very large number of poorly estimated feature weights corresponding to sparse indicator features. In this work, we overcome this drawback by using

© Springer International Publishing Switzerland 2015
X.-L. Li et al. (Eds.): PAKDD 2015, LNCS 9441, pp. 261–272, 2015.
DOI: 10.1007/978-3-319-25660-3_22

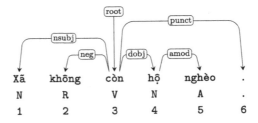

**Fig. 1.** An example of dependency tree.

dense features of distributed word representations, also called word embeddings. Low-dimensional and dense word embeddings, being produced by a continuous skip-gram model under a neural network architecture, are integrated in a greedy, transition-based dependency parsing framework to create a good dependency parser. Experiments on a Vietnamese dependency treebank show that the parser not only works faster but also achieves better accuracy in comparison to a conventional transition-based dependency parser.

The remainder of this paper is structured as follows. Section 2 describes a background on transition-based dependency parsing and distributed word representation. Section 3 gives our approach, including details of the greedy dependency parsing algorithm which is used in our framework, how the distributed word representations are produced, and the statistical classifier in use. Section 4 presents the experimental setups and results. Section 5 discusses related work and Sect. 6 concludes the paper.

## 2 Background

### 2.1 Transition-Based Dependency Parsing

There are two dominant approaches for data-driven dependency parsing. The first approach parameterizes models over dependency graphs and learns these parameters to globally score correct graphs above incorrect ones. Inference is also global in that systems attempt to find the highest scoring graph among the set of all graphs. Such systems are called graph-based parsing models. The second approach parameterizes models over transitions from one state to another in an abstract state-machine. Parameters in these models are typically learned using standard classification techniques that learn to predict one transition from a set of permissible transitions given a state history. Inference is local in that systems start in a fixed initial state and greedily constructing the graph by taking the highest scoring transitions at each state entered until a termination condition is met. Such systems are called transition-based parsing models [1].

In practical applications, the speed of a class of transition-based dependency parsers which employs a greedy inference algorithm has been very appealing. In greedy parsing, we use a classifier to predict the most probable transition based on features extracted from the configuration. This class of parsers is of great interest because of their efficiency, although they tend to perform slightly worse than the search-based parsers because of subsequent error propagation. However, some greedy parser can achieve comparable accuracy with a very good speed [2]. We give details of our transition-based parsing system in subsect. 3.1.

## 2.2 Distributed Representations

Supervised lexicalized natural language processing approaches usually use the one-hot representation of words, in that each word is converted into a symbolic identifier, which is then transformed into a feature vector of the same length of the vocabulary. In this representation, only one dimension of each feature vector is on. However, the one-hot representation of a word suffers from data sparsity. That is, the parameters corresponding to rare or unknown words are poorly estimated. This limitation of the one-hot word representation has motivated unsupervised methods for inducing word representations over large, unlabeled corpora.

Recently, distributed representations of words have been shown to be advantageous in many natural language processing tasks. A distributed representation is dense, low dimensional and real-valued. Distributed word representations are called word embeddings. Each dimension of the embedding represents a latent feature of the word which hopefully captures useful syntactic and semantic similarities [3].

Word embeddings are typically induced using neural language models, which use neural networks as the underlying predictive model. Historically, training and testing of neural language models has been slow, scaling as the size of the vocabulary for each model computation [4]. However, many approaches have been recently proposed to speed up the training process, allowing scaling to very large corpora [5–8].

# 3 Approach

## 3.1 Transition-Based Dependency Parsing

In this work, we employ the arc-eager algorithm, which is a transition-based dependency parsing algorithm introduced by [9,10]. In an arc-eager system, a *configuration* $c = (\sigma, \beta, A)$ consists of *a stack $\sigma$, a buffer $\beta$ and a set of dependency arcs $A$.* The initial configuration for a sentence $s = w_1, w_2, \ldots, w_n$ is $\sigma = [\text{ROOT}], \beta = [w_1, \ldots, w_n]$ and $A = \emptyset$. A configuration $c$ is terminal if the buffer is empty and the stack contains a single element ROOT. We use the notation $v|\beta$ to indicate that the first element of the buffer is the word $v$; the notation $\sigma|u$ to indicate that the top element of the stack is the word $u$; and $A_c = \{(x, y)\}$ where $x, y$ are words of a sentence being parsed to indicate the set of dependency arcs of a configuration $c$.

The arc-eager parsing algorithm defines four types of transitions as shown in Table 1. In the labeled version of parsing, there are in total $|\mathcal{T}| = 2N_l + 2$ transitions where $N_l$ is the number of different arc labels. The preconditions of the four transition types are explained as follows:

**Table 1.** Four transition types of the arc-eager parsing algorithm.

| Name | Operation | Precondition |
|------|-----------|--------------|
| LEFT-ARC | $(\sigma\|u, v\|\beta, A) \Rightarrow (\sigma, v\|\beta, A \cup \{(v, u)\})$ | $\nexists k : (k, u) \in A$ |
| RIGHT-ARC | $(\sigma\|u, v\|\beta, A) \Rightarrow (\sigma\|u\|v, \beta, A \cup \{(u, v)\})$ | $\nexists k : (k, v) \in A$ |
| REDUCE | $(\sigma\|u, \beta, A) \Rightarrow (\sigma, \beta, A)$ | $\exists v : (v, u) \in A$ |
| SHIFT | $(\sigma, v\|\beta, A) \Rightarrow (\sigma\|v, \beta, A)$ | |

- The precondition of LEFT-ARC $u \leftarrow v$ is that there does not exist any arc coming to $u$; in other words, $u$ has not been a dependent of another word. After this transition, the parsing of $u$ is done and popped from the stack.
- The precondition of RIGHT-ARC $u \rightarrow v$ is that there does not exist any arc coming to $v$. After this transition, the word $v$ is pushed onto the stack to consider next word. Note that there can be multiple arcs coming out of $u$.
- The REDUCE transition pops the stack and presupposes that the top element has already been attached to its head in a previous RIGHT-ARC transition.
- The SHIFT transition extracts the first element of the buffer and pushes it onto the stack. This transition does not require any precondition.

Figure 2 illustrates an example of one transition sequence from the initial configuration to a terminal one.

| Transition | Stack | Buffer | A |
|------------|-------|--------|---|
| | [ROOT] | [Xã không còn hộ nghèo .] | ∅ |
| SHIFT | [ROOT Xã] | [không còn hộ nghèo .] | |
| SHIFT | [ROOT Xã không] | [còn hộ nghèo .] | |
| LEFT-ARC (neg) | [ROOT Xã] | [còn hộ nghèo .] | +neg(còn,không) |
| LEFT-ARC (nsubj) | [ROOT] | [còn hộ nghèo .] | +nsubj(còn,Xã) |
| RIGHT-ARC (root) | [ROOT còn] | [hộ nghèo . ] | +root(ROOT,còn) |
| RIGHT-ARC (dobj) | [ROOT còn hộ] | [nghèo .] | +dobj(còn,hộ) |
| RIGHT-ARC (amod) | [ROOT còn hộ nghèo] | [.] | +amod(hộ,nghèo) |
| REDUCE | [ROOT còn hộ] | [.] | |
| REDUCE | [ROOT còn] | [.] | |
| RIGHT-ARC (punct) | [ROOT còn .] | [] | +punct(còn,.) |

**Fig. 2.** An example of arc-eager dependency parsing

It has been shown that the arc-eager parsing algorithm can derive any projective dependency tree $G$ for an input sentence $s$ and doing so always adds arc as early as possible. The essential step in the greedy parsing process is to predict a correct transition from $\mathcal{T}$. We can use a statistical classifier to predict the most probable transition with highest probability. In this setting, the prediction function is defined as $f : \mathcal{C} \rightarrow \mathcal{Y}$, where $\mathcal{C}$ is a set of all possible configurations and $\mathcal{Y}$ is the set of all possible transitions.

The algorithm guarantees termination after at most $2n$ transitions for a sentence of length $n$, which means the time complexity is $O(n)$ given that transitions can be performed in constant time. Furthermore, the dependency graph given at termination is guaranteed to be acyclic and projective [1].

## 3.2   Word Vector Representations

We use word embeddings produced by Mikolov's continuous skip-gram model using the neural network and source code introduced in [11]. The continuous skip-gram model itself is described in details in [8].

For our experiments we used a continuous skip-gram window of size 2, *i.e.* the actual context size for each training sample is a random number up to 2. The neural network uses the central word in the context to predict the other words, by maximizing the average conditional log probability

$$\frac{1}{T}\sum_{t=1}^{T}\sum_{j=-c}^{c}\log p(w_{t+j}|w_t),$$

where $\{w_i : i \in T\}$ is the whole training set, $w_t$ is the central word and the $w_{t+j}$ are on either side of the context. The conditional probabilities are defined by the softmax function

$$p(a|b) = \frac{\exp(o_a^\top i_b)}{\sum_{w \in \mathcal{V}} \exp(o_w^\top i_b)},$$

where $i_w$ and $o_w$ are the input and output vector of $w$ respectively, and $\mathcal{V}$ is the vocabulary. For computational efficiency, Mikolov's training code approximates the softmax function by the hierarchical softmax, as defined in [5]. Here the hierarchical softmax is built on a binary Huffman tree with one word at each leaf node. The conditional probabilities are calculated according to the decomposition:

$$p(a|b) = \prod_{i=1}^{l} p(d_i(a)|d_1(a)...d_{i-1}(a), b),$$

where $l$ is the path length from the root to the node $a$, and $d_i(a)$ is the decision at step $i$ on the path (for example 0 if the next node the left child of the current node, and 1 if it is the right child). If the tree is balanced, the hierarchical softmax only needs to compute around $\log_2 |\mathcal{V}|$ nodes in the tree, while the true softmax requires computing over all $|\mathcal{V}|$ words.

The training code was obtained from the tool word2vec[1] and we used frequent word subsampling as well as a word appearance threshold of 5. The output dimension is set to 50, *i.e.* each word is mapped to a unit vector in $\mathbb{R}^{50}$. This is deemed adequate for our purpose without overfitting the training data. Figure 3 shows the scatter plot of 100 Vietnamese words which are projected onto the first two principal components after performing the principal component analysis of all the word distributed representations. We can see that semantically related words are grouped closely togethser.

---

[1] http://code.google.com/p/word2vec/.

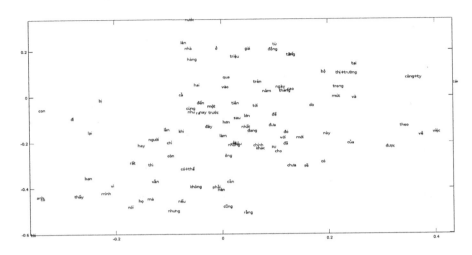

**Fig. 3.** One hundred Vietnamese words in two dimensions

## 3.3 Multinomial Logistic Classifier

Multinomial logistic regression (a.k.a maximum entropy model) is a general purpose discriminative learning method for classification and prediction which has been successfully applied to many problems of natural language processing. In contrast to generative classifiers, discriminative classifiers model the posterior $P(y|\mathbf{x})$ directly. One of the main advantages of discriminative models is that we can integrate many heterogeneous features for prediction, which are not necessarily independent. Each feature corresponds to a constraint on the model. In this model, the conditional probability of a label $y$ given an observation $\mathbf{x}$ is defined as

$$P(y|\mathbf{x}) = \frac{\exp(\theta \cdot \phi(\mathbf{x}, y))}{\sum_{y \in \mathcal{Y}} \exp(\theta \cdot \phi(\mathbf{x}, y))},$$

where $\phi(\mathbf{x}, y) \in \mathbb{R}^D$ is a real-valued feature vector, $\mathcal{Y}$ is the set of labels and $\theta \in \mathbb{R}^D$ is the parameter vector to be estimated from training data. This form of distribution corresponds to the maximum entropy probability distribution satisfying the constraint that the empirical expectation of each feature is equal to its true expectation in the model:

$$\widehat{\mathbb{E}}(\phi_j(h, t)) = \mathbb{E}(\phi_j(h, t)), \qquad \forall j = 1, 2, \ldots, D.$$

The parameter $\theta \in \mathbb{R}^D$ can be estimated using iterative scaling algorithms or some more efficient gradient-based optimization algorithms like conjugate gradient or quasi-Newton methods [12]. In this paper, we use the L-BFGS optimization algorithm [13] and $L_2$-regularization technique to estimate the parameters of the model, with smooth term is fixed at 1.0. This classification model is applied to build a classifier for the dependency parser where each observation $\mathbf{x}$ is a parsing configuration and each label $y$ is a transition type.

# 4  Experiments

## 4.1  Datasets

*Distributed Word Representations.* To create distributed word representations, we use a dataset consisting of 6.1GB of text from 1.8 million articles collected through the Vietnamese news portal at http://www.baomoi.com. The text is first normalized to lower case and all special characters are removed except these common symbols: the comma, the semicolon, the colon, the full stop and the percentage sign. All numeral sequences are replaced with the special token <number>, so that correlations between certain words and numbers are correctly recognized by the neural network.

Each word in the Vietnamese language may consist of more than one syllables with spaces in between, which could be regarded as multiple words by the neural network. Hence it is necessary to replace the spaces within each word with underscores to create full word tokens. The tokenization process follows the method described in [14].

After removal of special characters and tokenization, the articles add up to 920 million word tokens, spanning a vocabulary of $433,191$ unique tokens. We train the neural network with the full vocabulary to obtain the representation vectors, and then prune the collection of word vectors to the $5,000$ most frequent words, excluding special symbols and the token <number>, representing numeral sequences.

*Dependency Treebank.* We conduct our experiments on the Vietnamese dependency treebank dataset [15]. This treebank is derived automatically from the constituency-based annotation of the VTB treebank [16], containing $10,471$ sentences ($225,085$ tokens). We manually check the correctness of the conversion on a subset of the converted corpus to come up with a training set of $2,058$ sentences, and a test set of 685 sentences.

## 4.2  Feature Sets

Training data for the transition classifier were generated by parsing each sentence in the training set using the gold-standard dependency graph. For each parser configuration $c$ and transition $f(c)$ in the gold parse, a training instance $(\phi(c), f(c))$ was created, where $\phi(c)$ is the feature vector representation of the parser configuration $c$. Table 2 shows the feature templates used for the classifier. We use the notation $\ell_i$ to denote the $i$th element of the stack or buffer $\ell$, with $\ell_0$ for the first element (top element of the stack $\sigma$ or the first element the buffer $\beta$). The function $w(\cdot)$ and $d(\cdot)$ extract the word or the distributed representation of the word of a token, respectively. The base feature set $\Phi_0$ consists of the following feature templates:

- Part-of-speech tags of tokens on the buffer: $t(\beta_0), t(\beta_1), t(\beta_2), t(\beta_3)$
- Part-of-speech tags of tokens on the stack: $t(\sigma_0), t(\sigma_1)$

- Relation of the top token on the stack: $r(\sigma_0)$
- Seven joint features: $t(\sigma_0) + t(\beta_0)$, $t(\sigma_0) + r(\sigma_0)$, $t(\sigma_1) + t(\sigma_0) + t(\beta_0)$, $t(\beta_0) + t(\beta_1) + t(\beta_2)$, $t(\beta_1) + t(\beta_2) + t(\beta_3)$, $t(\sigma_0) + t(\beta_0) + t(\beta_1)$, $t(\sigma_1) + t(\sigma_0) + t(\beta_0)$.

Thus, feature set $\Phi_1$ consists of the features defined in $\Phi_0$, plus the four indicator word features: the top word on the stack, the first and the second word on the buffer, and the head word of the top word on the stack. Feature set $\Phi_2$ consists of the features defined in $\Phi_0$ like $\Phi_1$, but replaces indicator word features with their corresponding distributed representations. Finally, feature set $\Phi_3$ consists of all features defined in $\Phi_1$ and $\Phi_2$.

We fix a frequency cutoff for indicator features at 3 times in order to remove possibly noisy features from the training set. That is, if a generated feature has frequency less than 3, it is removed from the feature set.

**Table 2.** Feature sets for use in the transition classifier

| Feature Set | Feature Templates |
|---|---|
| $\Phi_1$ | $\Phi_0, w(\sigma_0), w(\beta_0), w(\beta_1), w(h(\sigma_0))$ |
| $\Phi_2$ | $\Phi_0, d(\sigma_0), d(\beta_0), d(\beta_1), d(h(\sigma_0))$ |
| $\Phi_3$ | $\Phi_1, \Phi_2$ |

### 4.3   Evaluation Metrics

The evaluation metrics used for parsing accuracy are the precision, recall and $F$-measure. The precision ($P$) is the proportion of labeled arcs identified by the parser which are correct; the recall ($R$) is the proportion of labeled arcs in the gold results which are correctly identified by the parser; and the $F$-measure is the harmonic mean of $P$ and $R$, that is $F = 2PR/(P + R)$. A labeled arc is correct if and only if its source vertex, its target vertex and its label are all correctly identified by the parser.

### 4.4   Results and Discussion

Table 3 shows the parsing accuracy for three feature sets $\Phi_0, \Phi_1, \Phi_2$. The best results are marked by a bold font. Not surprisingly the lowest accuracy is obtained with the simplest feature set $\Phi_0$ where word features are not used. It is interesting that the use of distributed representations of words gives about 0.57 % point higher than the use of the word identities ($F$ ratio of 56.359 % compared to 55.793 %). The feature set $\Phi_3$ gives the highest accuracy with $F$ ratio of 57.646 %. This result not only confirms the importance of word identities but also shows that discrete and distributed word features can work well together.

Another important factor when comparing the two feature sets $\Phi_1$ and $\Phi_2$ is the efficiency in terms of space and time. The feature set $\Phi_2$ produces a compact dense model with a much smaller number of features (and hence number of parameters to be computed) in comparison with the feature set $\Phi_1$. In particular,

**Table 3.** Parsing accuracy

| Feature Set | Dataset | $P$ | $R$ | $F$ |
|---|---|---|---|---|
| $\Phi_0$ | test | 53.416 % | 45.934 % | 49.393 % |
| | training | 63.667 % | 54.918 % | 58.970 % |
| $\Phi_1$ | test | 60.713 % | 51.610 % | 55.793 % |
| | training | 80.769 % | 69.786 % | 74.877 % |
| $\Phi_2$ | test | 61.454 % | 52.045 % | 56.359 % |
| | training | 75.773 % | 65.429 % | 70.222 % |
| $\Phi_3$ | test | **63.057 %** | **53.090 %** | **57.646 %** |
| | training | 83.480 % | 72.321 % | 77.501 % |

$\Phi_2$ generates a total of 200 real-valued features for lexical tokens, as each of the four tokens corresponds to a 50-dimensional real-valued vector of their distributed representations; while $\Phi_1$ generates thousands of indicator features on the training set. For this reason, the optimization algorithms run significantly faster with the $\Phi_2$-based model than with the $\Phi_1$-based one. In addition, as pointed out by [17], in modern dependency parsers, most of the running time is consumed not by the core parsing algorithm but in the feature extraction step. By using dense features in place of the sparse indicator features, the parser's running time is greatly reduced. As a result, the training and testing time with $\Phi_2$ is much slower than that with $\Phi_1$.

# 5 Related Work

Dependency parsing using feature-based discriminative statistical parser has seen enormous success in recent years. For well-studied languages, the average accuracy of dependency parsers developed for 13 languages is in the range of from 80 % to 82 % [1]. Most of the parsers use millions of indicator features and hence suffer from the problem of feature sparseness. From a statistical perspective, their corresponding parameters are poorly estimated because there is insufficient data to correctly estimate such parameters. To alleviate this problem, higher-support features such as word classes have been incorporated to improve parsing performance [18]. However, these parsers are still not perfect in terms of both speed and efficiency.

Recently, Chen and Manning [2] has proposed to use neural networks to train a dependency parser which is fast and accurate. They train a neural network classifier to make parsing decisions within a transition-based dependency parser. The neural network learns compact dense distributed representations of words, part-of-speech tags, and dependency labels. This parser gives good gains in parsing accuracy and speed on English and Chinese. Compared to this work, our parsing model is simpler in that we do not create and use distributed representations for part-of-speech tags and arc labels, only for words. In addition, we do not use a complicated neural network classifier but instead employ a multinomial regression classifier, which is simpler and easier to train. A neural network architecture is only used in a skip-gram model in order to obtain distributed word representations of Vietnamese words.

Previously, [19] applied incremental sigmoid belief networks to dependency parsing using a temporal restricted Boltzman machine. Despite of using a neural network, it is a very different architecture than that of [2] and is much less scalable and practical for large vocabulary.

For the Vietnamese language, it is not surprising that there have been few published works dealing with syntactic parsing in general and dependency parsing in particular. One of the main reason is that Vietnamese does not yet have vast and readily available constructed linguistic resources upon which to build effective statistical models, nor does it have reference works against which new ideas may be experimented.

To our knowledge, up to now there have existed few published works on the syntactic analysis of Vietnamese. The first report on parser performance is an empirical study of applying probabilistic context-free grammar parsing models, by [20] for Vietnamese, its best result on constituency analysis is $78\%$ on a test corpus; there is no reported result on dependency analysis. The most complete report on building and evaluating a syntactic parser using lexicalized tree-adjoining grammars for Vietnamese was presented in [21]. The best results obtained are $73.21\%$ (dependency accuracy) and $69.33\%$ ($F$-measure of constituency accuracy) on a test corpus. These results are better than the those described in this work. However, these results are not directly comparable since the parsing models are trained and tested on different corpus. Finally, it is not our goal in this work to present the most accurate dependency parser for Vietnamese but to demonstrate the usefulness of distributed word representations in dependency parsing. We believe that an integration of this type of word features into proven state-of-the-art feature sets for dependency parsing would give us the best parsing accuracy.

## 6    Conclusion

In this paper, we have presented a dependency parser for Vietnamese which is fast and accurate. The parser is fast because of two reasons. First, it uses a greedy, transition-based parsing algorithm to perform disambiguation deterministically. Second, it uses a compact dense feature model of distributed word representations instead of word indicator features. We have shown that the parser also achieves a better accuracy in comparison to a conventional transition-based dependency parser.

An interesting line of future work is to apply the technique described in this paper to more elaborate classifiers, such as support-vector machines and to more sophisticated parsing algorithms, such as those employed in two popular off-the-self dependency parsers (MaltParser and MSTParser). In addition, we plan to improve and compare our parser with the similar MaltParser on the same dataset.

Syntactic dependency representation of natural sentences has recently gained a wide interest in the natural language processing community and has been successfully applied to many problems and applications such as machine translation, ontology construction and automatic question answering. A primary advantage of dependency representation is its natural mechanism for representing discontinuous constructions or long distance dependencies which are common in Vietnamese. We think that the presence of a good dependency parser for Vietnamese will be very helpful in a wide range of tasks for Vietnamese processing.

**Acknowledgements.** This research is partly funded by the Vietnam National University, Hanoi (VNU) under project number QG.15.04. The last author is funded by Hanoi University of Science (HUS) under project number TN.15.04. The authors would like to thank Dr. Dang Hoang Vu of FPT Research for providing us the distributed representations of Vietnamese words. We are grateful to our anonymous reviewers for their helpful comments which helped us improve the quality of the article in terms of both presentation and content.

# References

1. McDonald, R., Nivre, J.: Analyzing and integrating dependency parsers. Comput. Linguist. **37**(1), 197–230 (2011)
2. Chen, D., Manning, C.D.: A fast and accurate dependency parser using neural networks. In: Proceedings of EMNLP, pp. 740–750. ACL (2014)
3. Turian, J., Ratinov, L., Bengio, Y.: Word representations: a simple and general method for semi-supervised learning. In: Proceedings of ACL, Uppsala, Sweden, pp. 384–394 (2010)
4. Bengio, Y., Ducharme, R., Vincent, P., Janvin, C.: A neural probabilistic language model. J. Mach. Learn. Res. **3**, 1137–1155 (2003)
5. Morin, F., Bengio, Y.: Hierarchical probabilistic neural network language model. In: Proceedings of AISTATS, Barbados, pp. 246–252 (2005)
6. Collobert, R., Weston, J.: A unified architecture for natural language processing: deep neural networks with multitask learning. In: Proceedings of ICML, New York, NY, USA, pp. 160–167 (2008)
7. Mnih, A., Hinton, G.E.: A scalable hierarchical distributed language model. In: Koller, D., Schuurmans, D., Bengio, Y., Bottou, L. (eds.) Advances in Neural Information Processing Systems 21, pp. 1081–1088. Curran Associates Inc. (2009)
8. Mikolov, T., Chen, K., Corrado, G., Dean, J.: Efficient estimation of word representations in vector space. In: Proceedings of Workshop at ICLR, Scottsdale, Arizona, USA (2013)
9. Nivre, J.: An efficient algorithm for projective dependency parsing. In: Proceedings of the 8th International Workshop on Parsing Technologies (IWPT 03), Nancy, France, pp. 149–160 (2003)
10. Nivre, J., Scholz, M.: Deterministic dependency parsing of English text. In: Proceedings of COLING 2004, Geneva, Switzerland (2004)
11. Mikolov, T., Sutskever, I., Chen, K., Corrado, G.S., Dean, J.: Distributed representations of words and phrases and their compositionality. In: Burges, C., Bottou, L., Welling, M., Ghahramani, Z., Weinberger, K. (eds.) Advances in Neural Information Processing Systems 26, pp. 3111–3119. Curran Associates Inc. (2013)

12. Andrew, G., Gao, J.: Scalable training of $l_1$-regularized log-linear models. In: Proceedings of ICML, Oregon State University, Corvallis, USA, pp. 33–40 (2007)
13. Nocedal, J., Wright, S.J.: Numerical Optimization, 2nd edn. Springer, New York (2006)
14. Le-Hong, P., Thi Minh Huyên, N., Roussanaly, A., Vinh, H.T.: A hybrid approach to word segmentation of Vietnamese texts. In: Martín-Vide, C., Fernau, H., Otto, F. (eds.) LATA 2008. LNCS, vol. 5196, pp. 240–249. Springer, Heidelberg (2008)
15. Nguyen, T.L., Ha, M.L., Nguyen, V.H., Nguyen, T.M.H., Le-Hong, P.: Building a treebank for Vietnamese dependency parsing. In: The 10th IEEE RIVF, Hanoi, Vietnam, pp. 147–151. IEEE (2013)
16. Nguyen, P.T., Xuan, L.V., Nguyen, T.M.H., Nguyen, V.H., Le-Hong, P.: Building a large syntactically-annotated corpus of Vietnamese. In: Proceedings of the 3rd Linguistic Annotation Workshop, ACL-IJCNLP, Suntec City, Singapore, pp. 182–185 (2009)
17. Bohnet, B.: Very high accuracy and fast dependency parsing is not a contradiction. In: Proceedings of COLING, Beijing, China, pp. 89–97 (2010)
18. Koo, T., Carreras, X., Collins, M.: Simple semi-supervised dependency parsing. In: Proceedings of ACL-HLT, Columbus, Ohio, USA, pp. 595–603 (2008)
19. Garg, N., Henderson, J.: Temporal restricted Boltzman machines for dependency parsing. In: Proceedings of ACL-HLT, Portland, Oregon, USA, pp. 11–17 (2011)
20. Collins, M.: Head-driven statistical models for natural language parsing. Comput. Linguist. **29**(4), 589–637 (2003)
21. Le-Hong, P., Roussanaly, A., Nguyen, T.M.H.: A syntactic component for Vietnamese language processing. J. Lang. Model. **3**(1), 145–183 (2015)

# Modeling Vietnamese Speech Prosody: A Step-by-Step Approach Towards an Expressive Speech Synthesis System

Dang-Khoa Mac and Do-Dat Tran[✉]

International Research Institute MICA, HUST-CNRS/UMI 2954-Grenoble INP,
Hanoi Vietnam
{dang-khoa.mac,do-dat.tran}@mica.edu.vn

**Abstract.** Attempts to add expressivity to synthesized speech is one of the main strategies in speech technologies. This paper summarizes our researches on modeling Vietnamese prosody, with the goal of improving naturalness of synthesized speech in Vietnamese, as well as integrating expressivities (i.e. emotion/attitude). Based on the concept of "rendez-vous" between linguistic levels and prosodic functions, the prosody of utterance is proposed to be decomposed into several components. Therefore, each component is step by step modeled by an independent model: a dynamic linear segment model for tones, a relative registers model for F0 level of syllable, a rule-based approach for phrasing modeling and a F0 stylization modeling for the expressive function. All proposed models were integrated in speech Text-to-speech systems and also were evaluated by perception experiments.

**Keywords:** Text-to-speech · Vietnamese · Prosody modeling · Tones · Phrasing · Attitude · Expressive speech

## 1 Introduction

Speech is one of the fundamental human behavior events that simultaneously conveys linguistic information as well as the speaker's affective variability (e.g., mental, intentional, attitudinal, emotional states). Attempts to add expressivity to synthesized speech have existed for more than a decade. For a tonal language like Vietnamese, acoustic parameters implied in the linguistic and affective functions of prosody (typically F0, intensity, timing) also play an important role at the phonemic level for lexical access. Moreover, the Vietnamese tones can imply some voice quality cues that have been shown to be used in the morphology of some attitudes (and emotions) in other languages [1].

The main task of the prosody generator of a TTS system is to provide an acoustic representation of prosody from linguistic information. It is well known that, for a tonal language like Vietnamese, Chinese, the fundamental frequency (F0) contour of a sentence always consists of local tonal components and the intonation of the sentence. Thus the variation of the F0 in the sentences for tonal languages seems more complicated than that of non-tonal languages. The Vietnamese prosodic contour could be generated

© Springer International Publishing Switzerland 2015
X.-L. Li et al. (Eds.): PAKDD 2015, LNCS 9441, pp. 273–287, 2015.
DOI: 10.1007/978-3-319-25660-3_23

automatically by using the Fujisaki model [2, 3] or a linear F0 model combined with relative registers [4]. But there is no model that can generate the prosodic contours of tones combined with expressive prosodic contours.

According to the prosodic model proposed in [6], the intonation is considered as a result of superimposed and independent prototypical gestures belonging to hierarchical linguistic levels: sentence, clause, group, sub-group etc. That concept is called the "rendez-vous" between linguistic levels and prosodic functions of utterance [6, 7]. This theoretical model allows the generation of complex prosodic contours using a superposition process directed by functions. It was applied in the speech synthesis for 3 modalities (declaration, question, surprise), in the automatic generation of 6 expressive prosodic attitudes for French [7] and in the prosody generation of tonal language such as Chinese [8].

Our approach to Vietnamese expressive speech production consists of applying the "rendez-vous" concept above to combine the variation of many prosodic functions such as tone, phrasing, sentences modality and expressivities (attitude/emotion). Each component is modeled by three separated model:

1. a dynamic linear segment model for tones;
2. a relative registers model for F0 height of syllable;
3. a rule-based approach for phrasing modeling and a F0 stylization modeling for the expressive function.

The next sections will present step by step our proposal models for these prosodic components. All proposed models were developed separately and evaluated in the speech different Text-to-speech system.

## 2 Modeling the Prosodic Contour of Vietnamese Tones in Continuous Speech

In order to build an intonation model for the Vietnamese language, we begun our studies with modeling F0 contours of tones of isolated words.

### 2.1 Overview

The Vietnamese language has 6 tones as shown in Fig. 1: level (1), falling (2), broken (3), curve (4), rising (5) and drop (6). Tone 5b and 6b correspond to tone 5 and 6 on a syllable ended by a stop consonant. Moreover the Vietnamese tonal system can employ some production of voice quality, within F0. That is the co-occurrence of glottalization during the production of tone 3 and tone 6: tone 3 is accompanied with harsh voice quality due to a glottal stop (or a rapid series of glottal stops) around the middle of the vowel; tone 6 has the same kind of harsh voice quality as tone 3; however, it is distinguished by dropping very sharply and it is almost immediately cut off by a strong glottal stop [9].

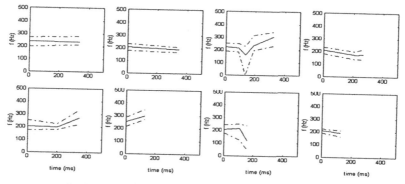

**Fig. 1.** Examples of contours of 8 Vietnamese tone representations from a female subject [9]. From the left to right, top to bottom: tone 1, 2, 3, 4, 5, 5b, 6, 6b.

In the continuous speech, the F0 contour of the Vietnamese tones with the influence of tonal coarticulation effect can be described by the linear F0 model (as in Fig. 2) combined with relative registers of Vietnamese tone, as proposed in. This method is used in our work to generate the prosodic contour in the syllable level, which correspond to the tonal function of prosody.

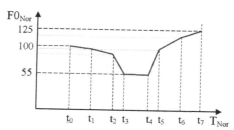

**Fig. 2.** The normalized linear contour of tone 3

## 2.2   Linear Segment Model of Vietnamese Tone

### 2.2.1   Vietnamese Tones Model in Isolated Mode

Several models of generation of F0 contour for Vietnamese tones were presented in the work of [2, 3, 10]. In study of [10] the average F0 contours are used as contour templates for tones. The speech synthesis systems presented in the work of [11, 12] employ the Fujisaki model to generate the F0 contours of 6 tones, but the systems meet difficulties in generating F0 contours of Tones 3 and 6 caused by phenomena of glottalization during their pronunciation. In addition, the three researches – were based on analysis of variation of F0 in voiced syllables, and on the hypothesis that the tone has an effect on the entire syllable. Under these conditions, the patterns of tones concern only voiced syllables. The results of these three studies did not indicate whether these patterns could be used for all types of Vietnamese syllables, particularly for syllables that begin with unvoiced consonants.

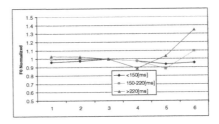

**Fig. 3.** Three variants of tone 3 in respect to the duration of the syllable

To build the F0 contour patterns for Vietnamese tones, we apply the results of a study [13] about the influence of tone on the syllable. The results showed that the initial consonant of the syllable does not carry the information of the tone, and the Vietnamese tone affects only the final part of the syllable.

Based on the results of [14] about the shapes of F0 contour of the six Vietnamese tones, we got average values of F0 contours of the six Vietnamese tones and then we constructed linear F0 contour models for the Vietnamese tones (Fig. 2 shows a linear contour model for Tone 3). These models only describe the F0 evolution of a final part of the Vietnamese syllable, this is different from studies [2, 10] which model the F0 contour of tones on the whole syllable.

The process of tone modeling composed of three phases:

- Calculating average values of F0 at specific points, the number of points N is dependent on the complexity of tone;
- Normalization of average values, the mean values are divided by the average value of the initial point;

$$FO_i^{Nor} = FO_i / FO_1 \quad i = 1 \dots N \tag{4.1}$$

- Connecting the points by the lines, the value of F0 of the middle points are calculated by the equation:

$$FO(t) = FO_i^{Nor} + \alpha_i * t \qquad \left( t = t_i - t_{i+1} \right) \tag{4.2}$$

To generate the F0 contour for a tone, the normalized F0 contour is firstly calculated, and then normalized values are multiplied by a specific factor, for example the average value of the fundamental frequency of the speaker.

The detail information on the F0 patterns and results of the perception tests is presented in [15].

### 2.2.2  Dynamic Model of Vietnamese Tones in Continuous Speech

Figure 3 presents three variants of Tone 3, which depend on the length of the syllable: it is easy to see that these three variants differ greatly from one another. In order to describe more clearly these differences, and also to compare with other tones, we normalized the F0 contours of the three variants (Fig. 4). The F0 value of 3th point was chosen as the reference value because of its stability.

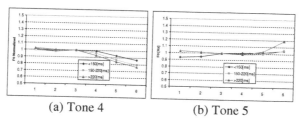

(a) Tone 4                              (b) Tone 5

**Fig. 4.** The normalized F0 contours of (a) tone 4 and (b) tone 5 with the different durations of the syllable

The F0 contours of variants of the five remaining tones were also normalized. Concerning Tones 4 and 5, three F0 contours change in a larger range (Fig. 4), they can be classified into two groups, and each group is represented by an only form.

The same process of tone modeling in isolated mode was carried out for Vietnamese tones in dynamic mode. But in this case, each tone can have more than one model; it depends on the duration of syllable carrying tone.

## 2.3 Generation of F0 Contour in Continuous Speech

Based on results from on variation of Vietnamese intonation in continuous speech, we believe that it is necessary to consider the four following factors when analyzing and modeling the contour of F0 an utterance in Vietnamese:

- Tones that make up the statement;
- Register for each tone;
- The influence of the phenomena of tonal coarticulation;
- The duration of the syllable;

A method for the generation of the F0 contours for Vietnamese text-to-speech based on the assumption: *"The tonal coarticluation effect takes place from begin to the end of each phrase, and after a pause it is cancelled"*.

Suppose that a phrase of N syllables ($S_1 S_2 \dots S_N$) will be synthesized. The F0 contour of the phrase is obtained through 3 steps (Fig. 5).

Step 1:  The register of all the syllables in the phrase is calculated, based on the phonetic information and position of syllable in the sentence

Step 2:  Generation of the tonal contour for each syllable by using tone patterns. The tonal contour is then placed on the register contour.

Step 3:  The F0 contour of the phrase is smoothed. For smoothing the discontinuity of the F0 contour, the transition pattern *Exclusive Carry-over* is applied.

And finally the normalized contour of F0 is scaled with a specific factor. For example, in the Fig. 5b, the value of factor equals to the initial F0 value (250 Hz) of the original phrase.

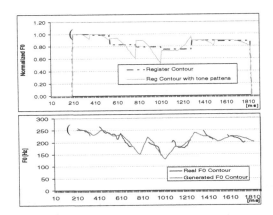

**Fig. 5.** (a) Generated register contour (dashed line) and the superimposed tone patterns. (b) F0 contour generated by the proposed model and the F0 contour of target speech.

## 2.4 Evaluation

In order to evaluate the performance of the proposed model on the natural characteristic of synthetic phrase, a perceptual test based on MOS test was performed. Thirty sentences were selected and re-synthesized in different ways. For each phrase, only the contour of F0 is manipulated by applying TD-PSOLA algorithm to have 4 variants. Thus, a speech corpus which contains 5 groups of 30 sentences was built:

- Group 1 contains 30 natural sentences.
- Group 2 includes 30 re-synthetic sentences. Their contour of F0 is generated by applying all of 3 steps the proposed method.
- Group 3 contains 30 re-synthetic sentences whose contour of F0 is generated by applying the first and second steps.
- Group 4 includes 30 re-synthetic sentences whose contour of F0 is generated by applying the second and the third steps. In these sentences, the relative registers of all tones equal 1.
- Group 5 contains 30 re-synthetic sentences whose F0 contour is generated by applying only the tone patterns (step 2). Like the sentences of group 4, the relative registers of all tones equal 1.

Twenty persons participated into the test. The listeners were asked to rate the natural quality of each perceptual sentence on a scale 1–5, where 1 is bad and 5 is completely natural.

Figure 6 presents the naturalness scores of the five groups. Group 1 which contains the natural sentences has the highest score; this is a predictable result. The next is Group 2 whose sentences are re-synthesized by applying all 3 steps. This is a good result for an intonation model. The lowest score group is belong to Group 5, which applies only the tone patterns. By comparison the score between Group 2 and Group 4, and the score between Group 3 and Group 5, we found that, by applying the relative tone register for the generation of the F0 contour, the naturalness score of synthetic sentences of Group 2 and 3 (3.84 and 3.72) is significantly higher than that of Group 4 and 5 (3.11 and 3.10).

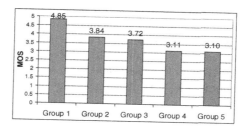

**Fig. 6.** MOS test result

With respect to the influence of the smoothing F0 contour on the naturalness of re-synthetic sentences, we can see a difference only in the sentences which have a quite natural quality. This is presented clearly when comparing the scores between Group 2 and 3 (3.84 vs. 3.72), and between Group 4 and 5 (3.11 vs. 3.10). Therefore, the obtained results show that, for a tonal language like Vietnamese, the relative tonal register is an important parameter for generation of F0 contour.

# 3   Vietnamese Phrasing Modeling

Phrasing modeling plays an important role in improving the naturalness for speech synthesis. Many researchers have been working on prosodic structure generation for Chinese [16, 17], pause/break modeling for French [18], German [19], Russian [20] or modeling style specific break [21, 22]. They may use rules or machine learning with lexical information (e.g. POS tagger) or contextual length. However, to the best of our knowledge, there is no such work for Vietnamese, a tonal language. It is believed that there is an interface between syntax and prosodic structure [23–27]. Recently, much effort has been devoted for Vietnamese syntax parsing with some has proven fruitful results [28–30].

## 3.1   Corpus Preparation

Resources of Vietnamese language is messy and lacking of unified and big-enough corpus, especially for speech processing [31]. To have a preliminary experiment for prosodic phrasing modeling, we adopted the existing corpus, "VNSpeechCorpus for speech synthesis" [32], for analyzing. In this corpus, there are 630 sentences that are recorded by a Vietnamese female broadcaster from Hanoi at 48 kHz and 16 bps (~37 min). Audio files in this corpus are transcribed, time-aligned at the syllable level, and annotated for perceived pauses. Text files are parsed and represented with syntax trees in XML format. These tasks are semi-automatically executed.

## 3.2  Proposal Syntactic Rules

From the corpus, we discover two types of rules: one between two constituents in phrase structure grammar and the other between two dependents in dependency grammar. Hypotheses are proposed for constituency syntactic rules (Table 1) and for dependency syntactic rules (Table 2) [33]. The IP (Intonation Phrase) boundaries are put for hypotheses either if the left constituent is or contains a clause (HC1, HC2) or both left and right dependents are predicates (HD1) or head elements (HD2). Other cases are made decision based on the syntactic information or number of syllables in the left or right element.

**Table 1.**  Constituency rules and intermediate boundaries

| # | Intermediate boundaries | Left constituent | Right constituent |
|---|---|---|---|
| HC1 | IP | a SBAR or a constituent whose child is a clause | any constituent |
| HC2 | | a S >= 6 syllables | any constituent |
| HC3 | PhP | any phrase >= 7 syllables | a phrase >=4 syllables |
| HC4 | | any phrase | a C following by a constituent >= 5 syllables |
| HC5 | | a PP >= 3 syllables | a C or AP/NP/VP |
| HC6 | | a S having 3 to 5 syllables or C following by S | any constituent |
| HC7 | | a C 'rằng' whose parent is a SBAR | any constituent |

**Table 2.**  Dependency rules and intermediate boundaries

| # | Boundary | Left dependent | Right dependent |
|---|---|---|---|
| HD1 | IP | a predicate | a predicate |
| HD2 | | a H element >= 4 syllables | a head element |
| HD3 | | an adjunct >= 3 syllables | any dependent that is a phrase |
| HD4 | C | a H element: 2-3 syllables | a head element |
| HD5 | | an adjunct having 2-3 syllables | a subject >= 2 syllables |

## 3.3  Evaluation

Based on the proposed model of prosodic phrasing and analysis results on the speech corpus (presented in detail [33]), two new prosodic features are introduced: break levels and syllable position relative to phrase. Table 3 presents our proposed break levels and syllable relative positions used as training features for an HMM-based TTS. The break levels "0", "1", "5" and "6" are easily identified by POS tags or punctuation marks at the end of sentence whereas others ("2", "3", "4") need syntactic rules for prediction. Syllable positions are distinguished for the boundaries above the Word (1) and above the Intonation phrase boundaries ("2").

**Table 3.** Break levels as training features

| Break level | Syllable position | Prosodic hierarchy | Rule |
|---|---|---|---|
| 0 | 0 | Within word | Between 2 consecutive pho-nemes in one word |
| 1 | 0 | Word | Between 2 consecutive words |
| 2 | 1 | Clitic group | HD4, HD5 |
| 3 | 1 | Phonological phrase | HC3, HC4, HC5, HC6, HC7 |
| 4 | 1 | Intonation phrase | After a punctuation mark in the middle of the sentence or HC1, HC2, HD1, HD2, HD3 |
| 5 | 2 | Utterance boundary | After punctuation marks at end of sentence, not of paragraph |
| 6 | 2 | Paragraph boundary | At the end of paragraph |

For evaluations, the MOS test was carried out with two versions of TTS system and a natural speech reference, presented in random order. 19 subjects (8 females) participated in the tests. All subjects are from the North of Vietnam, living for a long time in Hanoi. Participants were 20–35 years old and reported normal hearing. In the test corpus, 40 sentences are chosen so that each sentence covers only one hypothesis for ease of analysis. There are three to four examples designed for each hypothesis.

Subjects were asked to score "5-Excellent, *4-Good, 3-Fair, 2-Poor and 1-Bad*" for the naturalness after listening to an utterance. The experimental results illustrated in Fig. 7 show an increase of 0.35 on a 5 point MOS scale, for the new prosodic informed system (3.96/5) compared to the previous TTS system (3.61/5).

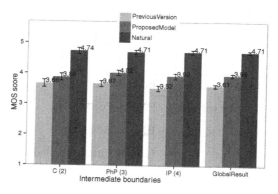

**Fig. 7.** Results of naturalness using MOS test.

# 4   Modeling Prosody of Attitude in Vietnamese

As mention above, our approach to Vietnamese expressive speech production consists of applying the "rendez-vous" concept in order to combine the local variation of tones and the global prosodic contours of attitude.

## 4.1 Vietnamese Attitude Corpus

Our first work is the construction of first corpus for Vietnamese attitudes. This corpus was not only constructed to be used in speech synthesis, but also to conduct fundamental studies on Vietnamese social affects. In the face-to-face interaction, attitudes are expressed within the multimodality of speech such as speech, face, gestures, etc. Thus this corpus was done not only in audio modality but also in visual modality, in order to investigate the relative contribution of audio and visual information in the generation and perception of Vietnamese attitude.

Based on research on attitudes in Vietnamese and other languages [34, 35], 16 attitudes have been represented for Vietnamese in our corpus (Table 4). To observe the effects of tone and tonal co-articulation on attitudinal expression, the corpus contains 8 sentences of one-syllable length, corresponding to the 8 types of Vietnamese tone, and 72 sentences of two-syllable length, which correspond to all combinations of two tones among the 8 Vietnamese tones. The remainder of the corpus is based on 45 sentences of 3- to 8-syllable length and systematically varied in their syntactic structure: single word, nominal group, verbal group and a simple structure "subject-verb-object". That means that the corpus is built from 125 sentences without specific affective meaning produced with all the 16 attitudes and balanced in terms of tone position. These sentences were recorded (both audio and video, but only audio is focused in this paper) by one male speaker native of the Hanoi dialect (standard pronunciation). The whole corpus thus contained 2000 sentences corresponding to more than 90 min of signal after post-processing.

**Table 4.** 16 selected Vietnamese attitudes, with their abbreviations

| Declaration | DEC | Irritation | IRR |
|---|---|---|---|
| Interrogation | INT | Sarcastic irony | SAR |
| Exclamation of neutral surprise | EXo | Scorn | SCO |
| Exclamation of positive surprise | EXp | Politeness | POL |
| Exclamation of negative surprise | EXn | Admiration | ADM |
| Obviousness | OBV | Infant-directed speech | IDS |
| Doubt-incredulity | DOU | Seduction | SED |
| Authority | AUT | Colloquial | COL |

## 4.2 Modeling

The prosodic contour of attitude represents the attitudinal function of prosody and it corresponds to the sentence level. According to [6], the forms of these contours are independent of others linguistic factors (syntax, tone) and depend only on the type of attitude. Therefore, we propose that the form of the prosodic contour of attitudes can be obtained by the mean value of prosodic contour of the neutral-tone sentences (all syllable produced with tone 1).

Figure 8 shows an example of the mean F0 contours of neutral-tone sentences with the length from 1 to 8 syllables. In observation the mean value of F0 contours, duration and intensity of all attitudes, we found that for each attitude, the F0 contour remains a common form when the number of syllables in the utterance increases. This common form can be divided into three parts: initial, middle and final part. The initial and final parts cover typically one or two syllables. The difference between F0 contours of 16 attitudes are mainly represented in these two parts. For all attitudes, the middle part is stable and can be simply represented by a line connecting the initial and the final part. For the duration and intensity, the differences between 16 attitudes are also mainly characterized by the duration and the mean intensity of the first and the last syllable.

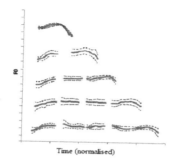

**Fig. 8.** Mean and deviation of F0 contours of 1–5 syllables sentences uttered with the attitude authority.

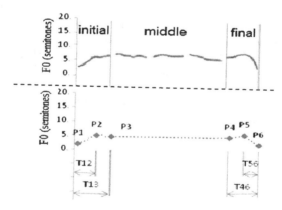

**Fig. 9.** An example of stylization F0 contour of attitude

The description given above enables us to stylize the prosody of attitudes when the number of syllables in the utterance increases:

- The F0 contour is stylized by 6 points as in Fig. 9. The mean values of 6 point and the relative distance between them represent the common form of F0 contour for each attitude.

- The duration and intensity of each attitude is characterized by the mean value of the first and the last syllable.

### 4.3   Perceptual Evaluation

An experiment was designed to perceptually evaluate the predicted prosody of attitudes, generated with the proposal model.

As mentioned above, in the face-to-face interaction, attitudes are expressed within the multimodality: audio and visual information. In this experiment, we aim to evaluate our prosodic model on the attitudes which are well transferred by the audio information. Using the result of the perception test on 16 attitudes with both of audio and visual modality (presented in [36]), we chose 4 attitudes well recognized with audio information for this experiment, they are: *Declaration, Exclamation of neutral surprise, Authority* and *Sarcastic irony*.

Four sentences (with tone and non-tone) from 3 to 8 syllables are used for this experiment. Using these sentences, the synthetic utterances corresponding to 4 selected attitudes above are generated generation with the speech synthesis system developed by the Institute MICA [5].

The prosody synthetic utterances (with 4 attitudes) are predicted by using the proposed model. The 32 synthetic utterances (4 attitudes, 4 sentences, 2 methods) above are then used in a perceptual test in order to examine whether the listeners can indicate the attitudes of synthetic utterances or not. Twenty Vietnamese listeners participated in this experiment. All subjects listened to each stimulus only one time.

Figure 10 presents the mean recognition rates of synthetic utterances (with tone and without tone) generated by re-synthesis method and by the MICA speech synthesis system. Overall, for both type of synthetic utterances and both type of sentence, the recognition rates are over 60 %. The sentences without tone are better recognized than the sentence with tone. That means that the local perturbation by tones increases the complexity of the global cues of prosody of the sentence. The perception result on the utterances generated by re-synthesis method is slightly better than on the utterances generated by MICA speech synthesis system.

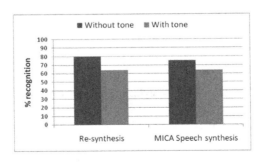

**Fig. 10.** The recognition rate (%) of synthetic utterances generated by re-synthesis method and by MICA speech synthesis system.

Figure 11 shows the recognition rates for 4 attitudes with difference lengths of sentence. Except in the case of Authority, the length of sentence shows no affect on the perception of attitude. The attitudes Declaration and Sarcastic irony have very good result (recognition rate >90 %). The attitude Authority has the lowest recognition rate (from 30 to 60 %).

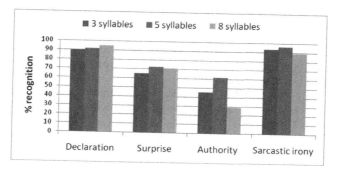

**Fig. 11.** The recognition rate (%) of synthetic utterances with four attitudes.

## 5   Conclusions and Perspectives

This paper presents our preliminary attempt of modeling the completed prosody of Vietnamese speech. Based on the concept of superposition the prosodic contour, a prosodic model was proposed to encode the attitudinal function of prosody for Vietnamese attitudes. This model was applied in generation the prosody of attitudes in Vietnamese. The predicted prosody of attitudes using this model was well recognized in the perception experiment. This result shows us the ability of applying the proposed model in generation the prosody of attitude for the tonal language such as Vietnamese. With this result, the hypothesis of global prosodic contours encoding speaker attitudes is also verified.

However, this work concerns only with the three basic parameters of prosody (F0, duration, intensity). The future work will also have to analyze the role of voice quality in the production and perception of attitudes, in order to characterize the voice quality of attitudes and to be applied in expressive speech synthesis for Vietnamese.

**Acknowledgment.**  We would like to thank Mrs. NGUYEN Thi Thu Trang for her contributions in the frame work of the paper and of the research group.

## References

1. Scherer, K.R., Ellgring, H.: Multimodal expression of emotion: affect programs or componential appraisal patterns? Emotion **7**(1), 158 (2007)
2. Nguyen, D.T., Luong, C.M., Vu, B.K., Mixdorff, H., Ngo, H.H.: Fujisaki model based F0 contours in vietnamese TTS. In: INTERSPEECH (2004)

3. Fujisaki, H., Gu, W.: Phonological representation of tone systems of some tone languages based on the command-response model for F0 contour generation. In: Tonal Aspects of Languages (2006)
4. Do Dat, T., Castelli, E., Hung, L.X., Serignat, J.-F., Van Loan, T.: Linear F0 contour model for Vietnamese tones and Vietnamese syllable synthesis with TD-PSOLA. In: Second International Symposium on Tonal Aspects of Languages (2006)
5. Trần, Ð.Ð.: Synthèse de la parole à partir du texte en langue Vietnamienne. INPG, Grenoble (2007)
6. Aubergé, V.: A gestalt morphology of prosody directed by functions: the example of a step by step model developed at ICP. In: International Conference on Speech Prosody 2002 (2002)
7. Morlec, Y., Bailly, G., Aubergé, V.: Generating the prosody of attitudes. In: Intonation: Theory, Models and Applications (1997)
8. Chen, G.-P., Bailly, G., Liu, Q.-F., Wang, R.-H.: A superposed prosodic model for Chinese text-to-speech synthesis. In: 2004 International Symposium on Chinese Spoken Language Processing, pp. 177–180 (2004)
9. Yên, P.T.N., Castelli, E., Cuong, N.Q.: Gabarits des tons vietnamiens. In: JEP 2002, Journées d'Etude Sur Parole XXIV, Nancy, France, pp 23–26 (2002)
10. Do, T.T., Takara, T.: Vietnamese text-to-speech system with precise tone generation. Acoust. Sci. Technol. 25(5), 347–353 (2004)
11. Mixdorff, H., Nguyen, B.H., Fujisaki, H., Luong, C.M.: Quantitative analysis and synthesis of syllabic tones in Vietnamese. In: EuroSpeech2003, Geneva, pp. 177–180 (2003)
12. Fujisakia, H., Gu, W.: Phonological representation of tone systems of some tone languages based on the command-response model for F0 contour generation. In: TAL2006, pp. 59–62 (2006)
13. Trần, Ð.Ð., Castelli, E., Serignat, J.-F., Trinh, V.L., Le, X.H.: Influence of F0 on Vietnamese syllable perception. Presented at the Interspeech 2005, Lisbon, Portugal, pp. 1697–1700 (2005)
14. Nguyen, Q.C.: Reconnaissance de la parole en langue Vietnamienne. Ph.D. thesis, INP-Grenoble, Grenoble, France (2002)
15. Trần, Ð.Ð., Castelli, E., Lê, X.H., Segrinat, J.F., Văn Loan, T.: Linear F0 contour model for Vietnamese tones and vietnamese syllable synthesis with TD-PSOLA. In: TAL2006, France, pp. 103–107 (2006)
16. Chou, F.-C., Tseng, C.Y., Lee, L.-S.: Automatic generation of prosodic structure for high quality Mandarin speech synthesis. In: ICSLP (1996)
17. Tao, J., Dong, H., Zhao, S.: Rule learning based Chinese prosodic phrase prediction. In: 2003 International Conference on Natural Language Processing and Knowledge Engineering. Proceedings, pp. 425–432 (2003)
18. Doukhan, D., Rilliard, A., Rosset, S., d' Alessandro, C.: Modelling pause duration as a function of contextual length. In: INTERSPEECH (2012)
19. Apel, J., Neubarth, F., Pirker, H., Trost, H.: Have a break! Modelling pauses in German speech. In: KONVENS (2004)
20. Chistikov, P., Khomitsevich, O.: Improving prosodic break detection in a Russian TTS system. In: Železný, M., Habernal, I., Ronzhin, A. (eds.) SPECOM 2013. LNCS, vol. 8113, pp. 181–188. Springer, Heidelberg (2013)
21. Jokisch, O., Kruschke, H., Hoffmann, R.: Prosodic reading style simulation for text-to-speech synthesis. In: Tao, J., Tan, T., Picard, R.W. (eds.) ACII 2005. LNCS, vol. 3784, pp. 426–432. Springer, Heidelberg (2005)
22. Parlikar, A.: Style-Specific Phrasing in Speech Synthesis. Carnegie Mellon University, Pittsburgh (2013)

23. Selkirk, E.O.: On Prosodic Structure and Its Relation to Syntactic Structure. Indiana University Linguistics Club, Bloomington (1980)
24. Selkirk, E.: The syntax-phonology interface. In: Goldsmith, J., Riggle, J., Yu, A.C.L. (eds.) The Handbook of Phonological Theory, pp. 435–484. Wiley, New York (2011)
25. Nespor, M., Vogel, I.: Prosodic structure above the word. In: Cutler, D.A., Ladd, D.D.R. (eds.) Prosody: Models and Measurements, pp. 123–140. Springer, Berlin Heidelberg (1983)
26. Hayes, B.: The prosodic hierarchy in meter. Phon. Phonol. **1**, 201–260 (1989)
27. Dehé, N., Feldhausen, I., Ishihara, S.: The prosody–syntax interface: focus, phrasing, language evolution. Lingua **121**(13), 1863–1869 (2011)
28. Viet, H.A., Thu, D.T.P., Thang, H.Q.: Vietnamese parsing applying the PCFG model. In: Proceedings of the Second Asia Pacific International Conference on Information Science and Technology, Vietnam (2007)
29. Nguyen, P.-T., Vu, X.-L., Nguyen, T.-M.-H., Nguyen, V.-H., Le, H.-P.: Building a large syntactically-annotated corpus of Vietnamese. In: Proceedings of the Third Linguistic Annotation Workshop, Suntec, Singapore, pp. 182–185 (2009)
30. Le, A.-C., Nguyen, P.-T., Vuong, H.-T., Pham, M.-T., Ho, T.-B.: An experimental study on lexicalized statistical parsing for Vietnamese. In: Proceedings of the 2009 International Conference on Knowledge and Systems Engineering, Hanoi, Vietnam, pp. 162–167 (2009)
31. Le, V.-B., Besacier, L.: Automatic speech recognition for under-resourced languages: application to Vietnamese language. IEEE Trans. Audio Speech Lang. Process. **17**(8), 1471–1482 (2009)
32. Tran, D.D., Castelli, E.: Generation of F0 contours for Vietnamese speech synthesis. In: Proceedings of the third International Conference on Communications and Electronics (ICCE), Nha Trang, Vietnam, pp. 158–162 (2010)
33. Trang, N.T.T., Rilliard, A., Trần, Đ.Đ., D'Alessandro, C.: Prosodic phrasing modeling for Vietnamese TTS using syntactic information. In: INTERSPEECH 2014, Singapore, pp. 2332–2336 (2014)
34. Le Thi, X.: Etude contrastive de l'intonation expressive en français et en vietnamien. Ph.D. thesis, Université Paris 3, Paris, France (1989)
35. Shochi, T., Aubergé, V., Rilliard, A.: How prosodic attitudes can be false friends: Japanese vs. French social affects. In: Speech Prosody, Dresden, pp. 692–696 (2006)
36. Mac, D.-K., Aubergé, V., Rilliard, A., Castelli, E.: Audio-visual prosody of social attitudes in Vietnamese: building and evaluating a tones balanced corpus. In: Tenth Annual Conference of the International Speech Communication Association (2009)

# Author Index

Printed in the United States
By Bookmasters